Pharmacy
Calculations

FOR TECHNICIANS

Don A. Ballington
Skye A. McKennon

Sixth Edition

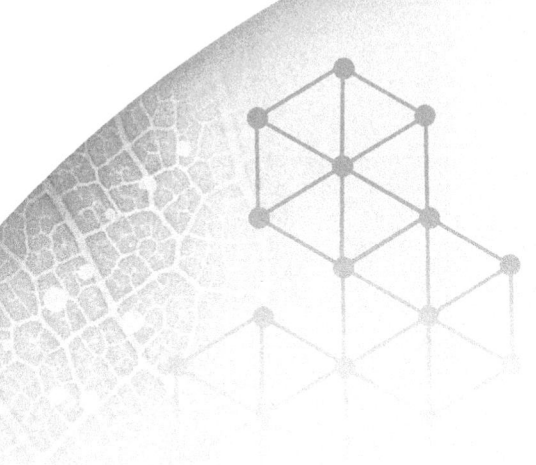

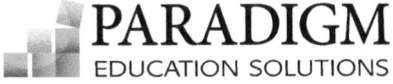
PARADIGM
EDUCATION SOLUTIONS

Minneapolis

Senior Vice President	Linda Hein
Managing Editor	Carley Fruzzetti
Project Manager	Lana Cox, QBS Learning
Developmental Editor	Jane Tufts, QBS Learning
Director of Production	Timothy W. Larson; Deb Sarkar, QBS Learning
Production Editor	Carrie Rogers
Copyeditor	Jana Sweeney, QBS Learning
Proofreader	Dudley Brooks, QBS Learning; Lauren Butler, QBS Learning
Cover and Text Designer	Dasha Wagner
Photo Researchers	Alicia DiPiero, QBS Learning
Indexer	Robert Swanson, QBS Learning
Vice President Sales and Marketing	Scott Burns
Director of Marketing	Lara Weber McLellan
Digital Projects Manager	Tom Modl
Digital Production Manager	Aaron Esnough
Web Developer	Blue Earth Interactive

Care has been taken to verify the accuracy of information presented in this book. However, the authors, editors, and publisher cannot accept responsibility for Web, e-mail, newsgroup, or chat room subject matter or content, or for consequences from application of the information in this book, and make no warranty, expressed or implied, with respect to its content.

Trademarks: Some of the product names and company names included in this book have been used for identification purposes only and may be trademarks or registered trade names of their respective manufacturers and sellers. The authors, editors, and publisher disclaim any affiliation, association, or connection with, or sponsorship or endorsement by, such owners.

Image Credits: Following the index.

We have made every effort to trace the ownership of all copyrighted material and to secure permission from copyright holders. In the event of any question arising as to the use of any material, we will be pleased to make the necessary corrections in future printings. Thanks are due to the authors, publishers, and agents listed in the Photo Credits for permission to use the materials therein indicated.

978-0-76386-845-1 (print)
978-0-76386-846-8 (digital)

BRIEF CONTENTS

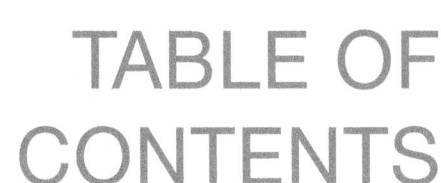

TABLE OF CONTENTS

PREFACE

Pharmacy Calculations for Technicians, 6e: What Makes This New Edition Exciting?

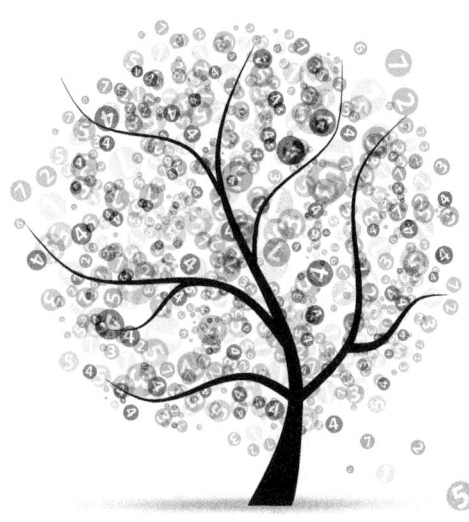

*P*harmacy Calculations for Technicians, Sixth Edition, provides the essential mathematics concepts and calculations skills that pharmacy technicians need to assist in the filling of drug doses in both community and institutional pharmacy practices as well as to preparing readers for certification exams. Guided by clear, complete examples and practice problems, students review basic mathematical concepts and learn about different calculation methods.

The text provides students with plenty of practice in pharmacy math calculations, conversions, measurements, and equations, including calculations required for the preparation of doses, parenteral solutions, and compounded products. These skills are taught using authentic medication labels and real-world applications. In addition, the text teaches business terms and supports calculations related to pharmacy operations. Students learn how to perform calculations for inventory applications, purchasing needs, profit margins, and insurance reimbursements. *Pharmacy Calculations for Technicians* provides pharmacy technicians with the knowledge, skills, and confidence to provide safe and effective care for the patients they serve. The sixth edition includes:

- Complete coverage of ASHP™ curriculum standard 12 which requires students to perform mathematical calculations essential to the duties of pharmacy technicians in a variety of settings
- Additional practice with compounding calculations, including weight-in-weight calculations and special dilutions
- Business-related calculations covering insurance processing, inventory management, and depreciation
- More practice using ratios, percents, and proportions
- Multiple approaches for solving examples
- Additional pediatric problems
- Work Wise marginalia tips covering professional habits and soft skills specific to pharmacy technician careers
- The web-based Navigator+ learning management platform to assemble all student and instructor resources in one easy-to-access location

Study Assets: A Visual Walk-Through

Print and eBook

1 **Accreditation-Targeted Learning Objectives**

establish clear goals to focus each chapter.

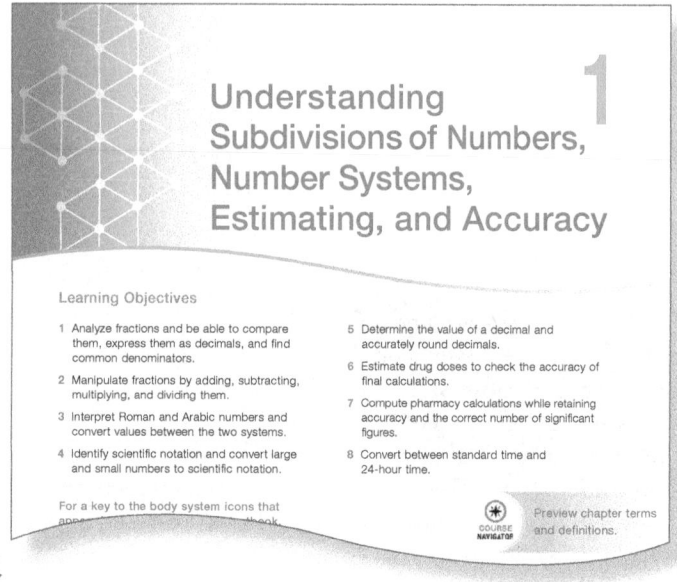

Understanding Subdivisions of Numbers, Number Systems, Estimating, and Accuracy — 1

Learning Objectives

1. Analyze fractions and be able to compare them, express them as decimals, and find common denominators.

2. Manipulate fractions by adding, subtracting, multiplying, and dividing them.

3. Interpret Roman and Arabic numbers and convert values between the two systems.

4. Identify scientific notation and convert large and small numbers to scientific notation.

5. Determine the value of a decimal and accurately round decimals.

6. Estimate drug doses to check the accuracy of final calculations.

7. Compute pharmacy calculations while retaining accuracy and the correct number of significant figures.

8. Convert between standard time and 24-hour time.

For a key to the body system icons that appear...

Preview chapter terms and definitions.

2 **"Take Note" Boxes**

identify important information related to the program and the art of pharmacy calculation.

NEW!

✓ TAKE NOTE

Rounding numbers can be a challenge in pharmacy calculations. In this text, rounding should generally not occur until the last step in the calculation. Please be aware that different work environments may have different rounding policies. Make sure to inquire about rounding policies at your practice location.

3 **Examples**

provide realistic problem statements and show clear, step-by-step solutions. Many include authentic medication labels so students can gain confidence in reading and accurately interpreting labels.

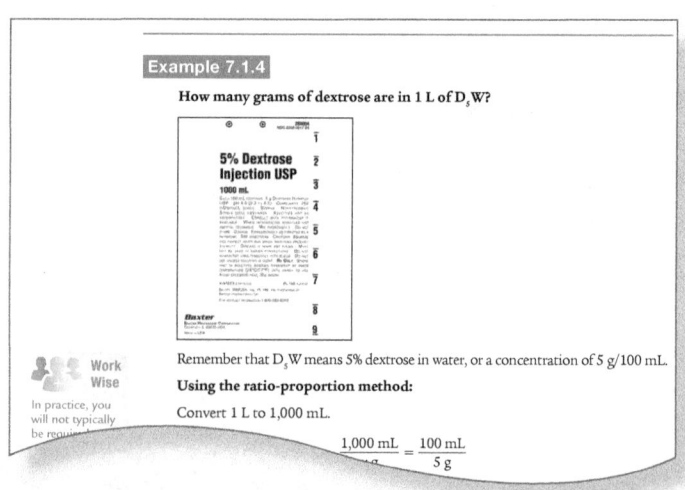

Example 7.1.4

How many grams of dextrose are in 1 L of D_5W?

5% Dextrose Injection USP
1000 mL

Baxter

Work Wise

In practice, you will not typically be required...

Remember that D_5W means 5% dextrose in water, or a concentration of 5 g/100 mL.

Using the ratio-proportion method:

Convert 1 L to 1,000 mL.

$$\frac{1{,}000 \text{ mL}}{g} = \frac{100 \text{ mL}}{5 \text{ g}}$$

enhance visual learning, aid memory, and provide study tools.

TABLE 4.4 Metric Unit Equivalents

Kilo	Base	Milli	Micro
0.001 kg	1 g	1,000 mg	1,000,000 mcg
0.001 kL	1 L	1,000 mL	1,000,000 mcL
0.001 km	1 m	1,000 mm	1,000,000 mcm

FIGURE 4.1 Levothyroxine

25 mcg orange	50 mcg white	75 mcg violet	88 mcg olive	100 mcg yellow	112 mcg rose	125 mcg brown	137 mcg turquoise	150 mcg blue	175 mcg lilac	200 mcg pink	300 mcg green

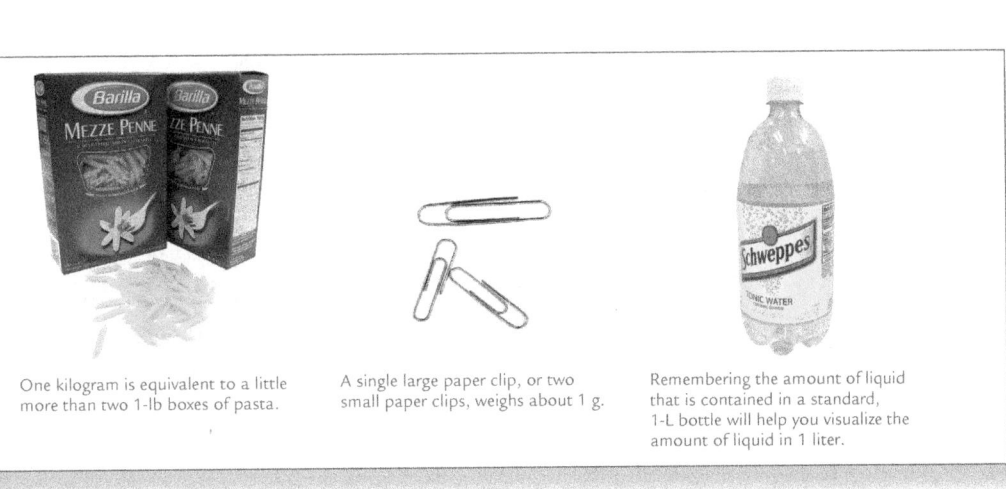

One kilogram is equivalent to a little more than two 1-lb boxes of pasta.

A single large paper clip, or two small paper clips, weighs about 1 g.

Remembering the amount of liquid that is contained in a standard, 1-L bottle will help you visualize the amount of liquid in 1 liter.

6. A patient is to receive 40 mg of morphine sulfate. The pharmacy has the following medication available. How many milliliters will be prepared for this patient?

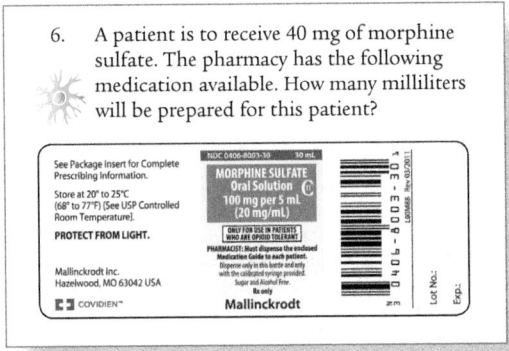

5 Attractive Margin Features

spotlight important information.

 Put Down Roots
Offers word origins to make terms memorable.

 Work Wise
Gives advice on professional and soft skills.

 Safety Alert
Calls out warnings to avoid problems.

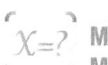 **Math Morsels**
Supply calculating hints.

For Good Measure
Assists in accuracy with measuring counsel.

 Name Exchange
Reminds about items with two names, such as brand and generic drugs.

6 Body System Icons

identify connections between drugs and the body systems they are prescribed to treat.

 Anti-Infective

 Cancer

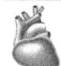 Cardiovascular System

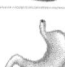 Digestive System

 Endocrine System

 Immune System

 Integumentary System

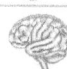 Mental Health/Substance Abuse

 Pediatrics

 Musculoskeletal System

 Nervous System

 Nutrition

 Pain and Pyrexia

 Reproductive System

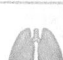 Respiratory System

 Sensory System

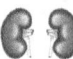 Urinary System

7 Problem Sets

reinforce chapter content and provide opportunities for students to practice their skills and gain confidence in their abilities. Answers can be found in Appendix A.

1.4 Problem Set

Use rounding to estimate the dollar amounts to the nearest whole dollar, and then calculate the actual value.

1. $12.53 − $6.15 =

2. $6.28 + $1.99 + $3.98 =

3. $40 − $34.81 =

4. $100 − $18.29 =

5. $100 − $17.52 − $31.90 =

Estimate the products by rounding the two numbers and then multiplying them. Also calculate the actual value.

6. $6.8 \times 7,656 =$

7. $4.02 \times 350.07 =$

8. $598.4 \times 0.015 =$

9. $4,569 \times 0.0972 =$

10. $6,183 \times 18 =$

11. $1,253 \times 9.1 =$

Estimate the quotients by rounding the two numbers and then dividing them. Also calculate the actual value.

12. $185 \div 18 =$

13. $18,015 \div 56 =$

14. $584.0 \div 8 =$

15. $844.23 \div 4.4 =$

16. $123 \div 14 =$

8 Chapter Summaries

reinforce key points in
each chapter.

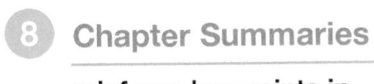

📖 CHAPTER SUMMARY

🔑 KEY TERMS

accuracy the correctness of a number in its
  representation of a given value

Arabic numbers numbers in a numbering
  system that uses symbols to indicate
  numbers, fractions, and decimals; uses the
  numerals 0, 1, 2, 3, 4, 5, 6, 7, 8, 9

common denominator a number into which
  each of the unlike denominators of two or
  more fractions can be divided evenly

mixed number a whole number and
  a fraction

numerator the number in the top part of a
  fraction

place value the location of a numeral in a
  string of numbers that describes the numeral's relationship to the decimal point

product th
  by anoth

proper frac
  than 1 (t
  than the

of a whole.

r in a fraction is the numerator.

r in a fraction is the denominator.

ubtracting fractions, you need to have a common denominator.

fractions, you multiply the numerators together and the

9 Key Terms

are highlighted in bold,
and defined in context,
and also included in
the chapter glossaries.

🔗 CHAPTER REVIEW

Finding Solutions

To gain practice in handling challenging situations in the workplace, consider the following real-world scenarios
and then use the guiding questions to help you formulate your responses.

Note: *To indicate your answer for Scenario D, Question 9, ask your instructor for the handout depicting a*
dosing spoon.

5. How many milligrams did she receive from
   the ingestion of the ½ tablet?

How many total milligrams of medication

10 Chapter Reviews

provide Finding Solutions activities that present
challenging situations and real-world scenarios
for each chapter.

11 Appendices

Appendices provide important resources
for pharmacy technician students.

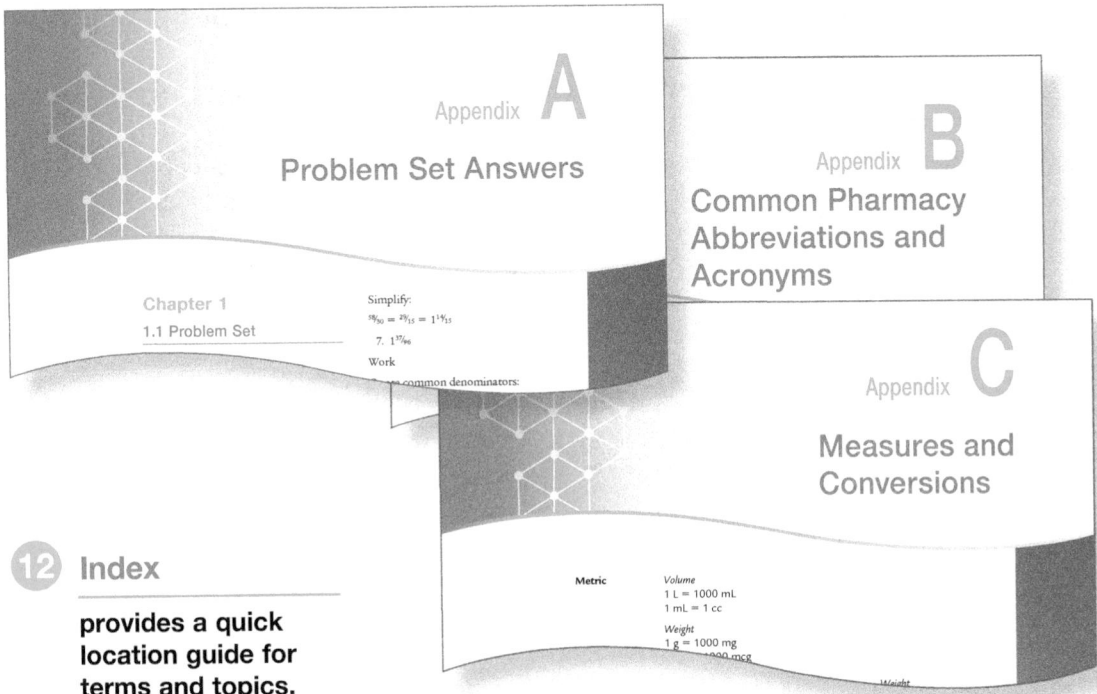

Appendix **A**

Problem Set Answers

Chapter 1

1.1 Problem Set

Simplify:

⁸⁸/₃₀ = ²⁸/₁₅ = 1¹³/₁₅

7. 1³⁷/₉₆

Work

common denominators:

Appendix **B**

**Common Pharmacy
Abbreviations and
Acronyms**

Appendix **C**

**Measures and
Conversions**

Metric | Volume
     1 L = 1000 mL
     1 mL = 1 cc

    Weight
     1 g = 1000 mg
     1000 mcg

12 Index

provides a quick
location guide for
terms and topics.

Student Resources Available on the Navigator+

- **Animated Walkthrough Tutorials** present textbook instruction and examples in a more engaging and dynamic way.
- **End-of-Chapter Exercises** allow for an automated check of a student's chapter comprehension.

  > **Assessing Comprehension** multiple choice exercises based on the chapter content
  >
  > **Sampling the Certification Exam** chapter-specific challenges in the style of the certification exam

- **Flashcards** make it easy to study key terms.
- **Games** provide a fun way to practice key terms and chapter concepts.
- **Practice Test Handouts** provide printable, chapter-specific assessment opportunities for students; tests could be used as chapter pre-tests if desired to assess prior knowledge.
- **Chapter Student Exams** provide the opportunity to check chapter comprehension and receive automatic feedback.
- **Additional Resources** give access to study resources (such as a complete program glossary) and supplements, including a supplement on the apothecary system and the Canadian Pharmacy Technician supplement. The Canadian Pharmacy Technician Supplement addresses topics specific to Canadian pharmacy by Dr. Shahriar Siddiq, updated by Melissa Bleier, BscPharm, RPh.
- **Glossary** document provides the complete program's set of key terms and definitions.

Instructor Resources Available on the Navigator+ and through the Instructor eResources

- **Course Planning Documents** provide essential course planning materials including course information, lesson plans, and syllabus models.
- **Course Delivery Documents** provide resources, such as PowerPoint presentations, to demonstrate and reinforce classroom instruction.
- **Assessment** materials evaluate student performance and track student progress, including question banks organized in pre-built chapter tests that are provided in RTF format and cartridges (Blackboard, Canvas, Common Cartridge, and D2L).

Paradigm's Comprehensive Pharmacy Technician Series

In addition to *Pharmacy Calculations for Technicians,* Sixth Edition, Paradigm Education Solutions offers additional courseware designed specifically for the pharmacy technician curriculum:

- *Pharmacy Labs for Technicians,* Third Edition
- *Pharmacy Practice for Technicians,* Sixth Edition
- *Pharmacology for Technicians,* Sixth Edition
- *Pocket Drug Guide: Generic Brand Name Reference* available in print, eBook, or an app*!
- *Certification Exam Review for Pharmacy Technicians,* Fourth Edition
- *Sterile Compounding and Aseptic Technique,* Second Edition

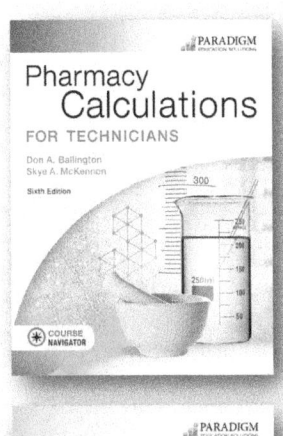

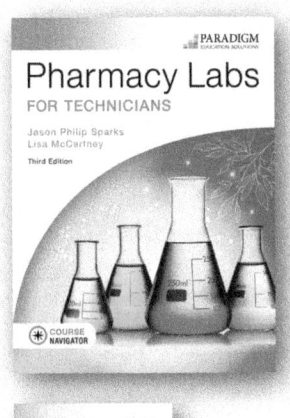

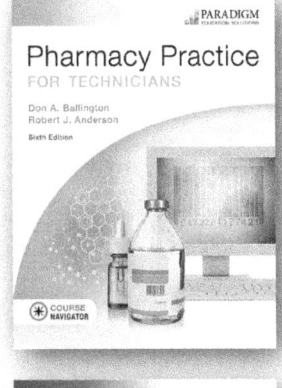

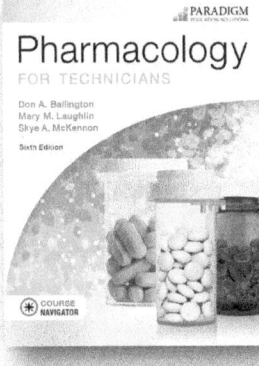

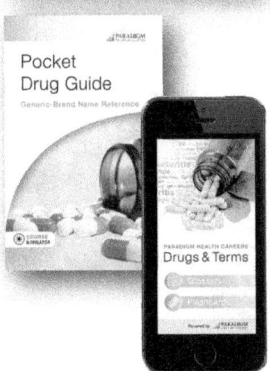

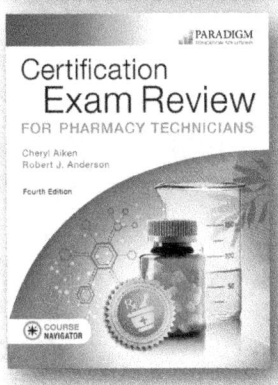

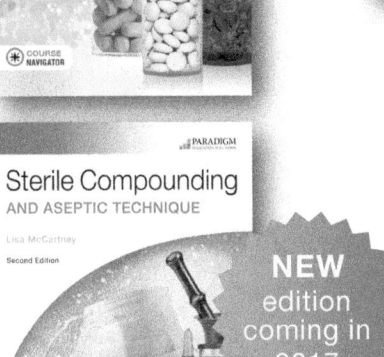

NEW edition coming in 2017

* For more information on Paradigm's new SmartPhone App on drugs and terms, see page xviii.

Related Health Career Titles

Paradigm offers additional health career courseware that is particularly useful for pharmacy technicians:

- *What Language Does Your Patient Hurt In?: A Practical Guide to Culturally Competent Care,* Third Edition
- *Medical Terminology: Connecting through Language*
- *Pharmacology Essentials for Allied Health*

- *Exploring Electronic Health Records*
- *Deciphering Procedural Coding*
- *Introduction to Health Information Management*

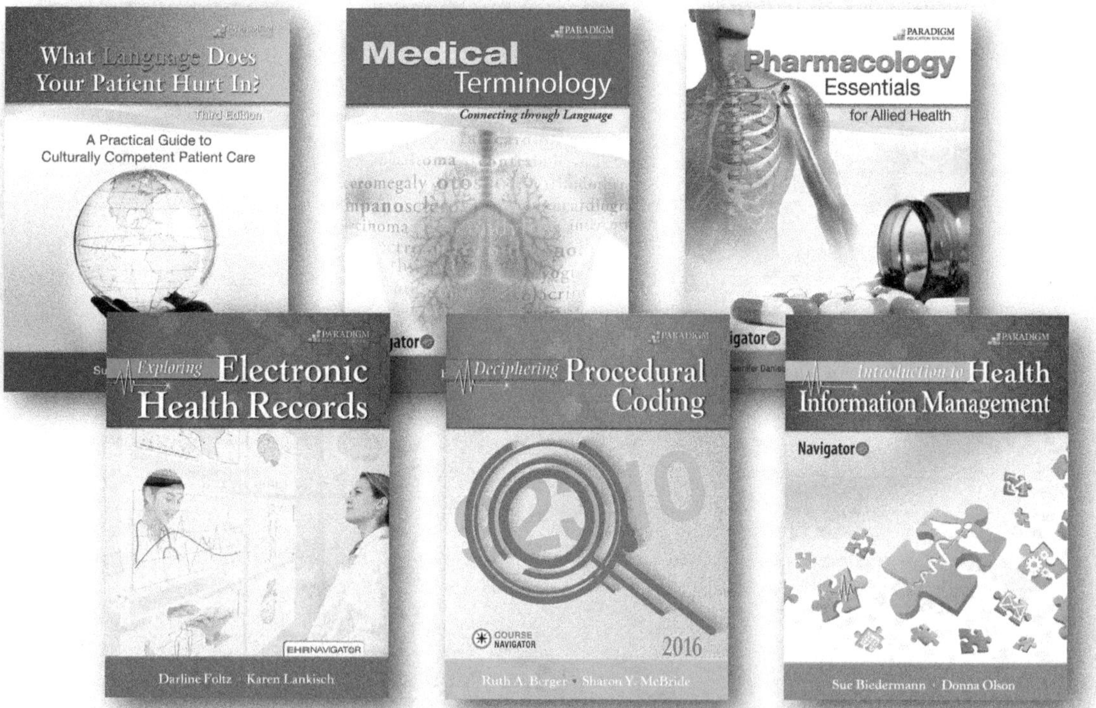

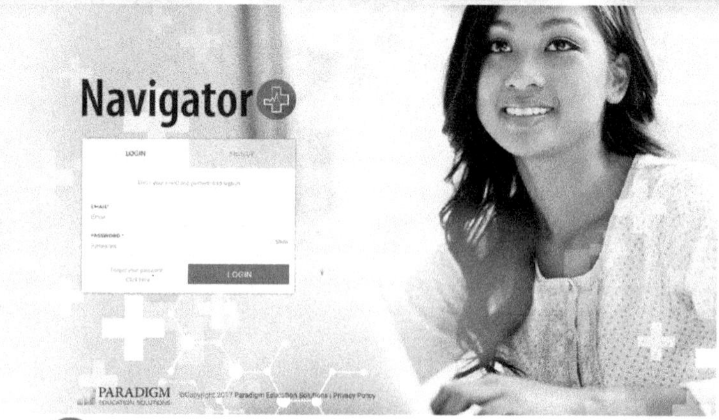

 Navigator+ resources accompany all new editions.

About the Authors

Don A. Ballington

Don A. Ballington, MS, has been a leader in the pharmacy technician profession. He was a founding member of the Pharmacy Technicians Educators Council (PTEC) and served as its president. As a dynamic professor and program director, he coordinated the pharmacy technician training program at Midlands Technical College in Columbia, South Carolina, for 27 years. In 2005, he received the Council's Educator of the Year Award. Mr. Ballington has conducted site visits for pharmacy technician accreditation and helped develop education curriculum standards with the American Society of Health-System Pharmacists (ASHP). He has also been a consulting editor for the *Journal of Pharmacy Technology*. Over the course of his career, he has developed a set of high-quality training materials for pharmacy technicians. These materials became the foundation for Paradigm's *Pharmacy Technician Series*.

Skye McKennon

Skye A. McKennon is a licensed pharmacist, board-certified pharmacotherapy specialist (BCPS), group exercise instructor, certified lifestyle coach, and preventionist. Dr. McKennon received her bachelor's degree and doctor of pharmacy (PharmD) degree from Washington State University. She also completed postdoctoral residency training at Swedish Medical Center in Seattle, Washington.

After residency, Dr. McKennon practiced in the institutional and ambulatory pharmacy settings. In 2009, her passion for teaching and education led her to a faculty position at the University of Washington School of Pharmacy. Courses designed and directed by Dr. McKennon include applied pharmacotherapeutics, institutional pharmacy practice, and diabetes prevention. She has been both an instructor and a guest lecturer of various courses for pharmacy and other health science students, including therapeutics, pharmacotherapy for older adults, global health brigades, and law and ethics. In 2015, Dr. McKennon relocated to Salt Lake City and is currently an associate instructor at the University of Utah. Her role includes teaching pharmacotherapy and preventive medicine to health professional students and practicing in an ambulatory clinic.

Dr. McKennon has presented her work at international and national symposiums such as the Seventh International Conference on Interprofessional Practice and Education and the American Association of Colleges of Pharmacy annual meeting. She is also a contributor to her regional pharmacy community and regularly provides live and online continuing education. Her education research has been published in the *American Journal of Pharmacy Education*.

About the Experts

Several exceptional instructors and content specialists reviewed and contributed to this program's textbook and digital resources to help ensure accuracy and appropriate instructional approaches. Special thanks are due to these individuals who shared their vast expertise and passion for the profession:

Content Area Experts and Contributing Writers

Jennifer Babin, PharmD, BCPS—Assistant professor with the University of Utah College of Pharmacy (Clinical) (Salt Lake City, UT); Clinical Pharmacist in internal medicine at University of Utah Hospital. As a faculty member and clinical pharmacist, Babin trains students in both the classroom and experiential settings to provide high quality, evidence-based patient care. Babin is the contributing writer for Chapters 6 and 7.

Lisa McCartney, MEd, CPhT, PhTR—Department chair for the ASHP/ACPE accredited pharmacy technician program at Austin Community College. She also serves as the CPE administrator for the department's ACPE accredited providership, which offers a variety of continuing pharmacy education activities for pharmacists and technicians. McCartney was the contributing writer for Chapters 7 and 8 in the fifth edition.

Shelina Hardwick-Moses, MBA, MSHCA, CPhT, PhTR—Educator with Thomas Nelson Community College (Business) in Hampton, VA; Former Pharmacy Technician and Healthcare Administration/Management Instructor. As a faculty member and certified pharmacy technician, Moses has trained students and educators in both the classroom and educational settings to provide high quality training and instruction. Moses is the contributing writer for Chapter 9.

Expert Reviewer for Textbook and Assessment Banks

Nikki Ratliff, BS, CPhT—Former pharmacy technician instructor from the Tennessee College of Applied Technology and part-time retail pharmacy technician. Ratliff has been PTCB-certified since 2003 and was a 2016 finalist for the Pharmacy Technician Certification Board's CPhT of the Year.

Expert Reviewers for Textbook

Nicole Lewis, CPhT, CPI (NCCT)—Health studies division manager with San Joaquin Valley College (Modesto campus); former pharmacy technician with Wal-Mart; Lewis will receive her MEd from Concordia University-Portland in 2017 and is a certified post-secondary instructor. Lewis reviewed Chapter 9 of the text.

Shannon Bui, BPharm, RPh—Certified SCAT Instructor with 26 years of hospital pharmacist experience. Bui works as an associate professor at Austin Community College Pharmacy Technology Program (Austin, TX), teaching specialty courses in Chemotherapy, Total Parenteral Nutrition, and Pediatrics. In addition, she serves as a preceptor for pharmacy students at the University of Texas at Austin College of Pharmacy. Bui reviewed Chapter 7 and 8 of the text.

Assessment Banks Writer

Ashanti C. La Roché, BA, AS, CPhT, SCAT-Certified—Pharmacy Technician and Delgado Community College Pharmacy Technician Program Assistant Professor, City Park Campus (New Orleans, LA). La Roché earned degrees in Philosophy and General Science along with certification in Sterile Compounding and Aseptic Technique (SCAT). She has over nine years teaching experience in Allied Health related subjects and was also nominated for NISOD Excellence in Teaching in 2015.

Canadian Supplement Updater

Melissa Bleier, BScPharm, RPh—Instructor for the Pharmacy Technician Program and the National Pharmacy Technician Bridging Program at the School of Health and Human Services at Selkirk College, in Castlegar, BC. (Canada's National Pharmacy Technician Bridging Program is for existing pharmacy technicians to upgrade their skills for the growing responsibilities of contemporary technicians.)

Acknowledgements

The quality of this body of work is a testament to the many contributors and reviewers who participated in the creation of *Pharmacy Calculations for Technicians*, Sixth Edition. We would like to thank Tova Wiegand-Green for her contributions and work on the previous edition. In addition, we offer a heartfelt thank-you to all contributors, instructors, and survey-respondents for their commitment to producing high-quality instructional materials for pharmacy technicians.

Hope Ballard, BS, CPhT, KCST
Fortis Institute (Cookeville, TN)

Debra Blasco, BS CDI College (Vancouver, British Columbia, Canada)

Keith Binion, BS, CPhT Wayne County Community College (Detroit, MI)

April Henry, Pharmacy Assistant Instructor TriOS College (London, Ontario)

Modesty Joy Isaguirre, CPhT, MAED-AET American Career College (Anaheim, CA)

Marlen P. Jimenez, BA Biological Sciences Alvin Community College (Alvin, TX)

Della Khoury, CPhT, BS, BA, MA LARE Institute (Andover, MA)

Marcy May, MEd, CPhT, PhTR
Austin Community College (Austin, TX)

Laurisa McKissack, MBA, CPhT, RPhT Virginia College (Pensacola, FL)

James J. Mizner, Jr., MBA, BS Pharmacy Panacea Solutions Consulting (Reston, VA)

Elina Pierce, MSP, CPhT Southeast Community College (Lincoln, NE)

Charity Sapp, MBA, CPhT, RPT Southeastern College (Tampa, FL)

Joanne Stafford, BSc Pharm, RPh Red Deer College (Red Deer, Alberta, Canada)

Brooke Stokely, BS, CPhT Palmetto School of Career Development and Pharmacy Technician Educators Council (Rock Hill, SC)

Paradigm's Health Career Drugs and Terms App

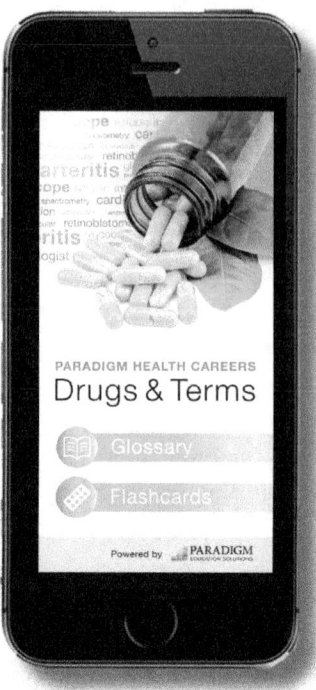

This valuable tool identifies more than 3,000 drugs and terms. Students are able to:

- Search the terms database by drug class or body system.
- Use flashcards included in the app to review Schedule II drug classes and common medical terminology.
- Create their own flashcards to practice identifying drugs and terms.

This app also offers audio functionality to help students master pronunciation.

Canadian Pharmacy Technician Supplement

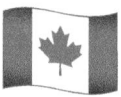 This supplement assists Canadian students in understanding the differences between US and Canadian pharmacy practice. The supplement has four parts that can be read alongside specific chapters in this textbook:

- Part 1: Scope of Practice of Pharmacy Technicians in Canada (Chapter 1: The Profession of Pharmacy)
- Part 2: Drug Regulation in Canada (Chapter 2: Pharmacy Law, Regulations, and Standards)
- Part 3: Controlled Substances (Chapter 2: Pharmacy Law, Chapter 7: Community Pharmacy Dispensing, and Chapter 14: Medication Safety)
- Part 4: Top 100 Drugs Dispensed in Canadian Pharmacies (Chapter 4: Introducing Pharmacology)

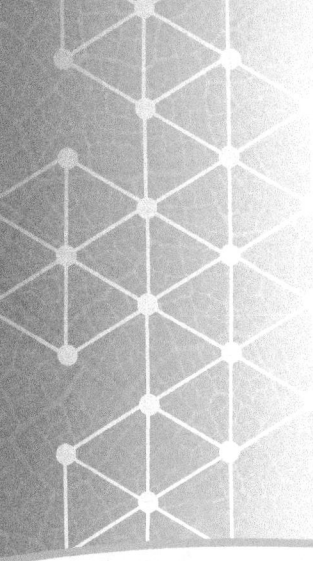

1

Understanding Subdivisions of Numbers, Number Systems, Estimating, and Accuracy

Learning Objectives

1 Analyze fractions and be able to compare them, express them as decimals, and find common denominators.

2 Manipulate fractions by adding, subtracting, multiplying, and dividing them.

3 Interpret Roman and Arabic numbers and convert values between the two systems.

4 Identify scientific notation and convert large and small numbers to scientific notation.

5 Determine the value of a decimal and accurately round decimals.

6 Estimate drug doses to check the accuracy of final calculations.

7 Compute pharmacy calculations while retaining accuracy and the correct number of significant figures.

8 Convert between standard time and 24-hour time.

For a key to the body system icons that appear in each chapter of this textbook, refer to the Preface.

 Preview chapter terms and definitions.

1.1 Fractions

When something is divided into parts, each part is a **fraction** of the whole. For example, a pie might be divided into eight equal slices, each of which is a fraction, or $\frac{1}{8}$, of the whole pie. The pie is still whole but has been divided into eight slices. If we select one slice, it is one eighth of the whole pie, or 1 (the number of slices in the selection) over 8 (the number of slices in the whole pie). In the fraction $\frac{3}{8}$, the selection is 3 of the 8 slices (see Figure 1.1).

FIGURE 1.1
Fractions of the Whole Pie

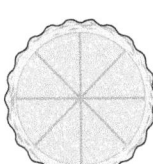 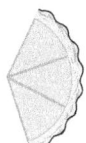

8 slices = 1 whole pie = $\frac{8}{8}$ of the whole pie   3 slices = $\frac{3}{8}$ of the whole pie   1 slice = $\frac{1}{8}$ of the whole pie

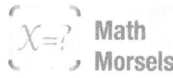
A common fraction is composed of a **numerator** (top number) and a **denominator** (bottom number). The denominator represents the number of equal pieces the whole pie is broken into (8, in this case) and the numerator represents the number of those pieces which are selected (1 of the pieces).

$$\text{numerator} \longrightarrow \frac{1}{8} \longleftarrow \text{denominator}$$

Just as a pie can be divided into parts, so can a tablet. Dividing a tablet is a common procedure for both pharmacist and patient. Figure 1.2 shows how cutting a tablet into smaller parts relates to fractions.

FIGURE 1.2 Fractions of a Tablet

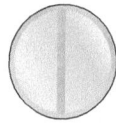
1 tablet = 1,000 mg

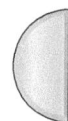
$\frac{1}{2}$ tablet = 500 mg

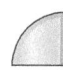
$\frac{1}{4}$ tablet = 250 mg

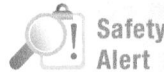
A fraction with the same numerator and denominator has a value of 1.

$$\frac{8}{8} = \frac{5}{5} = \frac{3}{3} = \frac{10}{10} = \frac{15}{15} = 1$$

A fraction with a value less than 1 (numerator less than denominator) is called a **proper fraction**.

$$\frac{1}{4} \quad \frac{2}{3} \quad \frac{7}{8} \quad \frac{9}{10}$$

A fraction with a value greater than or equal to 1 (numerator greater than or equal to the denominator) is called an **improper fraction**.

$$\frac{6}{5} \quad \frac{7}{5} \quad \frac{9}{6} \quad \frac{15}{8}$$

A **mixed number** consists of a whole number and a fraction. A mixed number can be converted to an improper fraction by multiplying the whole number by the denominator and adding the numerator.

$$5\frac{1}{2} = \frac{(5 \times 2) + 1}{2} = \frac{11}{2}$$

A fraction in which the numerator, the denominator or both, contain a fraction is called a **complex fraction**.

$$\frac{\frac{1}{4}}{\frac{1}{8}}$$

Equivalent fractions are fractions that may look different, but have the same overall value. For example, ½ = ²⁄₄ or ³⁄₅ = ¹⁵⁄₂₅. Two fractions are equivalent (equal) only if the product of the numerator (*a*) of the first fraction and the denominator (*d*) of the other fraction is equal to the product of the denominator (*b*) of the first fraction and the numerator (*c*) of the other fraction.

$$If \frac{a}{b} = \frac{c}{d} \text{ then } a \times d = b \times c$$

Consider the fractions ¾ and ⁹⁄₁₂. The two fractions are only equal if 3 × 12 = 4 × 9. When you multiply the numbers you see that 3 × 12 = 36 and 4 × 9 = 36. Therefore, ¾ and ⁹⁄₁₂ are equivalent fractions. If two fractions are equivalent, they are then proportionate (see section 2.3 for more details). The concept and relationship of equivalent fractions and proportions are important tools in pharmacy calculations.

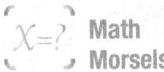
Math Morsels

The symbol > means "is greater than," and the symbol < means "is less than."

Comparing Fractions

When comparing fractions with the same numerator, the fraction with the smaller denominator has the larger value.

$$\frac{1}{10} > \frac{1}{25}$$

If two fractions have the same denominator, the fraction with the larger numerator has the larger value.

$$\frac{3}{6} > \frac{2}{6}$$

If two fractions have different numerators and denominators, you must thoughtfully assess their values. This can be done by converting the fractions to equivalent fractions with the same denominator and then compare. Both methods are described in detail in the next pages. When medications are dosed using fractions, it is important to recognize which strengths are largest and smallest.

Example 1.1.1

 Which of the following nitroglycerin tablets is the smallest dose?

$$\frac{3}{10} \text{ mg tablet} \qquad \frac{4}{10} \text{ mg tablet} \qquad \frac{6}{10} \text{ mg tablet}$$

The ³⁄₁₀ mg tablet is the smallest dose, because when fractions have the same denominator, the fraction with the smallest numerator has the smallest value.

Example 1.1.2

 Which of the following nitroglycerin tablets is the largest dose?

$$\frac{1}{200} \text{ grain tablet} \qquad \frac{1}{150} \text{ grain tablet} \qquad \frac{1}{100} \text{ grain tablet}$$

The ¹⁄₁₀₀ grain tablet is the largest dose, because when fractions have the same numerator, the fraction with the smallest denominator has the largest value.

Adding and Subtracting Fractions

When adding or subtracting fractions with unlike denominators, it is necessary to create a **common denominator**, a number into which each of the unlike denominators can be divided evenly. Think of it as making both fractions into "pieces of pies" with equal slices. Creating a common denominator requires transforming each fraction by multiplying it by a fraction that is equal to 1.

Multiplying a number by 1 does not change the value of the number ($5 \times 1 = 5$). Therefore, if you multiply a fraction by a fraction that equals 1 (such as $\frac{5}{5}$), you do not change the value of the fraction. This mathematical rule allows for the conversions in the following examples.

Example 1.1.3

Find the sum of $\frac{1}{2} + \frac{3}{5}$.

The lowest number that can be divided evenly by both 2 and 5 is 10. A quick way to determine a possible common denominator is to multiply the denominators ($5 \times 2 = 10$). Thus, 10 will be the common denominator for the two fractions, and each fraction must be converted to tenths.

To convert $\frac{1}{2}$ to tenths, multiply $\frac{1}{2}$ by $\frac{5}{5}$. The product is $\frac{5}{10}$.

$$\frac{1}{2} = \frac{1}{2} \times \frac{5}{5} = \frac{5}{10}$$

To convert $\frac{3}{5}$ to tenths, multiply $\frac{3}{5}$ by $\frac{2}{2}$. The product is $\frac{6}{10}$.

$$\frac{3}{5} = \frac{3}{5} \times \frac{2}{2} = \frac{6}{10}$$

Then add $\frac{5}{10} + \frac{6}{10}$. The sum is $\frac{11}{10}$, which in turn can be written as 1 and $\frac{1}{10}$.

$$\frac{5}{10} + \frac{6}{10} = \frac{11}{10} = 1\frac{1}{10}$$

Example 1.1.4

Find the sum of $\frac{1}{4} + \frac{3}{7}$.

The common denominator is 28, because $4 \times 7 = 28$.

$$\frac{1}{4} = \frac{1}{4} \times \frac{7}{7} = \frac{7}{28} \qquad \frac{3}{7} = \frac{3}{7} \times \frac{4}{4} = \frac{12}{28}$$

$$\frac{7}{28} + \frac{12}{28} = \frac{19}{28}$$

$$\frac{1}{4} + \frac{3}{7} = \frac{19}{28}$$

Sometimes, especially when there are three or more fractions, multiplying the denominators is not the most efficient method for finding a common denominator. When there are three or more fractions, follow the steps in Table 1.1.

TABLE 1.1 Steps for Finding a Common Denominator

Step 1. Find the prime* factors of each denominator.

$$\frac{1}{15} \quad \frac{5}{6} \quad \frac{11}{36}$$

$$15 = 3 \times 5$$
$$6 = 2 \times 3$$
$$36 = 2 \times 2 \times 3 \times 3$$

Summarized below.

Denominator	Prime Factors
15	3, 5
6	2, 3
36	2, 2, 3, 3

Step 2. Count the number of times each prime number appeared when you found the prime factors for the denominators.
- The count of primes in 15 is one 3 and one 5.
- The count of primes in 6 is one 2 and one 3.
- The count of primes in 36 is two 2s and two 3s.

Step 3. For each prime number, take the largest of these counts.
- The largest count of the 2s is two.
- The largest count of the 3s is two.
- The largest count of the 5 is one.

Step 4. The least common denominator is the product of all the prime numbers listed in Step 3.

$$2 \times 2 \times 3 \times 3 \times 5 = 180$$

*A number that is divisible only by 1 and itself (such as 2, 3, 5, 7)

After two fractions have been converted to fractions with a common denominator and added together, it may be necessary to reduce the fraction. This process requires canceling. To understand why this works, remember that multiplying or dividing a fraction by 1 will not change its value.

$$\frac{a}{b} \times 1 = \frac{a}{b}$$

Determine the largest number c that goes into both a and b. Subsequently write a as some number (call it p) times c and write b as some other number (call it q) times c.

$$\frac{a}{b} = \frac{pc}{qc} = \frac{p}{q}$$

We have used the fact that $c/c = 1$ to cancel out c. Once the largest number possible has been canceled out of the numerator and denominator, the fraction is reduced to lowest terms.

Example 1.1.5

Simplify the fraction $\dfrac{3}{27}$.

$$\frac{3}{27} = \frac{1 \times 3}{9 \times 3} = \frac{1}{9} \times \frac{3}{3} = \frac{1}{9}$$

Another way to simplify $^3/_{27}$ is to divide both the numerator and denominator by a common factor (in this case 3).

$$\frac{3}{27} = \frac{3 \div 3}{27 \div 3} = \frac{1}{9}$$

Example 1.1.6

Simplify the fraction $\dfrac{2}{12}$.

$$\frac{2}{12} = \frac{1 \times 2}{6 \times 2} = \frac{1}{6} \times \frac{2}{2} = \frac{1}{6}$$

Another way to simplify $^2/_{12}$ is to divide both the numerator and denominator by a common factor (in this case 2).

$$\frac{2}{12} = \frac{2 \div 2}{12 \div 2} = \frac{1}{6}$$

When adding or subtracting fractions that have the same denominator, add or subtract the numerators and place the number over the common denominator. It may be necessary to reduce the answer fraction if it is not in lowest terms.

Example 1.1.7

Perform the following subtraction.

$$\frac{5}{6} - \frac{3}{6}$$

Because these fractions have a common denominator 6, subtract the numerators.

$$\frac{5}{6} - \frac{3}{6} = \frac{2}{6}$$

Reduce: $\dfrac{\cancel{2} \times 1}{\cancel{2} \times 3} = \dfrac{1}{3}$

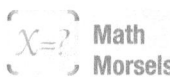
Example 1.1.8

Simplify the following subtraction.

$$3\frac{3}{4} - \frac{1}{2}$$

Change the mixed number to an improper fraction.

$$3\frac{3}{4} = \frac{(3 \times 4) + 3}{4}$$

In the subtraction, replace the mixed fraction with the improper fraction, and confirm that the denominators are the same. Because the denominator of the second fraction is 2, the second fraction must be changed to a fraction with a denominator of 4. To do this, multiply the numerator and denominator by 2.

$$\frac{1}{2} \times \frac{2}{2} = \frac{2}{4}$$

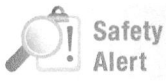
Then, $3\frac{3}{4} - \frac{2}{4} = \frac{15}{4} - \frac{2}{4}$ (Both denominators are 4.)

Solve the problem by subtracting the numerators.

$$\frac{15}{4} - \frac{2}{4} = \frac{13}{4}$$

Change the improper fraction to a mixed fraction by dividing 13 by 4.

$$\frac{13}{4} = 3\frac{1}{4}$$

When subtracting fractions that have different denominators, find the least common denominator and convert to equivalent fractions. Then subtract the numerators and place the number over the denominator. It may be necessary to reduce the answer fraction to lowest terms.

Example 1.1.9

Perform the following calculation.

$$\frac{3}{4} - \frac{2}{3}$$

The least common denominator is 12. To convert to equivalent fractions, multiply $\frac{3}{4}$ by $\frac{3}{3}$ and $\frac{2}{3}$ by $\frac{4}{4}$.

$$\frac{3}{4} = \frac{9}{12}$$
$$\frac{2}{3} = \frac{8}{12}$$

Replace the original fractions and subtract the numerators.

$$\frac{9}{12} - \frac{8}{12} = \frac{1}{12}$$

Example 1.1.10

Subtract the following:

$$2\frac{1}{2} - \frac{6}{3}$$

Change the mixed number to a fraction.

$$2\frac{1}{2} = \frac{(2 \times 2) + 1}{2} = \frac{5}{2}$$

Replace the mixed number with the improper fraction.

$$2\frac{1}{2} - \frac{6}{3} = \frac{5}{2} - \frac{6}{3}$$

The least common denominator is 6. Convert to equivalent fractions.

$$\frac{5}{2} \times \frac{3}{3} = \frac{15}{6}$$

$$\frac{6}{3} \times \frac{2}{2} = \frac{12}{6}$$

Rewrite the original problem and subtract the numerators.

$$\frac{15}{6} - \frac{12}{6} = \frac{3}{6}$$

Simplify the answer.

$$\frac{3}{6} = \frac{1}{2}$$

Therefore, $2\frac{1}{2} - \frac{6}{3} = \frac{1}{2}$.

Multiplying and Dividing Fractions

To multiply fractions, multiply numerators by numerators and denominators by denominators. Then reduce to lowest terms.

$$\frac{1}{8} \times \frac{1}{2} = \frac{1 \times 1}{8 \times 2} = \frac{1}{16}$$

$$\frac{1}{8} \times \frac{1}{2} \times \frac{2}{3} = \frac{1 \times 1 \times \cancel{2}}{8 \times \cancel{2} \times 3} = \frac{1}{24}$$

$$5 \times \frac{3}{4} = \frac{5}{1} \times \frac{3}{4} = \frac{15}{4} = 3\frac{3}{4}$$

When partial doses, such as ½ tablet or ¾ teaspoonful, are prescribed, it may become necessary to multiply fractions to determine the amount of medication to dispense. The following examples demonstrate these calculations.

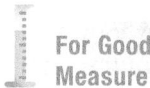
Example 1.1.11

A patient needs to take ¹/₂ of a furosemide 40 mg tablet each day for 30 days. How many tablets will the patient need to last 30 days?

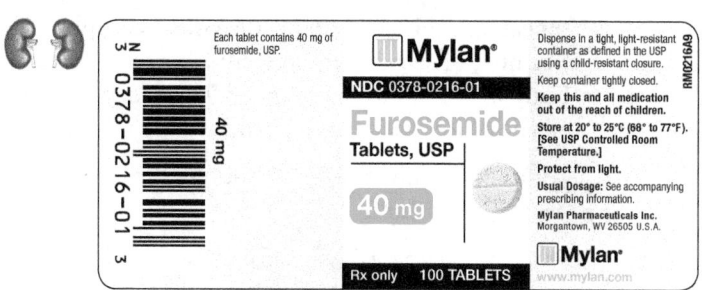

This problem may be solved by multiplying the number of days by the amount of medication taken per day.

$$\frac{30 \text{ days}}{1} \times \frac{\frac{1}{2} \text{ tablet}}{\text{day}} = \frac{30}{1} \times \frac{1}{2} = \frac{30 \times 1}{2 \times 1} = \frac{30}{2} = 15 \text{ tablets}$$

Introduction to Dimensional Analysis

In the previous example, you may notice how the units "days" were canceled out leaving the desired ending units of "tablets". This technique is called **dimensional analysis** (or the factor-label method or unit factor method). Dimensional analysis is a problem-solving method that uses the fact that any number can be multiplied by 1 without changing its value. Dimensional analysis involves multiplication and division of fractions. Chapter 4 gives further instruction on the use of dimensional analysis.

To understand dimensional analysis, you must first understand equal fractions.

$$If\ a = b, \text{ then } \frac{a}{b} = 1 \text{ and } \frac{b}{a} = 1.$$

Therefore any equality ($a = b$) can form two fractions ($^a/_b = 1$, $^b/_a = 1$). This principle allows you to solve problems by setting them up as fractions that are multiplied by other fractions. You must set up the problems so that the starting units cancel one another out and you are left with the desired units.

$$\text{starting units} \times \frac{\text{desired units}}{\text{starting units}} = \text{desired units}$$

Using dimensional analysis, calculate the number of minutes in one hour.

The desired units (the units you want to find) are minutes and the starting units (the units you are given) are hours.

$$1 \text{ hour} \times \frac{60 \text{ minutes}}{1 \text{ hour}} = 60 \text{ minutes}$$

The starting units of hours are canceled out and leave the desired units as minutes.

Consider calculating the number of minutes in one day. There are 24 hours in a day and 60 minutes in an hour. The desired units are minutes per day (minutes/day). Set up fractions to solve for minutes/day by canceling out the hour units.

$$\frac{24 \text{ hours}}{1 \text{ day}} \times \frac{60 \text{ minutes}}{1 \text{ hour}} = \frac{1,440 \text{ minutes}}{\text{day}} = 1,440 \text{ minutes per day}$$

You can use this method to solve more complex calculations. Consider calculating the number of seconds in one day. There are 60 seconds in one minute, 60 minutes in one hour, and 24 hours in one day. The desired units are seconds per day (seconds/day), and the units that must be canceled are minutes and hours.

$$\frac{60 \text{ seconds}}{1 \text{ minute}} \times \frac{60 \text{ minutes}}{1 \text{ hour}} \times \frac{24 \text{ hours}}{1 \text{ day}} = \frac{86,400 \text{ seconds}}{\text{day}} = 86,400 \text{ seconds per day}$$

Dimensional analysis is useful in performing some types of math calculations, and you may find this problem-solving method to be helpful in your pharmacy studies.

Example 1.1.12

How many milligrams are in $\frac{1}{2}$ of a furosemide tablet shown in the following label? Use dimensional analysis to solve the problem.

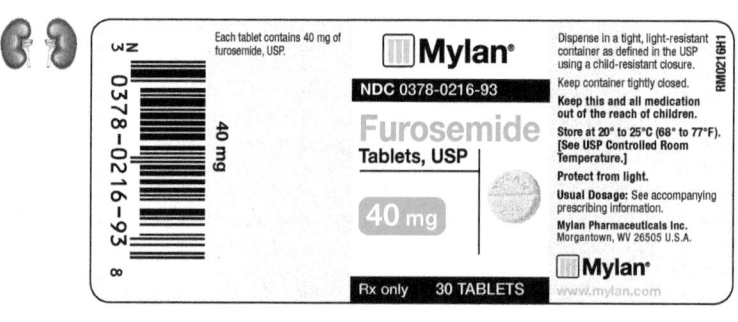

$$\frac{40 \text{ mg}}{1 \text{ tablet}} \times \frac{\frac{1}{2} \text{ tablet}}{1} = \frac{40}{1} \times \frac{1}{2} = \frac{40}{2} = 20 \text{ mg}$$

Alternatively, you can divide the strength of the tablet by 2, because $\frac{2}{1}$ is the reciprocal (or inverse) of $\frac{1}{2}$.

$$40 \text{ mg} \div 2 = 20 \text{ mg}$$

Tables 1.2 and 1.3 list guidelines for multiplying and dividing fractions. To divide by a fraction, change the "÷" (division sign) to "×" (multiply sign) and invert the number to the right of the operation sign. The inverted number is called the reciprocal. Then multiply the fractions and reduce as necessary.

TABLE 1.2 Guidelines for Multiplying Fractions

1. Multiplying the numerator by a number, while multiplying the denominator by 1, increases the value of a fraction.

$$\frac{1}{4} \times \frac{2}{1} = \frac{1 \times 2}{4 \times 1} = \frac{2}{4} = \frac{1}{2}$$

2. Multiplying the denominator by a number, while multiplying the numerator by 1, decreases the value of a fraction.

$$\frac{1}{4} \times \frac{1}{2} = \frac{1 \times 1}{4 \times 2} = \frac{1}{8}$$

3. The value of a fraction is not altered by multiplying both the numerator and the denominator by the same number.

$$\frac{1}{4} \times \frac{4}{4} = \frac{1 \times 4}{4 \times 4} = \frac{4}{16} = \frac{1}{4}$$

TABLE 1.3 Guidelines for Dividing Fractions

1. Dividing the denominator by a number is the same as multiplying the numerator by that number.

$$\frac{3}{\frac{20}{7}} = \frac{3 \times 7}{20} = \frac{21}{20} \text{ because } 3 \div \frac{20}{7} = 3 \times \frac{7}{20} = \frac{21}{20}$$

2. Dividing the numerator by a number is the same as multiplying the denominator by that number.

$$\frac{\frac{3}{4}}{6} = \frac{3}{4 \times 6} = \frac{3}{24} = \frac{1}{8} \text{ because } \frac{3}{4} \div 6 = \frac{3}{4} \times \frac{1}{6} = \frac{3}{24} = \frac{1}{8}$$

1.1 Problem Set

Circle the fraction with the greatest value.

1. $\frac{1}{2}$ $\frac{1}{3}$ $\frac{1}{4}$

2. $\frac{3}{10}$ $\frac{3}{12}$ $\frac{3}{8}$

Circle the fraction with the lowest value.

3. $\frac{3}{1}$ $\frac{4}{1}$ $\frac{2}{1}$

4. $\frac{2}{6}$ $\frac{3}{6}$ $\frac{4}{6}$

5. $\frac{1}{10}$ $\frac{1}{8}$ $\frac{1}{6}$

Solve.

6. $\frac{5}{6} + \frac{7}{10} + \frac{2}{5} =$

7. $\frac{21}{32} + \frac{1}{12} + \frac{31}{48} =$

Reduce the following fractions to lowest terms and rewrite as a mixed number, if necessary.

8. $\frac{25}{100}$

9. $\frac{67}{10}$

10. $\frac{11}{5}$

11. $\frac{27}{30}$

12. $\frac{12}{30}$

13. $\frac{90}{100}$

14. A patient has taken ¼ tablet, ½ tablet, 1½ tablets, and ¾ tablet. In total, how many tablets has the patient taken?

15. Which dose contains the largest amount of medication: one tablet containing ¹/₁₅₀ grain or two tablets containing ¹/₁₀₀ grain in each tablet?

16. You are to measure ¼ grain of medication each into unit dose oral containers. Your bulk container holds 375 grains. How many unit dose oral containers will be prepared?

Table sugar is needed for making simple syrup. One formula calls for ½ lb to make enough syrup, a second formula requires ⅘ lb, a third formula requires ¼ lb, and the last formula requires 2½ lb. You need to make one batch of all four formulas.

17. How many bags of sugar should you buy if it is packaged in 2 lb bags?

18. How many bags of sugar must be purchased if it is packaged in 5 lb bags?

Self-check your work in Appendix A.

1.2 Decimals

A fraction in which the denominator is a power of 10 (such as 10, 100, 1,000, etc.) is a decimal fraction or, more simply, a **decimal**. In decimal fractions, the denominator is not written but is represented by the location of the number in relation to the decimal point. For example, ²/₁₀ is a decimal fraction. The Arabic representation of ²/₁₀ is 0.2. Notice the 10 in the denominator is not written, but represents the location of the 2 relative to the decimal point.) The decimal point separates the whole number part from the decimal fraction part of a number. Numbers written to the right of the decimal point are decimal fractions and have a value of less than 1. Numbers written to the left of the decimal point have a value of 1 or greater (whole numbers).

An understanding of decimals is *crucial* to pharmacy calculations because most medication orders are written using the metric system, which uses decimals. Remember that numbers to the left of the decimal point are whole numbers, and numbers to the right of the decimal point are decimal fractions (parts of a whole).

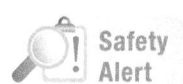

Safety Alert

For a decimal value less than 1, use a leading zero to prevent errors.

Reading and Writing Decimals

A decimal is read by first reading the whole number to the left of the decimal point, if there is one, then the decimal point (say "and" or "point"), and then the decimal fraction, to the right of the decimal point. For example, the number 2.375 is read as "two point three seven five" or "two and three hundred seventy-five thousandths."

A decimal is written as a whole number or a zero, then a decimal point, and then the fractional portion. The values to the right of the decimal point are powers of one-tenth: tenths, hundredths, thousandths, ten thousandths, and so on. Figure 1.3 illustrates this relationship in terms of medication.

When there is no whole number, a zero should be placed to the left of the decimal point. This zero is called a **leading zero**. Using a leading zero helps prevent errors by ensuring that the reader does not overlook the decimal point.

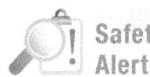

For Good Measure

The size of a tablet or capsule does not always represent the amount of active drug within it. Many tablets and capsules contain large amounts of inactive ingredients (fillers) to make the medication a size or flavor that is more conducive to the patient.

Safety Alert

Medication labels for nitroglycerin tablets—a medication prescribed for chest pain—may contain either decimals or fractions. Therefore, be sure to check the label carefully before preparing the medication.

TABLE 1.4　Writing and Reading Decimals

Fraction	Writing the Decimal	Reading the Decimal
$1\frac{1}{2}$ or $\frac{3}{2}$	1.5	"One point five" or "One and five tenths"
$\frac{3}{4}$	0.75*	"Zero point seven five" or "Seventy five hundredths"
$\frac{1}{8}$	0.125*	"Zero point one two five" or "One hundred twenty five thousandths"

*notice the presence of the leading zero

Adding and Subtracting Decimals

When adding or subtracting decimals, place the numbers in columns so that the decimal points are aligned vertically. Add or subtract from the far-right column to the far-left column.

$$
\begin{array}{r} 20.4 \\ +21.8 \\ \hline 42.2 \end{array}
\qquad
\begin{array}{r} 11.2 \\ 13.6 \\ +16.0 \\ \hline 40.8 \end{array}
\qquad
\begin{array}{r} 15.36 \\ -3.80 \\ \hline 11.56 \end{array}
$$

Multiplying and Dividing Decimals

Multiply two decimals as you would whole numbers. Then add the total number of decimal places that are in the two numbers being multiplied (which is the number of decimal places in your answer), count that number of places from right to left in the answer, and insert a decimal point.

$$
\begin{array}{r} 1.23 \\ \times 2.3 \\ \hline 369 \\ +2460 \\ \hline 2.829 \end{array}
$$

(2 decimal places)
(1 decimal place)

(A zero is added to align the columns.)
(Answer has three decimal places.)

To divide decimal numbers, change both the divisor (the number you are dividing by) and the dividend (the number being divided) to whole numbers by moving their decimal points the same number of places to the right. If the divisor and the dividend have a different number of digits after the decimal point, choose the one that has more digits and move its decimal point a sufficient number of places to make it a whole number. Then move the decimal point in the other number the same number of places, adding a zero at the end if necessary. In the first example below, the divisor has more digits after the decimal point, so move its decimal point three places to the right to make it a whole number. Then move the decimal point in the dividend the same number of places, adding a zero at the end. In the second example below, the dividend has more digits after the decimal point, so move its decimal point three places to the right to make it a whole number. Then move the decimal point in the divisor three places to the right also.

$$1.45 \div 3.625 = 0.4 \qquad 1.617 \div 2.31 = 0.7$$

$$\frac{1.45}{3.625} = \frac{1{,}450}{3{,}625} = 0.4 \qquad \frac{1.617}{2.31} = \frac{1{,}617}{2{,}310} = 0.7$$

Rounding Decimals

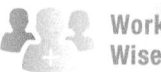 **Work Wise**

The terms "drug" and "medication" may be used interchangeably in your practice setting, especially when related to pharmacy calculations. Pharmacy technicians should be accustomed to hearing and using both terms.

Rounding is the process of simplifying a number by increasing or decreasing its value. Rounding numbers is essential for daily use of mathematical operations. The purpose of rounding is to make numbers easy to work with. It is important to recognize, however, that rounding will affect the **accuracy** to which a medication can be measured. In some cases, it may be appropriate to calculate a dose to the nearest whole milliliter and, in other cases, to round to the nearest tenth or hundredth of a milliliter. Depending on the medication and strength prescribed, it may not be possible to accurately measure a very small quantity such as a hundredth of a milliliter.

When numbers with decimals are used to calculate a volumetric (or volume related) dose, a number with multiple digits beyond the decimal often results. It is not practical to retain all of these digits, as a dose cannot be accurately measured beyond the hundredths or thousandths place for most medications. Most commonly, the dose is rounded to the nearest tenth. It is common practice to round the weight of a dose to the hundredths or thousandths place, or as precisely as the particular measuring device (or medication) will permit.

To round an answer to the nearest tenth, carry the calculation out two places, to the hundredths place. If the digit in the hundredths place is 5 or greater, add 1 to the tenths place number. If the digit in the hundredths place is less than 5, round the number down by omitting the digit in the hundredths place.

$$5.65 \text{ becomes } 5.7 \qquad 4.24 \text{ becomes } 4.2$$

The same procedure may be used when rounding to the nearest hundredths place or thousandths place.

3.8421 = 3.84	(hundredths place)
41.2674 = 41.27	(hundredths place)
0.3928 = 0.393	(thousandths place)
4.1111 = 4.111	(thousandths place)

As mentioned earlier, when rounding numbers used in pharmacy calculations, it is common to round to the nearest tenth. However, there are times when a dose is very small and rounding to the nearest hundredth or thousandth may be more appropriate.

The exact dose calculated is 0.08752 g
Rounded to nearest tenth: 0.1 g
Rounded to nearest hundredth: 0.09 g
Rounded to nearest thousandth: 0.088 g

Rounding numbers can be a challenge in pharmacy calculations. In this text, rounding should generally not occur until the last step in the calculation. Please be aware that different work environments may have different rounding policies. Make sure to inquire about rounding policies at your practice location.

Example 1.2.1

Round the answer of the following to the nearest tenth.

$$3.46 \times 7.1 = 24.566$$

Answer = 24.6

Example 1.2.2

Round the answer of the following equation to the nearest tenth.

$$0.3563 \times 1.3 = 0.46319$$

Answer = 0.5

In most cases, a zero occurring at the end of a string of digits after the decimal point is not written. This zero is called a **trailing zero**. The exception to this rule occurs when rounding results in a zero as the last place value. When the last digit resulting from rounding is a zero, this zero should be written because it is considered significant to that particular problem or dosage. In such cases, the amount can be measured out to an exact zero as the place value.

Example 1.2.3

Round 9.98 to the nearest tenth.

Answer = 10.0

Example 1.2.4

Round 0.599 to the nearest hundredth.

Answer = 0.60

1.2 Problem Set

Write the following decimals.

1. seven hundred eighty-four and thirty-six hundredths

2. nine tenths

Express the following fractions in decimal form.

3. $\dfrac{1}{5}$

4. $\dfrac{1}{20}$

5. $4\dfrac{2}{4}$

6. $\dfrac{30}{100}$

7. $\dfrac{1}{200}$

8. $\dfrac{1}{500}$

9. $1\dfrac{8}{10}$

10. $\dfrac{1}{25}$

11. $\dfrac{1}{125}$

Add the following decimals.

12. $0.34 + 1.54 =$

13. $1.39 + 1.339 =$

Subtract the following decimals.

14. $15.36 - 0.987 =$

15. $3.09875 - 0.00045 =$

16. $12.901 - 0.903 =$

Multiply the following decimals and round to the nearest hundredth.

17. $21.62 \times 21.62 =$

18. $0.9 \times 500 =$

Divide the following decimals and round to the nearest thousandth.

19. $12 \div 6.5 =$

20. $0.8 \div 0.6 =$

Round the following to the nearest hundredth.

21. 3.872

22. 0.138

23. 0.076

Round the following to the nearest thousandths.

24. 0.1961

25. 0.0488

Multiply the following and round to the nearest tenth.

26. $6.7 \times 5.21 =$

27. $0.45 \times 3.1 =$

Applications

28. Using the prescription below, answer the following questions.
Note: TID means "three times a day."

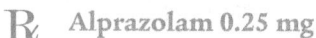 **Alprazolam 0.25 mg**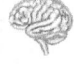
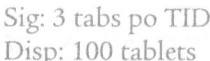
Sig: 3 tabs po TID
Disp: 100 tablets

a. How many milligrams is the patient taking with each dose?

b. How many milligrams is the patient taking each day?

c. How many tablets will the patient need for 14 days?

d. Is the prescription written for enough tablets to last the patient until the next office visit in two weeks?

e. The pharmacy plans to charge $7.59 plus the cost of the medication. The available products include:

alprazolam 0.25 mg #100/$14.95
alprazolam 0.5 mg #100/$17.46
alprazolam 1 mg #100/$23.87

Select the appropriate product and calculate the price for the patient. Based on the prescription provided, the pharmacy can only dispense 100 tablets.

29. The physician changes the prescription at the patient's next visit. The new prescription is shown below.

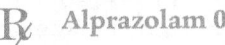 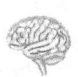

Rℂ **Alprazolam 0.25 mg**

Sig: 4 tabs po TID
Disp: 175 tablets

The available products include:

alprazolam 0.25 mg #100/$14.95
alprazolam 0.5 mg #100/$17.46
alprazolam 1 mg #100/$23.87

a. How many milligrams at each dose is this?

b. How much would #125 alprazolam 0.5 mg tablets cost the pharmacy?

c. How much would #50 alprazolam 1 mg tablets cost the pharmacy?

d. How many days would #50 alprazolam 1 mg tablets taken TID last?

30. Sterile water comes in bottles of 1 L. You will need to pour out 120 mL bottles for each patient.

a. How many 120 mL bottles will you get from a 1 L bottle? (1 L = 1,000 mL)

b. How much will be left over?

31. How many total milliliters will need to be dispensed for the following prescription? Round you answer to the nearest whole mililiter

Note: bid means "twice a day."

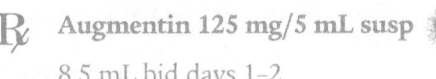

Rℂ **Augmentin 125 mg/5 mL susp**

8.5 mL bid days 1–2
5.75 mL bid days 3–7

32. Round the following to the nearest whole dollar.

a. $46.92

b. 12 @ $1.26

c. $7.37 divided by 2

33. Calculate the following dollar amounts and round to the nearest cent.

a. $5.84 × 12 =

b. $0.415 × 269 =

34. Calculate the following to the nearest hundredth.

a. 34 ÷ 38

b. 51 ÷ 60

c. 83 ÷ 90

Self-check your work in Appendix A.

1.3 Number Systems

Two types of numbers are used in pharmaceutical calculations: Roman and Arabic. The Arabic system is more commonly used in health care, although the Roman system is also used.

Roman Numerals

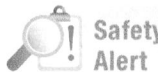
The Roman numbering system can be traced back to ancient Rome. This system uses letters to represent quantities or amounts, whereas the Arabic system uses numbers, fractions (such as $\frac{3}{8}$), and decimals. **Roman numerals** are expressed as either lowercase letters (particularly in calculations) or as capital letters. The most frequently used numerals are the uppercase I, V, and X, which represent 1, 5, and 10, respectively. In writing prescriptions, however, the lowercase letter i is often used to represent the number one, ii to represent two, and so on. To prevent errors in interpretation, a line is drawn above the letters, with the dot above the line (for example: $\bar{i}, \bar{ii}, \bar{iii}$). The symbol for $\frac{1}{2}$, if placed after a Roman numeral, is ss (for example, $5\frac{1}{2}$ is vss). Roman numerals are used to record amount or quantity but have little use in calculations.

Table 1.5 lists the common symbols and their values in the Roman system. The example that follows the table shows a prescription that uses Roman numerals to indicate both the amount to take at each dose and the quantity to dispense.

TABLE 1.5 Comparison of Roman and Arabic Numerals

Roman		Arabic	Roman		Arabic
ss	=	½	L or l	=	50
I or i or ɨ	=	1	C or c*	=	100
V or v	=	5	D or d	=	500
X or x	=	10	M or m	=	1,000

*be aware that cubic centimeter is abbreviated as cc.

Example 1.3.1

The following prescription is received in the pharmacy. How many tablets are in a daily dose and how many tablets are to be dispensed?

℞   metformin 850 mg

     Sig: ī tab daily with food
     Disp: C tablets

Determine the dose.

$$\bar{i} \text{ tablet per day} = 1 \text{ tablet}$$

Determine the quantity to dispense.

$$C \text{ tablets} = 100 \text{ tablets}$$

Roman numerals may be grouped together to express different quantities. To interpret these numbers, addition and subtraction must be used, as specified in the guidelines shown in Table 1.6. Example 1.3.2 demonstrates how to read groups of Roman numerals.

TABLE 1.6   Guidelines for Interpreting Roman Numerals

1. When a numeral is repeated or a smaller numeral follows a larger one, the values are added together.

ii or II = 1 + 1 = 2   VII = 5 + 2 = 7
LVII = 50 + 5 + 1 + 1 = 57   XXI = 10 + 10 + 1 = 21
CXIII = 100 + 10 + 1 + 1 + 1 = 113   LXV = 50 + 10 + 5 = 65

2. When a smaller numeral comes before a larger numeral, subtract the smaller value.

IV = 5 − 1 = 4   IX = 10 − 1 = 9
CD = 500 − 100 = 400

3. Numerals are never repeated more than three times in sequence.

III = 3   IV = 4   XXX = 30   XL = 40

4. When a smaller numeral comes between two larger numerals, subtract the smaller numeral from the numeral that follows.

XIX = 10 + (10 − 1) = 19   XIV = 10 + (5 − 1) = 14

 Example 1.3.2

The following prescription is received in the pharmacy. How many milligrams are in a dose, and how many tablets are to be dispensed?

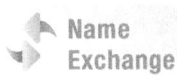 **Name Exchange**

Diphenhydramine is generic for Benadryl. The oral dosage form is an over-the-counter (OTC) medication, but the injectable form requires a prescription.

℞   diphenhydramine XXV mg
      Sig: ii tab each night
      Disp: XXXII tablets

To calculate the number of milligrams in a dose, start by calculating the number of milligrams in a tablet. Add the Roman numerals on the prescription.

$$\frac{XXV \text{ mg}}{1 \text{ tablet}} = 10 + 10 + 5 = \frac{25 \text{ mg}}{1 \text{ tablet}}$$

Then, determine the number of tablets taken each night.

$$\text{ii tab} = 1 + 1 = 2 \text{ tablets}$$

Determine the daily dose by multiplying the number of milligrams in each tablet by the number of tablets taken each night.

$$\frac{25 \text{ mg}}{1 \text{ tablet}} \times 2 \text{ tablets} = 50 \text{ mg}$$

Calculate the number to dispense by adding the Roman numerals on the prescription.

XXXII tablets = 10 + 10 + 10 + 1 + 1 = 32 tablets

The Arabic Number System

The Arabic number system is also called the decimal system. Ten figures are used: 0, 1, 2, 3, 4, 5, 6, 7, 8, 9. The decimal point serves as the anchor. Each place to the left of the decimal point signals a tenfold increase, and each place to the right signals a tenfold decrease. Figure 1.3 illustrates the relative value of each place. Memorize the **place values**, which describe each numeral's relationship to the decimal point.

FIGURE 1.3
Decimal Units and Values

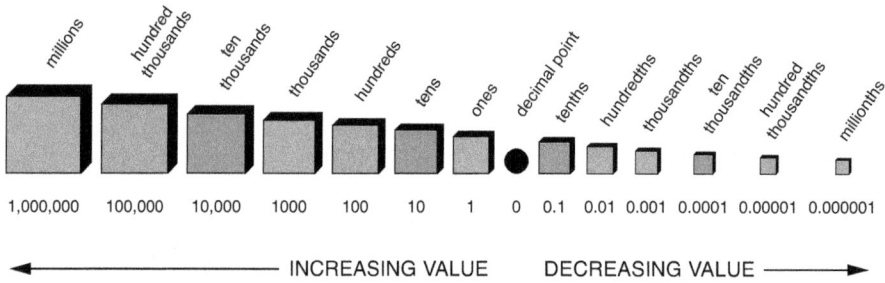

In expressions using **Arabic numbers**, whole numbers are to the left of the decimal point, whereas fractions are to the right. The positions for the numbers to the right of the decimal point are called decimal places. Table 1.7 on the following page provides guidelines for interpreting Arabic numbers.

Scientific Notation

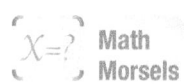

Math Morsels

Exponents can be positive or negative. For example, a number with a positive exponent is 10^2, and a number with a negative exponent is 10^{-2}. $10^2 = 100$, and $10^{-2} = 0.01$.

Scientific notation is a method used to write numbers that have a very large or very small numerical value. Because of space issues as well as readability, it is not practical to write out numbers that have a large number of zeros, such as 5,200,000,000,000, or very small numbers, such as 0.00000025. These two numbers are written in **decimal notation**. To change decimal notation to scientific notation, you can rewrite the number as a group of significant figures multiplied by 10 with an exponent. An exponent is a number placed above and to the right of another number to show it has been raised to a power. Significant figures are all the digits of a number that signify accuracy. The number in the exponent indicates how many places the decimal has been moved, and the sign of the exponent (positive or negative) indicates the direction the decimal was moved. A positive exponent indicates a number greater than 1, and a negative exponent indicates a number less than 1. Table 1.8 shows examples of values written in Arabic numbers and in scientific notation.

TABLE 1.7 Guidelines for Interpreting Arabic Numbers

1. The numerals to the left of the decimal point represent the whole number part of the fraction. If there is no number to the left of the decimal point, place a 0 to the left of the decimal point. This is called a leading 0.

2. If whole number parts are different, whichever has the larger whole number part has the higher value.

   8.2 > 6.2

   20.1 > 14.6

   3.08 > 0.39

3. If the whole numbers parts are identical (including if both are 0), look at the numerals to the right of the decimal point, starting with the tenths (the first one) and proceeding to the right.

4. If the tenths are different, the fraction with the greatest tenth has the higher value.

   0.4 > 0.3

   2.41 > 2.39

5. When the tenths are identical, a number with a decimal fraction that is greatest in hundredths has the greater value.

   0.17 > 0.15

   0.35 > 0.30

   10.66 > 10.64

6. If the hundredths are also identical, then the value is determined by the thousandths (and so on).

   0.125 > 0.124

   7.0097 > 7.0092

7. The total value of a number is the sum of the different parts.

467.43 represents	400.00	=	four hundreds
	+60.00	=	six tens
	+ 7.00	=	seven ones
	+ 0.40	=	four tenths
	+ 0.03	=	three hundredths

   You say this number as "four hundred sixty-seven and forty-three hundredths."

TABLE 1.8 Scientific Notation Equivalences

Arabic Number	Decimal Place Movement	Scientific Notation
6,500	3 places to the left	6.5×10^3
120,000	5 places to the left	1.2×10^5
921,000,000	8 places to the left	9.21×10^8
4,800,000,000,000	12 places to the left	4.8×10^{12}
0.109	1 place to the right	1.09×10^{-1}
0.000587	4 places to the right	5.87×10^{-4}
0.00000026	7 places to the right	2.6×10^{-7}
0.000000000049	11 places to the right	4.9×10^{-11}

1.3 Problem Set

Give the equivalent Arabic number for each of the following Roman numerals.

1. X

2. V

3. DCXXIV

4. MML

5. XLVIII

Give the equivalent Roman numeral for each of the following Arabic numbers.

6. 17

7. 67

8. 1,995

In each group of numbers, circle the highest value.

9. 3.1   1.7   4.1

10. 0.5   0.56   0.6

In each group of numbers, circle the lowest value.

11. 2.02   2.12   2.1

12. 0.16   0.167   0.017

Using the following number, list the value of each numeral in the named places.

92,375.046

13. tenths place

14. thousandths place

15. hundreds place

State the place value of the underlined digit.

16. 18,240.6

17. 7.2391

18. 621.508

19. 0.98

20. 40. 023

Write the following numbers as Arabic numbers.

21. 6.8×10^4

22. 1.87×10^6

23. 1.03×10^7

24. 8.4×10^{-4}

25. 7.68×10^{-3}

26. 6.239×10^{-5}

Write the following numbers using scientific notation.

27. 0.00000000329

28. 390,000,000,000

29. 0.0038

30. 52,000,000,000,000,000

31. 3,779,000

32. 0.000000000202

Applications

33. A patient is to take "VIIss tablets three times daily." How many tablets must be dispensed to last seven days?

34. Using the prescription below, answer the following questions.

R_x ASA gr X

Sig: i po daily
Disp: C

Note: po (or PO) means "by mouth."

a. What is the strength of the tablet?

b. What is the daily dose?

c. What is the quantity to be dispensed?

35. Using the prescription below, answer the following questions.

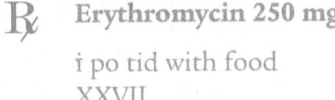

R_x **Erythromycin 250 mg**

  i po tid with food
  XXVII

Note: tid (or TID) means "three times a day."

a. How many tablets will be dispensed?

b. How many days will the prescription last?

36. Using the prescription below, answer the following questions.

R_x **Glucotrol tablet 5 mg**

  ii po q am
  i po with lunch
  ii po 8 pm
  30 days' supply

a. How many tablets are taken each day?

b. How many tablets will be dispensed?

c. How long would C tablets last?

Self-check your work in Appendix A.

1.4 Estimates

Estimating an answer before calculating the solution is a simple way of checking to see whether the answer you arrive at is reasonable. Estimating can be used in both simple mathematical equations and more complicated algebraic equations.

There are no set mathematical rules for estimating. Most commonly, estimating is performed by rounding to the nearest whole unit that makes sense for the numbers involved. This may be the ones place, tens place, hundreds place, or even larger. Rounding to the nearest whole dollar while shopping is an example of estimating.

Estimating Sums

A **sum** is the result of adding two or more numbers. When estimating sums, it is common to round the numbers to be added to the nearest ten, hundred, or thousand and then add the rounded numbers. When rounding and then adding, the values in the ones place and lower are often ignored. The following calculations compare an actual sum with a corresponding estimate.

Actual $73.8 + 42.03 + 18.3 + 87.32 = 221.45$
Estimate $70 + 40 + 20 + 90 = 220$

Actual $623 + 1{,}493 + 1{,}631 + 794 + 86 = 4{,}627$
Estimate $600 + 1{,}500 + 1{,}600 + 800 + 100 = 4{,}600$

Actual $6{,}425 + 2{,}652 + 2{,}328 + 4{,}490 = 15{,}895$
Estimate $6{,}000 + 3{,}000 + 2{,}000 + 4{,}000 = 15{,}000$

Safety Alert

Estimated values can be used to double-check doses but should never be relied on for accuracy.

Estimating is a process that becomes easier with practice. A small list of numbers will often generate a fairly accurate estimate, whereas longer lists of numbers may require more practice and may be less accurate. The sum determined by estimating cannot be relied on for accuracy when dispensing prescriptions.

Estimating Products and Quotients

A **product** is the result of multiplying two numbers. A **quotient** is the result of dividing one number by another number. One way to estimate products or quotients is common to round each of the original numbers, divided by the place value of its leftmost column, to the nearest whole number. The rounded numbers can be quickly multiplied or divided, and the appropriate number of zeros can be added to the answer.

Example 1.4.1

Estimate the product of 325 × 618.

First, round the two numbers. 325 is closer to 300 than 400 and should be rounded to 300. 616 is closer to 600 than 700 and should be rounded to 600.

Then divide each number by the place value of its leftmost column. The value of the leftmost column both numbers is hundreds.

$$300 \div 100 = 3$$
$$600 \div 100 = 6$$

Now multiply the rounded numbers.

$$3 \times 6 = 18$$

Last, add the appropriate number of zeros to the answer. Two zeros should be added for the hundreds place of 325 and two zeroes should be added for the hundreds place of 618.

$$180,000$$

Compare the estimate to the actual product, which is 200,850.

Example 1.4.2

Estimate the product of 843 × 41.

First, round the two numbers. 843 is rounded to 800 and 41 is rounded to 40.

Then divide each number by the place value of its leftmost column. The value of the leftmost column of 800 is hundreds and the value of the leftmost column of 40 is tens.

$$800 \div 100 = 8$$
$$40 \div 10 = 4$$

Now multiply the rounded numbers.

$$8 \times 4 = 32$$

Last, add the appropriate number of zeros to the answer. Two zeros should be added for the hundreds place of 843 and one zero should be added for the tens place of 41.

$$32,000$$

Compare the estimate to the actual product, which is 34,563.

Example 1.4.3

Estimate the product of 843 × 56.

First, round the two numbers. 843 is rounded to 800 and 56 is rounded to 60.

Then divide each number by the place value of its leftmost column. The value of the leftmost column of 800 is hundreds and the value of the leftmost column of 60 is tens.

$$800 \div 100 = 8$$
$$60 \div 10 = 6$$

Now multiply the rounded numbers.

$$8 \times 6 = 48$$

Last, add the appropriate number of zeros to the answer. Two zeros should be added for the hundreds place of 843 and two zeroes should be added for the tens place of 56.

$$48,000$$

Compare the estimate to the actual product, which is 47,208.

Example 1.4.4

Estimate the quotient of 5,355 ÷ 4.79.

First, round the two numbers. 5,355 is closer to 5,000 than 6,000 and should be rounded to 6,000. 4.79 is closer to 5 than 4 and should be rounded to 5.

Then divide each number by the place value of its leftmost column. The value of the leftmost column of 5,000 is the thousands and the value of the leftmost column of 5 is ones.

$$5,000 \div 1,000 = 5$$
$$5 \div 1 = 5$$

Now divide the rounded numbers.

$$5 \div 5 = 1$$

Last, add the appropriate number of zeros to the answer. Three zeros should be added for the thousands place of 5,355. No zeros should be added for the ones place of 4.79. Do not add zeros for the numbers to the right of the decimal place in 4.79.

$$1,000$$

Compare the estimate to the actual quotient, which is 1,117.95.

Example 1.4.5

Estimate the product of 14.3 × 0.19.

First, round the two numbers. 14.3 is rounded to 10 and 0.19 is rounded to 0.2.

Then divide each number by the place value of its leftmost column. The value of the leftmost column of 10 is tens and the value of the leftmost column of 0.2 is tenths.

$$10 \div 10 = 1$$
$$0.2 \div 0.1 = 2$$

Now multiply the rounded numbers.

$$1 \times 2 = 2$$

Round the two numbers.

$$14.3 \text{ is rounded to } 14$$
$$0.19 \text{ is rounded to } 0.2$$

To avoid the decimal in the estimate operation, simplify 0.2 to 2. The decimal point will be inserted after you have multiplied the two rounded numbers.

$$14 \times 2 = 28$$

Last, add the appropriate number of zeros to the answer. One zero should be added for the tens place of 14.3. One zero should be subtracted for the tenths place of 0.19. Therefore, no zeros should be added to the final answer.

Compare the estimate to the actual product, which is 2.717.

In other cases, it may make sense to round to the nearest ten, hundred, or even larger.

Actual	$18.79 × 6 = $112.74
Estimate	$20.00 × 6 = $120.00
Actual	$424.00 × 2 = $848.00
Estimate	$420.00 × 2 = $840.00
Actual	4,326 ÷ 3.78 = 1,144.44
Estimate	4,000 ÷ 4 = 1,000
Actual	820 ÷ 42 = 19.52
Estimate	800 ÷ 40 = 20

Example 1.4.6

A patient needs to take 3.75 mL daily for 30 days. Estimate the total number of milliliters needed. The pharmacy technician can select between a 120 mL bottle and 180 mL bottle for dispensing this liquid medication. Which bottle should the technician use?

Estimate   4 mL × 30 days = 120 mL for 30 days
Actual   3.75 mL × 30 days = 112.5 mL for 30 days

Because the 120 mL bottle has more than enough room, the 180 mL bottle is not necessary, and the 120 mL bottle will be used to dispense the medication.

Estimating a Drug Dose

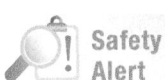

Safety Alert

As stated before, an estimated value can be used to double-check a dose but cannot be relied on for accuracy.

Estimating a drug dose before calculating the actual dose is helpful because the estimate can be used to double-check the accuracy of the calculated actual dose. If the actual dose is not close to the estimated dose, then the calculations should be rechecked. When estimating a drug dose, the first step is to determine whether the dose is going to be more or less than the unit dose or available drug strength. Continue estimating the dose by rounding the given dose to simplify the problem and dividing this rounded dose by the available drug strength.

Work Wise

Estimating can help you prevent dispensing errors by giving you an approximation of the amount of product that you expect to dispense. If the amount you prepare appears to be more or less than your estimate, it should prompt you to double check your work for accuracy.

Example 1.4.7

An order for 12.5 mg of a drug needs to be filled using a 5 mg tablet. Estimate the number of tablets needed for this dose.

The medication on hand has 5 mg of the drug for each tablet. Because the order is for 12.5 mg of the drug, the dose to be measured out will be larger than 1 tablet.

Simplify the estimation by rounding 12.5 mg down to 10 mg. This will make it easier to use the available dose to estimate the required number of tablets.

$$10 \, \text{mg} \; (\text{estimated requested amount}) \times \frac{1 \text{ tablet}}{5 \text{ mg}} \; (\text{available amount}) = 2 \text{ tablets}$$

Therefore, the estimate indicates that the dose will be at least 2 tablets.

The actual calculated dose of 2.5 tablets can then be checked by comparing it with the estimate. If an actual dose of 0.25 tablet or 25 tablets was calculated instead, then a quick comparison with the estimated dose of 2 tablets would immediately indicate that the actual dose was calculated incorrectly.

In addition to drug doses, the volume to be dispensed and the size of the container needed can be useful estimates when preparing a drug for dispensing.

Example 1.4.8

 The pharmacy receives an order for a 10-day supply of a liquid antibiotic to be taken in a dose of 8.5 mL of medication three times a day. The pharmacy has 100 mL, 200 mL, and 300 mL bottles of this antibiotic in stock. Which size bottle of antibiotic should be dispensed?

Begin by simplifying the problem, rounding the dose of 8.5 mL/dose to 10 mL/dose. It is important to round up to make sure the patient has enough of the medication.

Using this rounded value, calculate the amount of the medication needed per day by multiplying the estimated dose by the number of doses each day.

$$\frac{10 \text{ mL}}{1 \text{ dose}} \times \frac{3 \text{ doses}}{1 \text{ day}} = \frac{30 \text{ mL}}{1 \text{ day}}$$

In other words, the patient will need about 30 mL of the medication per day.

Because the patient needs to take this medication for 10 days, multiply the amount of the medication per day by the number of days of therapy.

$$\frac{30 \text{ mL}}{\text{day}} \times 10 \text{ days} = 300 \text{ mL}$$

Therefore, the patient will need about 300 mL of the medication. The actual amount needed is 255 mL, but the 300 mL bottle is the correct choice to fill this prescription.

1.4 Problem Set

Use rounding to estimate the dollar amounts to the nearest whole dollar, and then calculate the actual value.

1. $12.53 − $6.15 =

2. $6.28 + $1.99 + $3.98 =

3. $40 − $34.81 =

4. $100 − $18.29 =

5. $100 − $17.52 − $31.90 =

Estimate the products by rounding the two numbers and then multiplying them. Also calculate the actual value.

6. 6.8 × 7,656 =

7. 4.02 × 350.07 =

8. 598.4 × 0.015 =

9. 4,569 × 0.0972 =

10. 6,183 × 18 =

11. 1,253 × 9.1 =

Estimate the quotients by rounding the two numbers and then dividing them. Also calculate the actual value.

12. 185 ÷ 18 =

13. 18,015 ÷ 56 =

14. 584.0 ÷ 8 =

15. 844.23 ÷ 4.4 =

16. 123 ÷ 14 =

Applications

Round and estimate to find the following.

17. Employees of the pharmacy are being sent to the grocery store to buy the following items. Estimate how much petty cash they will need.

Food dye	$1.89
Sugar, 2 bags @	$4.25/bag
Baking soda	$0.79
Cherry flavoring	$2.39
1 gallon bleach	$1.97
Distilled water, 4 gal	$0.89/gal

18. Estimate how much sterile water for injection (SWFI) you will need for the following reconstitutions: 3.2 mL, 7.6 mL, 1.6 mL, and 4.1 mL. Choose the appropriate vial from the available vials (15 mL SWFI, 30 mL SWFI, and 50 mL SWFI).

19. A patient is receiving the following fluids: IV fluids, 1,723 mL; juice, 150 mL; coffee, 126 mL. Estimate the patient's intake to the nearest 10 mL.

20. The following is a patient's parenteral fluid intake for the first 24 hours of admittance: 780 mL normal saline (NS), 3 × 50 mL piggybacks, 250 mL NS, 3 × 1,000 mL NS. Estimate the total to the nearest 100 mL amount.

Self-check your work in Appendix A.

1.5 Significant Figures and Measurement Accuracy

Rounding and estimating have been discussed as a practical way of using numbers to calculate and measure a dose. In the process, you should not lose sight of the mathematical principle that each numerical value has a certain number of **significant figures**. These significant figures consist of those that are known to be accurate plus the digit in the lowest place value, which is approximate.

The **lowest known place value** is the last digit on the right of a written numeral. This lowest known value is approximate because of many sources of error including the limitation of the instrument used to measure, operator error, temperature variation, and the need to round at a certain point to make the number practical for calculations.

Significant figures are digits that have a practical meaning or value. A leading zero that marks the place of the decimal is not significant because it only marks the place value of the numbers that follow the decimal. Counting of significant figures begins at the first nonzero digit. Table 1.9 provides a short list of rules to follow when counting significant figures. Table 1.10 shows several numbers and indicates how many significant figures they have.

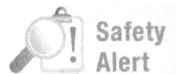 **Safety Alert**

Do not use a trailing zero unless it indicates accuracy of a number (i.e., is significant).

TABLE 1.9 Rules for Counting Significant Figures

Rule 1. Begin counting at the first nonzero digit.

Rule 2. Continue counting to the right until you reach the place value that is last (or rounded).

Rule 3. Zeros that are located between digits are significant and should be counted.

Rule 4. Do not count zeros that are placed to the left of the first digit. They only mark the place of the decimal.

Rule 5. One or more final zeros may or may not be significant depending on the accuracy to which the number is held.

TABLE 1.10 Counting Significant Figures

Number	Number of Significant Figures	Rule Applied
1.8	2	1, 2
18.3	3	1, 2
183	3	1, 2
1.832	4	1, 2
1,832	4	1, 2
0.183	3	1, 2, 4
0.108	3	1, 2, 3, 4
0.0108	3	1, 2, 3, 4
0.01	1	1, 2, 4
0.8	1	1, 2, 4
8	1	1, 2

In certain cases, when the accuracy of the measurement is known, the trailing zero to the right of the apparent last significant figure may also be considered significant. For example, if the device used to measure a substance is accurate to the nearest tenth, the tenths place may be considered significant even if the last digit is a zero. The zero may be retained to indicate the accuracy of the number. For example,

1.0 has two significant figures.

Larger numbers have significant figures based on their accuracy to the nearest factor of 10. If a very large amount of a substance is measured, at some point the person doing the measuring must estimate the closest amount represented by the device being used. As a result, the last digit recorded cannot be considered to be accurate and is thus not significant. For example, if 2,788 is only known for sure to be between 2,780 and 2,790, it has only three significant figures. Similarly, if 8,341,274 is only known for sure to be between 8,341,270 and 8,341,280, it has only six significant figures.

When the degree of accuracy is known to a certain place value, the significant figures are counted only to that place value. Knowing the level of accuracy is important when considering the weighing capacity and sensitivity of a scale or balance in the pharmacy.

Example 1.5.1

An item is weighed on a balance with a degree of accuracy to the nearest tenth when measuring milligrams. The balance indicates that an item weighs 1.459 mg. How many significant figures does this weight have? What would the rounded value be?

Because the accuracy of the scale can only be relied on to the tenths place, the number of significant figures is two. The "59" is not considered significant because of the sensitivity of the scale being used.

The weight would be rounded to 1.5 mg.

More significant digits indicate a greater accuracy of known values. A number that is accurate to within two figures has a practical 5% error from the actual measurement. Table 1.11 demonstrates these accuracy translations.

TABLE 1.11 Accuracy Ranges

Accuracy Level	Example
Two-figure accuracy is within 5%.	100 mg is in the range of 95 mg to 105 mg.
Three-figure accuracy is within 0.5%.	100 mg is in the range of 99.5 mg to 100.5 mg.
Four-figure accuracy is within 0.05%.	100 mg is in the range of 99.95 mg to 100.05 mg.
Five-figure accuracy is within 0.005%.	100 mg is in the range of 99.995 mg to 100.005 mg.

In studying mathematics, numbers may be considered accurate for an infinite number of figures. However, it is important to recognize that a quantity measured to a certain degree of accuracy has a number of significant figures that are more relevant than a number that quantity may be multiplied or divided by. The resulting product when multiplying two numbers is typically considered accurate only to the number of significant figures of the number with the fewer significant figures. In pharmacy, we recognize the measured dose as the more important of the two factors. For example, if 6.25 mg is measured exactly and then multiplied by 2 for a twice a day administration, the resulting daily dose is exactly 12.5 mg. In pharmacy applications, it is typical to treat number of tablets, number of days—in fact, number of anything—as exact numbers. Exact numbers can be thought of as having infinitely many significant digits. Therefore we only count the significant digits in the measured (inexact) quantities, such as dosages.

Numbers greater than 100 have significant figures based on the relative accuracy of the measurement. If a number over 100 is accurate to the nearest 10, the zero in the ones place is considered an estimate and thus not significant. Only the digits to the left of that are considered significant. Significant digits are counted similarly for numbers that are accurate to the nearest 100 or larger. For example, if the following numbers are accurate to the nearest 10, they will have the indicated number of significant figures.

200 has two significant figures

1,800 has three significant figures

30,000 has four significant figures

Similarly, if the following numbers are accurate to the nearest 100, they will have the indicated number of significant figures.

200 has one significant figure

1,800 has two significant figures

30,000 has three significant figures

When multiplying or dividing, the answer should have the same number of significant digits as the original inexact number which has the fewest significant digits. (Remember that we don't worry about the significant digits in exact numbers.)

Example 1.5.2

Determine the product of 6.75 × 3 using the appropriate number of accurate and significant figures.

Note the number of significant figures and the level of accuracy for each number: 6.75 has three significant figures and is accurate to the tenths place, whereas 3 has one significant figure and is accurate to the ones place.

Now, determine the product of the two numbers.

$$6.75 \times 3 = 20.25$$

Because 3 has one significant figure, we 20.25 needs to be rounded to the tens place. The answer 20, has one significant figure.

Example 1.5.3

Determine the product of 12.59 × 1,572 using the appropriate number of accurate and significant figures.

Note the number of significant figures and the accuracy of the numbers. Both factors have four significant figures.

Now, determine the product of the two numbers.

$$12.59 \times 1,572 = 19,791.48$$

Since the number of significant digits in either number in the problem is four, the answer can only have four significant digits, so the acceptable answer is 19,790.

1.5 Problem Set

Identify the number of significant figures in the following numbers. Assume that all final zeros in numbers without decimals are not significant.

1. 15.4324 grains

2. 1,500 mL

3. 0.21 mg

4. $1.07

5. 100,000 mcg

6. 507.2 mg

7. 1.0 kg

8. 0.001 mg

9. 21,204.075 mcg

10. 100 mL

Round the following numbers to three significant figures.

11. 42.75

12. 100.19

13. 0.04268

14. 18.426

15. 0.003918

Round the following numbers to two decimal places and state how many significant figures each has.

16. 0.3479

17. 0.056921

18. 1.9947

19. 0.00986

20. 1.0277

Calculate the following and retain the correct number of significant figures in the answers.

21. $0.67 \times 95.2 =$

22. $1.26 \times 24 =$

23. $325 \times 0.5 =$

Applications

24. You are to prepare capsules that contain 0.125 g of a drug. You have four partial containers of medication, which weigh 3.2 g, 1.784 g, 2.46 g, and 5.87 g. Assume you have weighed each of the four containers with the same scale, and the accuracy is known to the hundredth gram.

    a. Which amount will need to be rounded?

    b. Which amount is not as accurate as it should be?

    c. What is the amount of the medication that will be left over after making as many 0.125 g capsules as possible?

25. A unit dose of an oral medication requires 21.65 mg. You are to prepare 45 doses.

    a. How many milligrams will you need?

    b. How many significant figures does this amount have?

Self-check your work in Appendix A.

1.6 Time of Day

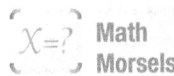

Math Morsels

Computer systems do not always permit the use of a colon when entering time. Consequently, you may see a time entry as a four-digit entry—for example, 0430 rather than 04:30. Be aware that both time entries indicate 4:30 a.m.

Telling time is a skill that you learn as a child. For many individuals, this skill was taught using a clock with movable hands: one hand indicating the hours and one hand indicating the minutes. In addition to these traditional clocks, digital clocks that display the hours and minutes as numbers separated by a colon are also used to tell time. Digital clocks are commonly seen on computer software programs. Both types of clocks typically indicate what is known as **standard time**—a system of time that relates to the natural day and is based on a 12-hour format. Standard time, also known as *civilian time*, uses the designations of a.m. and p.m.

However, the pharmacy profession uses a different method to indicate time: military time. **Military time** is based on a 24-hour format and, as its name indicates, is used among military personnel to avoid confusion between a.m. and p.m. In fact, most countries—with the exception of the United States and Canada—have adopted the military time system as their official time standard. The military time system is now commonly referred to as the *24-hour system* (see Table 1.12).

In the healthcare setting, the 24-hour system is used for accuracy. This system prevents ambiguity and provides a simple means of documenting the precise time in a 24-hour day. The 24-hour system may be used to document what time a medication is to be administered, what time an event (such as an adverse reaction) occurs, or what time an intravenous (IV) medication runs out. Precise minutes are also used, so if a medication is to be given at 6:30 a.m., it would be recorded as 0630 to indicate the exact time.

TABLE 1.12   Standard Time and 24-Hour Time (Military Time) Equivalents

Standard Time	24-Hour Time	Standard Time	24-Hour Time
1:00 a.m.	0100 hours	1:00 p.m.	1300 hours
2:00 a.m.	0200 hours	2:00 p.m.	1400 hours
3:00 a.m.	0300 hours	3:00 p.m.	1500 hours
4:00 a.m.	0400 hours	4:00 p.m.	1600 hours
5:00 a.m.	0500 hours	5:00 p.m.	1700 hours
6:00 a.m.	0600 hours	6:00 p.m.	1800 hours
7:00 a.m.	0700 hours	7:00 p.m.	1900 hours
8:00 a.m.	0800 hours	8:00 p.m.	2000 hours
9:00 a.m.	0900 hours	9:00 p.m.	2100 hours
10:00 a.m.	1000 hours	10:00 p.m.	2200 hours
11:00 a.m.	1100 hours	11:00 p.m.	2300 hours
12:00 p.m. (noon)	1200 hours	12:00 a.m. (midnight)	2400 hours

The 24-hour system uses the numbers 0–24 to represent the 24-hour day. To provide consistency and prevent confusion, the 24-hour system uses two digits for the hour and then two digits for the minutes. If seconds are indicated, a colon will be added between the digits for hours and the digits for minutes. Another colon will be used to separate the digits for minutes and the digits for seconds. Times less than 10:00 a.m. will often be preceded by one or two leading zeros so that the hour has two digits.

The start of each day is designated as 0000, and midnight is designated as 2400. These two designations are actually the same time, so some computer systems will accept times up to 2400 and then require the first minute after midnight to be entered as 0001, thereby skipping the 0000 time display.

It is important for pharmacy personnel to become familiar with the time equivalents and be able to accurately convert times without looking at a chart. The times that occur in the morning hours are simple and straightforward because they are similar to the display on a typical digital clock. The times that occur in the afternoon and evening (1:00 p.m. to 12:00 a.m.) have numbers that many individuals are not accustomed to seeing when telling time: 1300 to 2400. For these 24-hour times, remember this simple rule: These designations can quickly be converted back to standard time by subtracting 1200. Therefore, for example, if you subtract 1200 from 1900 hours, you get 7:00—the standard time designation for 7:00 p.m.

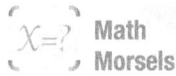

Math Morsels

Depending on which type of time conversion you are doing, for times in the afternoon and evening, you will either add or subtract 12 hours.

Example 1.6.1

Convert the following times from standard time to 24-hour time using the conversion chart:

3:45 a.m.	becomes 0345
9:20 a.m.	becomes 0920
6:13 p.m.	becomes 1813
11:56 p.m.	becomes 2356
12:10 a.m.	becomes 0010

Example 1.6.2

Convert the following times from 24-hour time to standard time using the conversion chart:

0128	becomes 1:28 a.m.
0456	becomes 4:56 a.m.
1530	becomes 3:30 p.m.
2215	becomes 10:15 p.m.

Example 1.6.3

According to her electronic health record, a patient has received medication at the following times: 0700, 1300, and 1900. Convert these 24-hour times to standard times.

0700	becomes 7:00 a.m.
1300	becomes 1:00 p.m.
1900	becomes 7:00 p.m.

1.6 Problem Set

Convert the followng standard times to 24-hour times:

1. 7:30 a.m.

2. 4:28 p.m.

3. 12:45 a.m.

4. 9:20 p.m.

5. 2:24 a.m.

6. 10:58 p.m.

7. 11:50 p.m.

8. 1:20 a.m.

9. 12:03 a.m.

10. 12:20 p.m.

Convert the following 24-hour times to standard times:

11. 1730

12. 2349

13. 1522

14. 0034

15. 1204

16. 0355

17. 2245

18. 1719

19. 1300

20. 0145

Applications

21. Sun Ng, a patient who arrived in the emergency room around midnight, stated that he took his pain medication three times during the day: at 8:15 in the morning, at 1:15 with his lunch, and at 7:00 in the evening. Using the 24-hour system, what times should be reflected in the patient's health record?

22. A prescription states that Lucy Andrews, a pediatric patient in the intensive care unit, is to take medication three times a day, every eight hours, beginning at 5:00 a.m. Using the 24-hour system, what time should the medication therapy begin?

23. Dr. Dominic Estores has written a prescription for a patient to take a preoperative medication at 2200 on the evening before his scheduled surgery. Using the standard time system, what time should you tell the patient to take his medication?

24. The IV medications prepared each afternoon for overnight administration have to be delivered to the floors between 1800 and 1900. According to the clock in the pharmacy, when should you deliver the medications?

25. Mrs. Singh has just been brought to the hospital via ambulance. During admittance, she said that before calling for an ambulance she had taken two sublingual nitroglycerin tablets for chest pain: one at 3:00 p.m. and one at 3:05 p.m. Because her pain didn't go away, she reported that she took a third nitroglycerin tablet five minutes later. Using 24-hour time, at what times did she take the medication?

Self-check your work in Appendix A.

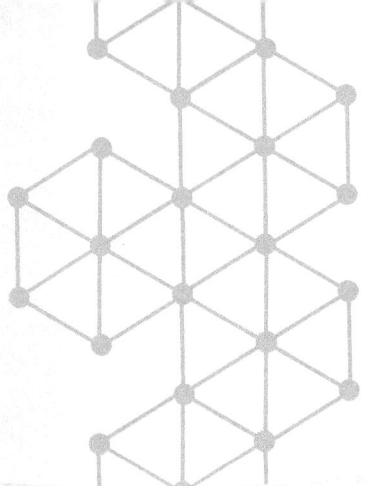

CHAPTER SUMMARY

- Fractions are part of a whole.

- The upper number in a fraction is the numerator.

- The lower number in a fraction is the denominator.

- When adding or subtracting fractions, you need to have a common denominator.

- When multiplying fractions, you multiply the numerators together and the denominators together.

- When dividing fractions, you multiply the first fraction by the reciprocal of the second fraction.

- Common denominators can be found by factoring the denominators and comparing them.

- Roman numerals are used on prescriptions, and they may be written as either uppercase or lowercase letters.

- Roman numerals are never repeated more than three times in sequence.

- Roman numerals that have a smaller value in front of Roman numerals that have a larger value should be subtracted to determine the final value.

- Arabic numbers use a decimal point to show the place value of digits in the number.

- Scientific notation is a way to write very large or very small numbers.

- Decimals may use a leading zero in front of the decimal point to avoid calculation errors.

- A trailing zero should only be used when indicating accuracy or significant figures.

- Estimation is helpful in double-checking results, but an estimate should never be considered accurate.

- Significant figures can be used to determine accuracy.

- Time can be recorded using a standard time system or a 24-hour system, also known as military time.

- The 24-hour system uses the numbers 0–24 to designate the 24 hours of a day.

- Hours before 10:00 a.m. have a leading zero in the 24-hour system.
- Hours and minutes may be separated by a colon.

KEY TERMS

accuracy the correctness of a number in its representation of a given value

Arabic numbers numbers in a numbering system that uses symbols to indicate numbers, fractions, and decimals; uses the numerals 0, 1, 2, 3, 4, 5, 6, 7, 8, 9

common denominator a number into which each of the unlike denominators of two or more fractions can be divided evenly

complex fraction a fraction in which the numerator, the denominator, or both are fractions

decimal a fraction value in which the denominator is 10 or some power of 10

denominator the number in the bottom part of a fraction

Dimensional analysis a problem-solving method that uses the fact that, when multiplying or dividing, units can be cancelled just like numbers.

Equivalent fractions are fractions that may look different, but have the same value.

fraction a portion of a whole that is represented as one number divided by another number

improper fraction a fraction with a value greater than or equal to 1 (the value of the numerator is larger than or equal to the value of the denominator)

leading zero a zero that is placed to the left of the decimal point, in the ones place, in a number that is less than 1 and is being represented by a decimal value

lowest known place value the last digit on the right of a written numeral

military time a system of time based on a 24-hour format

mixed number a whole number and a fraction

numerator the number in the top part of a fraction

place value the location of a numeral in a string of numbers that describes the numeral's relationship to the decimal point

product the result of multiplying one number by another

proper fraction a fraction with a value of less than 1 (the value of the numerator is smaller than the value of the denominator)

quotient the result of dividing one number by another

Roman numerals a numbering system that uses alphabetic symbols to indicate a quantity; uses the letters I, V, and X to represent 1, 5, and 10, respectively

scientific notation a method used to write numbers that have a very large or very small numerical value; uses "$\times 10$" with an exponent

significant figures the figures in a numeral that are known values and have not been rounded or estimated in the process of mathematical calculation, plus the digit in the lowest place value, which is approximate

standard time a system of time that relates to the natural day and is based on a 12-hour format

sum the result of adding two or more numbers together

trailing zero a zero that appears at the end of a decimal string and is not needed except when considered significant, that is, to indicate accuracy

Finding Solutions

To gain practice in handling challenging situations in the workplace, consider the following real-world scenarios and then use the guiding questions to help you formulate your responses.

Note: *To indicate your answer for Scenario D, Question 9, ask your instructor for the handout depicting a dosing spoon.*

Scenario A: A patient has brought in the following prescription:

 Lasix 40 mg

Sig: Take ī tablet by mouth each M, W, F and īī tablets on other days.

Dispense: 30-day supply

Refills: 2

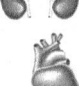

1. How many tablets per day does the patient take on MWF?

2. Estimate how many tablets a patient will need to last 30 days.

3. Calculate exactly how many tablets the patient will need in a 30-day period if the patient picks up the medication on a Sunday.

Scenario B: The maximum dose for an OTC medication is 4,000 mg per day. A patient tells you that she has taken 4 whole tablets and ½ tablet today but wants to know if she can take more. The package indicates that there are 500 mg in each tablet.

4. How many milligrams of medication did the patient receive from the ingestion of the whole tablets?

5. How many milligrams did she receive from the ingestion of the ½ tablet?

6. How many total milligrams of medication did the patient take?

7. How many more tablets can she take before she exceeds the maximum dose? Calculate to the nearest half tablet.

Scenario C: Dr. Ingrid Johansson has written a prescription for a patient to take an antibiotic three hours before a cardiac procedure. The operating room schedule indicates the procedure is slated for 1430.

8. What standard time will you tell the patient to take his medication?

Scenario D: A mother has come to the pharmacy and is confused about the markings on her daughter's dosage spoon. The prescription drug label states that she is to give ¾ of a teaspoon to her daughter.

9. On the handout that you obtained from your instructor, indicate the amount of medication that the mother should administer to her child.

Scenario E: A patient brings the following prescription to you:

R̠ **warfarin 5 mg**

sig: Take i̇ tablet by mouth on Tuesday, Thursday, and Saturday. Take ss tablets on all other days.

Dispense: 30 day supply

Refills: 5

10. How many tablets per day does the patient take on Monday, Wednesday, Friday, and Sunday?

11. How many tablets does the patient take on Tuesday, Thursday, and Saturday?

12. How many milligrams are ingested with Monday's dose?

13. Calculate exactly how many tablets the patient will need in a 30-day period if the patient begins taking the medication on Sunday.

Scenario F: A patient brings the following prescription to you:

R̠ **levothyroxine 125 mcg**

sig: Take i̇ tablet by mouth on Monday, Wednesday, Friday, and Saturday.

Dispense: 90 day supply

Refills: 1

14. How many tablets does the patient take per week?

15. How many milligrams of levothyroxine are taken each week?

16. How many tablets should you dispense if the patient's first fills the prescription on a Tuesday?

17. How many tablets would be dispensed if the patient received a 30 day supply and the first fill is on a Tuesday?

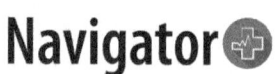

Navigator

Access interactive chapter review exercises, practice activities, flash cards, and study games.

2

Using Ratios, Percents, and Proportions

Learning Objectives

1 Describe the use of ratios and proportions in the pharmacy.

2 Compute pharmacy calculations by using ratios and proportions.

3 Define percent as it pertains to pharmacy calculations.

4 Convert percentages to decimals.

5 Compute pharmacy calculations using the ratio-proportion method.

6 Calculate percentage of error in measurements.

Preview chapter terms and definitions.

2.1 Numerical Ratios

A **ratio** is a numerical representation of the relationship between two parts of a whole or of the relationship of one part to the whole. Ratios may be written with a colon (:) between the numbers, which may be read as *per, of, to,* or *in.* The ratio 1:2 could mean that the second part has twice the value (e.g., size, number, weight, volume) of the first part, or it could mean that one part is something within a total of two parts. Ratios may also be written as fractions, and it is the ratio in fraction form that is most useful to the pharmacy technician.

$x=?$ **Math Morsels**

The ratio written in the form of a fraction is most useful in pharmacy calculations.

1:2	is read as	1 part to 2 parts	and may also be written as	$\frac{1}{2}$
3:4	is read as	3 parts to 4 parts	and may also be written as	$\frac{3}{4}$
1:20	is read as	1 part to 20 parts	and may also be written as	$\frac{1}{20}$
1:10	is read as	1 part to 10 parts	and may also be written as	$\frac{1}{10}$

In the above ratios, any unit of description may be substituted for the word *part* or *parts*. For example, you say there are 250 mg per tablet. Other common unit labels include capsule, bottle, gram, milligram, microgram, and liter.

A ratio can be any numerical relation you need to show. With medications, you commonly use a ratio to express the weight or strength of a drug per dose or volumetric measurement. Ratios are commonly used to express concentrations of a medication in solution. For example, a 1:100 concentration of a medication means that there is 1 part of the medication in 100 parts of the solution (1 g per 100 mL). It is also common to reverse the order of the values written in a ratio.

250 mg:1 tablet	or	1 tablet:250 mg
1 g:100 mL	or	100 mL:1 g
500 mg:20 mL	or	20 mL:500 mg

The ratio may be manipulated by multiplying or dividing both parts of the ratio by the same factor. Pharmacists and pharmacy technicians use this process when calculating the volume of a medication to be given or, in some cases, the amount of a drug per volume of the medication given.

FIGURE 2.1
Ratios on an Ampule Label

Total volume of ampule — 20 mL

AMPULE

AMINOPHYLLINE

INJECTION, USP

500 mg / 20 mL

A-1320E

(25 mg/mL)
Anhydrous Theophylline 19.7 mg/mL
FOR SLOW INTRAVENOUS USE

Amount of medication in ampule

Concentration of medication in anhydrous theophylline

Amount of medication in 1 mL

Some medication labels, especially those of injectable medications, have more than one ratio listed. For example, the aminophylline label shown in Figure 2.1 includes three ratios, each descriptive of the medication's concentration. The first ratio, 500 mg/20 mL, represents the total amount of medication in the ampule. The second ratio, 25 mg/mL, represents the amount of medication in 1 mL. The third ratio, 19.7 mg/mL, describes the concentration of the medication in its anhydrous-theophylline state. The pharmacist may use this concentration to further analyze the dosage. The ratio indicating the total amount of medication in the ampule is of the most importance to the pharmacy technician. Typically, this ratio is the most prominent one on the label, as is the case for this label.

Medication labels indicate the ratio of the active ingredient and, as described in Chapter 1, the ratio may be manipulated by multiplying or dividing both parts of the ratio by the same factor. If the dose needs to be increased, you multiply the ratio by a factor. If the dose needs to be decreased, you divide the ratio by a factor.

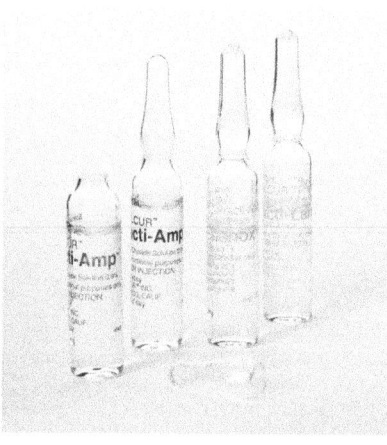

Ampules are small, single-dose containers of medication that are opened at the time of use.

Please refer to the label shown in Figure 2.1 when working on the following examples.

Example 2.1.1

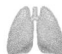 **How many milligrams of aminophylline were ordered if two ampules were administered and each ampule contained 500 mg/20 mL?**

For two ampules, you multiply both parts of the ratio by 2.

$$\frac{500 \text{ mg} \times 2}{20 \text{ mL} \times 2} = \frac{1{,}000 \text{ mg}}{40 \text{ mL}}$$

Therefore, 1,000 mg were given.

Example 2.1.2

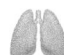 **How many milligrams of aminophylline were ordered if half an ampule was administered and each ampule contained 500 mg/20 mL?**

For half of an ampule, you divide both parts of the ratio by 2.

$$\frac{500 \text{ mg} \div 2}{20 \text{ mL} \div 2} = \frac{250 \text{ mg}}{10 \text{ mL}}$$

or

$$\frac{500 \text{ mg} \times \frac{1}{2}}{20 \text{ mL} \times \frac{1}{2}} = \frac{250 \text{ mg}}{10 \text{ mL}}$$

Therefore, 250 mg were given.

Example 2.1.3

The physician has ordered that a patient take ½ of a 137 mcg tablet of levothyroxine. How many micrograms will the patient take?

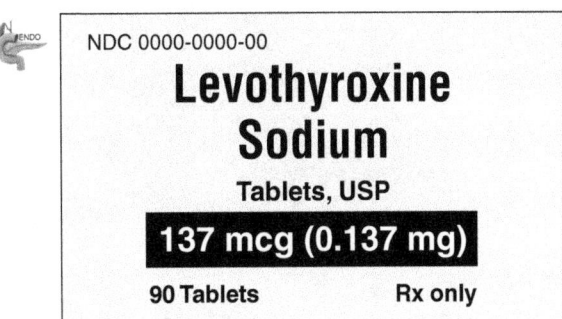

Using multiplication and division:

Multiplication Method

$$137 \text{ mcg} \times \frac{1}{2} = 68.5 \text{ mcg}$$

Division Method

$$137 \text{ mcg} \div 2 = 68.5 \text{ mcg}$$

$$\frac{137 \text{ mcg}}{2} = 68.5 \text{ mcg}$$

Using dimensional analysis (described in Chapter 1):

$$\frac{137 \text{ mcg}}{1 \text{ tablet}} \times \frac{0.5 \text{ tablet}}{1} = 68.5 \text{ mcg}$$

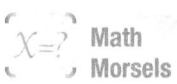 **Math Morsels**

When the dose is written as a typical ratio (1:1,000), the amount of medication is very small.

Some medications are ordered in concentrations that are expressed as a ratio. Typically, these medications are available in a very small percentage (less than 1%). The dose form will influence the ratio. A common dosage form is a **solution** (a liquid mixture in which the minor component, the solute, is uniformly distributed within the major component, the solvent). A similar dosage form is a **suspension**. A suspension is a mixture in which solute particles are mixed with, but not dissolved, in a fluid. The following examples use a 1:10,000 ratio.

1 g active ingredient:10,000 g product for a solid such as a cream

1 g active ingredient:10,000 mL solution for a solution

1 mL active ingredient:10,000 mL mixture for a liquid

Example 2.1.4

A 1:100 solution has 1 g active ingredient in 100 mL. How much active ingredient is present in 300 mL of this solution?

Set up a ratio and solve for x. In this problem, x equals the active ingredient.

$$\frac{x \text{ g}}{300 \text{ mL}} = \frac{1 \text{ g}}{100 \text{ mL}}$$

Because these fractions are equivalent, you can cross multiply and the equations will still equal one another.

$$x \text{ g } (100 \text{ mL}) = 300 \text{ mL } (1 \text{ g})$$

Now solve for x by dividing each side of the equation by 100 mL.

$$\frac{x \text{ g } (100 \text{ mL})}{100 \text{ mL}} = \frac{300 \text{ mL } (1 \text{ g})}{100 \text{ mL}}$$

This leaves us with

$$x \text{ g} = \frac{300 \ (1 \text{ g})}{100}$$

and $x = 3$ g.

Therefore, there are 3 g of active ingredient in 300 mL of solution.

You can also solve this problem using dimensional analysis.

$$\frac{1\text{ g}}{100\text{ mL}} \times \frac{300\text{ mL}}{1} = 3\text{ g}$$

$$\frac{(300\text{ mL})\,x\text{ g}}{300\text{ mL}} = \frac{(300\text{ mL})\,1\text{ g}}{100\text{ mL}}$$

$$x\text{ g} = 3\text{ g}$$

Therefore, there are 3 g of active ingredient in 300 mL of this solution.

2.1 Problem Set

Express the following ratios as fractions and reduce to lowest terms.

1. 3:7

2. 8:6

3. 3:4

4. 4:6

5. 1:7

Reduce the following fractions to lowest terms and express each as a ratio.

6. $\dfrac{2}{3}$

7. $\dfrac{6}{8}$

8. $\dfrac{5}{10}$

9. $\dfrac{1}{9}$

10. $\dfrac{1}{10,000}$

Applications

State the ratio for the following doses.

11. 30 mg capsule Cymbalta

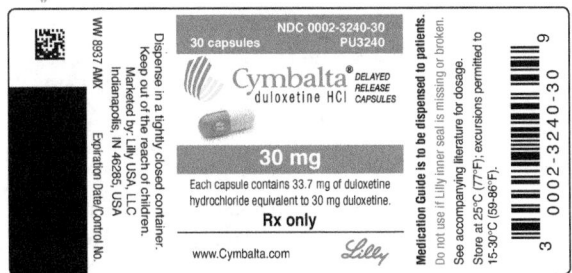

12. 100 mg capsule Dilantin

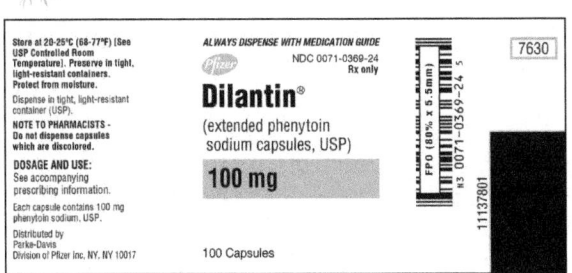

13. 5 mL dose of oral suspension containing 250 mg amoxicillin

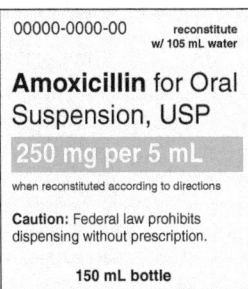

Use the ratios calculated in the preceding problems to calculate the amount of medication in the following doses. Write your answer as a ratio.

14. 3 capsules of Cymbalta

15. 2 capsules of Dilantin

16. 15 mL of amoxicillin suspension, 250 mg in 5 mL

Fill in the blanks.

17. A 10:1,000 solution contains _____ g of active ingredient in _____ mL of product, and 100 mL of that solution contains _____ g.

18. A 1:100 solution contains _____ g of active ingredient in _____ mL of product, and 500 mL of that solution contains _____ g.

19. A 1:250 solution contains _____ g of active ingredient in _____ mL of product, and 1,000 mL of that solution contains _____ g.

20. A 1:1,000 solution contains _____ g of active ingredient in _____ mL of product, and 50 mL of that solution contains _____ g.

Self-check your work in Appendix A.

2.2 Percents

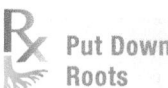
Put Down Roots

The word *percent* comes from the Latin term *per centum*, meaning "by the hundred." Therefore, *percent* literally means "per 100."

A percent expresses the number of parts compared with a total of 100 parts. The word *percent* means "per 100" or "hundredths." A percent is the same as a fraction in which the denominator is 100. Percent is represented by the symbol %. Percents can be visualized by comparing a stack of 100 pennies (equivalent to $1) next to smaller stacks of pennies (see Figure 2.2). A stack of 5 pennies equals 5 cents and represents 5% of a dollar. Similarly, a stack of 40 pennies equals 40 cents and represents 40% of a dollar.

A percent can be written as a ratio, a fraction, or a decimal. For example, 30% means there are 30 parts in a total of 100 parts.

$$30:100 \quad \text{or} \quad \frac{30}{100} \quad \text{or} \quad 0.30, \text{or } 30\%$$

FIGURE 2.2
Comparison of Percents

100% of a dollar

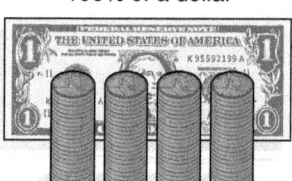

100 pennies

40% of a dollar

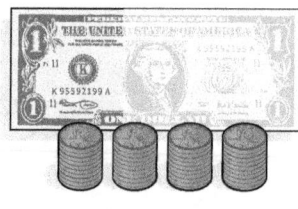

40 pennies

5% of a dollar

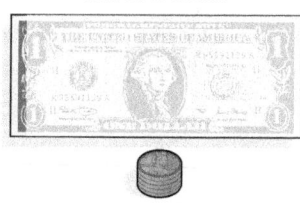

5 pennies

If a test has 100 questions and you receive a score of 89%, that means that you got 89 of the 100 questions correct.

$$89:100 \quad \text{or} \quad \frac{89}{100} \quad \text{or} \quad 0.89 \quad \text{or} \quad 89\%$$

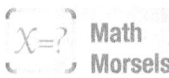 **Math Morsels**

The higher the percentage of a dissolved substance, the greater the strength.

Percent strengths are often used to describe intravenous (IV) solutions and topically applied medications. The higher the percentage of dissolved substances (in a solute or a topical medication), the greater the strength. Both of the following examples may be expressed as 1:100, $\frac{1}{100}$, or 0.01.

A 1% solution contains 1 g of medication per 100 mL of fluid.

A 1% hydrocortisone cream contains 1 g of hydrocortisone per 100 g of cream.

By multiplying the first number in the ratio (the solute) while keeping the second number unchanged, you can increase the strength. Conversely, by dividing the first number in the ratio while keeping the second number unchanged, you can decrease the strength.

Example 2.2.1

A 5% solution contains 5 g of solute per 100 mL of solution. If the patient is to receive a 200 mL of solution, how many grams of solute will at volume contain?

$$\frac{5 \text{ g}}{100 \text{ mL}} = \frac{x \text{ g}}{200 \text{ mL}}$$

$$x \text{ g} (100 \text{ mL}) = 5 \text{ g} (200 \text{ mL})$$

$$\frac{x \text{ g} (\cancel{100 \text{ mL}})}{\cancel{100 \text{ mL}}} = \frac{5 \text{ g} (200 \cancel{\text{ mL}})}{100 \cancel{\text{ mL}}}$$

$$x = 10 \text{ g}$$

Another way to solve this problem is by using dimensional analysis.

$$\frac{200 \cancel{\text{ mL}}}{1} \times \frac{5 \text{ g}}{100 \cancel{\text{ mL}}} = 10 \text{ g}$$

Example 2.2.2

A 2% solution contains 2 g of solute per 100 mL of solution. How many milliliters of this solution are needed to give a dose of 6 g of solute?

$$\frac{2 \text{ g}}{100 \text{ mL}} = \frac{6 \text{ g}}{x \text{ mL}}$$

$$x \text{ mL} (2 \text{ g}) = 100 \text{ mL} (6 \text{ g})$$

$$\frac{x \text{ mL} (\cancel{2 \text{ g}})}{\cancel{2 \text{ g}}} = \frac{100 \text{ mL} (6 \cancel{\text{ g}})}{2 \cancel{\text{ g}}}$$

$$x = 300 \text{ mL}$$

Another way to solve this problem is by using dimensional analysis.

$$\frac{6 \cancel{\text{ g}}}{1} \times \frac{100 \text{ mL}}{2 \cancel{\text{ g}}} = 300 \text{ mL}$$

Example 2.2.3

Convert the percent Xylocaine to a ratio and then convert the grams to milligrams.

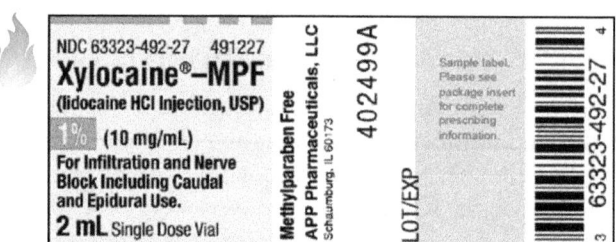

A 1% solution of Xylocaine contains 1 g of Xylocaine in 100 mL solution. This could also be written as 1,000 mg solute per 100 mL solution (1 g is equivalent to 1,000 mg). Equivalent to this ratio is the strength indicated on the label above (10 mg/mL). The label uses both percentage and milligrams per milliliter expressions to describe the concentration of the medication.

$$1\% = \frac{1 \text{ g}}{100 \text{ mL}} = \frac{1{,}000 \text{ mg}}{100 \text{ mL}} = \frac{10 \text{ mg}}{1 \text{ mL}}$$

When working in the pharmacy, the technician will need to know how to convert between ratios, percents, and decimals. The values in each row of Table 2.1 are equivalent. They are simply expressed in different ways.

TABLE 2.1 Equivalent Values

Percent	Fraction	Decimal	Ratio
45%	$\frac{45}{100}$	0.45	45:100
0.5%	$\frac{0.5}{100} = \frac{1}{200}$	0.005	0.5:100

Converting a Ratio to a Percent

Recall that percent is the number of parts compared to a total of 100. To convert 5:1 to a percent we need to make an equivalent fraction to $^5/_1$ with a denominator of 100. To achieve this, we multiply the numerator and denominator by 100.

$$\frac{5}{1} \times \frac{5 \times 100}{1 \times 100} = \frac{500}{100} = 500\%$$

A faster way to convert a ratio to a percent is to first rewrite the ratio as a fraction, then multiply by 100 , and finally add a percent sign.

$$5{:}1 \qquad \frac{5}{1} \times 100 = \frac{500}{1} = 500\%$$

$$1{:}5 \qquad \frac{1}{5} \times 100 = \frac{100}{5} = 20\%$$

$$1{:}2 \qquad \frac{1}{2} \times 100 = \frac{100}{2} = 50\%$$

Example 2.2.4

A prescriber ordered a 1:1,000 solution. You have a 1% solution, a 0.5% solution, and a 0.1% solution in stock. Will one of these work to fill the order?

$$1{:}1{,}000 = \frac{1}{1{,}000} \times 100 = \frac{100}{1{,}000} = 0.1\%$$

The 0.1% solution is the same concentration as the ordered 1:1,000 solution.

Converting a Percent to a Ratio

To convert a percent to a ratio, first change it to a fraction by dividing the percent by 100, and then reduce the fraction to lowest terms. Express this as a ratio by making the numerator the first number of the ratio and the denominator the second number.

$$2\% = 2 \div 100 = \frac{2}{100} = \frac{1}{50} = 1{:}50$$

$$10\% = 10 \div 100 = \frac{10}{100} = \frac{1}{10} = 1{:}10$$

$$75\% = 75 \div 100 = \frac{75}{100} = \frac{3}{4} = 3{:}4$$

$$\frac{1}{2}\% = \frac{1}{2} \div 100 = \frac{\frac{1}{2}}{100} = \frac{1}{2} \times \frac{1}{100} = \frac{1}{200} = 1{:}200$$

Example 2.2.5

A prescriber ordered a 0.02% solution. You have a 1:1,000 solution, a 1:5,000 solution, and a 1:10,000 solution in stock. Will one of these work to fill the order?

$$0.02\% = \frac{0.02 \text{ g}}{100 \text{ mL}}$$

We know that we can multiply any number by 1 (or a fraction that is equivalent to 1) without changing its value.

$$\frac{0.02 \text{ g}}{100 \text{ mL}} \times \frac{100}{100} = \frac{2 \text{ g}}{10{,}000 \text{ mL}}$$

We can reduce $^{2}\text{g}/_{10{,}000 \text{ mL}}$ to $^{1}\text{g}/_{5{,}000 \text{ mL}}$, which we know is 1:5000. Therefore a 0.02% solution is the same as a 1:5,000 solution. The supply of 1:5,000 solution can be used.

A solution commonly used for cleaning in healthcare facilities is a 1:10 solution of bleach and water. This solution is available commercially or may be made fresh daily using regular bleach. Figure 2.3 shows the recipe for making a 1:10 bleach solution. In the recipe, one part bleach is mixed with nine parts of water. The amounts can be adjusted, but the ratio should not change. Because it chemically degrades, a bleach solution prepared according to this recipe is good for only one day.

FIGURE 2.3
10% Bleach
Solution

1:10 Bleach Solution

Materials: Storage container, measuring cup or graduated cylinder,
bleach, water, label

Instructions: Measure one quantity of bleach (such as 1 cup) and
place it into the storage container. Measure the same quantity of
water nine times (in this case, 9 cups) and place it into the storage
container. Mix well, label, and date the container.

Example 2.2.6

**You have been asked to prepare a 480 mL (1 pt.) of 1:10 bleach
solution. How much bleach and water will you need to measure out?**

Determine the size of a "part" by dividing 10 parts into the total volume.

$$\text{total volume} \div \text{number of parts} = \text{volume per one part}$$

$$480 \text{ mL} \div 10 \text{ parts} = \frac{48 \text{ mL}}{1 \text{ part}}$$

You know from the recipe for a 10% bleach solution that the bleach volume is
equal to one part, or 48 mL. Determine the amount of water needed by subtracting the known amount of bleach from the total volume.

$$\text{total volume} - \text{bleach volume} = \text{water volume}$$
$$480 \text{ mL} - 48 \text{ mL} = 432 \text{ mL}$$

The following ratio and fractions show the relationship of the 1:10 solution.

$$1:10 = \frac{1 \text{ part bleach}}{10 \text{ parts water-bleach solution}} = \frac{48 \text{ mL bleach}}{480 \text{ mL water-bleach solution}}$$

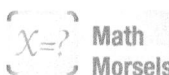 **Math
Morsels**

When convert-
ing a percent
to a decimal,
always remem-
ber to insert
zeros—including
a leading zero—if
necessary.

Converting a Percent to a Decimal

To convert a percent to a decimal, drop the percent symbol and divide the number by
100. Dividing a number by 100 is equivalent to moving the decimal point two places
to the left, inserting zeros if necessary.

$$4\% = 4 \div 100 = 0.04$$
$$15\% = 15 \div 100 = 0.15$$
$$200\% = 200 \div 100 = 2.0$$

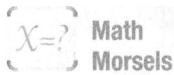 **Math Morsels**

When converting a decimal to a percent move the decimal point two places to the right.

Converting a Decimal to a Percent

To change a decimal to a percent, multiply by 100 or move the decimal point two places to the right. Then add a percent symbol.

$$0.25 = 0.25 \times 100 = 25\%$$
$$1.35 = 1.35 \times 100 = 135\%$$
$$0.015 = 0.015 \times 100 = 1.5\%$$

2.2 Problem Set

Express the following fractions as percents. Round to the nearest whole percent.

1. $\dfrac{6}{7}$

2. $\dfrac{5}{12}$

3. $\dfrac{1}{4}$

4. $\dfrac{2}{3}$

5. $\dfrac{0.5}{10}$

Express the following ratios as percents. Round to the nearest tenth of a percent.

6. 2:3

7. 1.5:4.65

8. 1:250

9. 1:10,000

10. 1:6

Convert the following percents to fractions; then reduce to lowest terms.

11. 50%

12. 2%

Convert the following percents to decimals.

13. 6%

14. 12.5%

15. 126%

Calculate the following, rounding to the nearest hundredth when necessary.

16. 5% of 20

17. 20% of 60

18. 19% of 63

19. 110% of 70

20. 0.2% of 50

Fill in the missing values.

	Percent	Fraction	Ratio	Decimal
21.	33%	$\dfrac{1}{3}$	_____	_____
22.	2.5%	_____	1:40	_____
23.	_____	$\dfrac{1}{2}$	_____	0.5
24.	_____	_____	1:100	0.01
25.	90%	_____	_____	0.90
26.	67%	_____	_____	0.67
27.	_____	$\dfrac{1}{500}$	1:500	_____
28.	0.45%	_____	_____	0.0045
29.	5%	_____	1:20	_____
30.	20%	$\dfrac{1}{5}$	_____	_____

Applications

Choose the appropriate solution from the available stock.

31. A 1:10,000 solution has been ordered. You have a 0.05% solution, a 0.01% solution, and a 1% solution in stock. Which will you choose?

32. A 1:20 solution has been ordered. You have a 5% solution, a 10% solution, and a 20% solution in stock. Which will you choose?

33. A 1:25 solution has been ordered. You have a 0.4% solution, a 0.05% solution, and a 4% solution in stock. Which will you choose?

34. A 1:800 solution has been ordered. You have a 0.01% solution, a 0.125% solution, and a 1.25% solution in stock. Which will you choose?

35. A 1:10 solution has been ordered. You have a 0.09% solution, a 0.01% solution, and a 10% solution in stock. Which will you choose?

Self-check your work in Appendix A.

2.3 Proportions

A **proportion** is an expression of equality between two ratios. A proportion can be visualized by thinking of two triangles that have the same shape but are different sizes. The triangles in Figure 2.4 have equal proportions.

FIGURE 2.4
Triangles with Equal Proportions

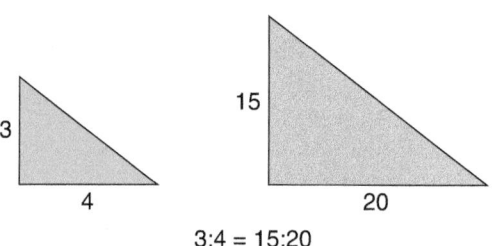

3:4 = 15:20

A proportion is notated by an equal sign or a double colon (::) between the ratios. It can also be noted by using fractions.

$$3:4 = 15:20 \qquad \text{or} \qquad 3:4 :: 15:20 \qquad \text{or} \qquad \frac{3}{4} = \frac{15}{20}$$

In a proportion, the first and fourth, or outside, numbers are called the *extremes*. The second and third, or inside, numbers are called the *means*.

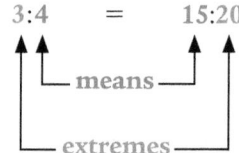

The product of the means must always equal the product of the extremes in a proportion. You can check for the correctness of the proportion by using this formula.

Given a proportion

$$a:b = c:d$$

the product of means = the product of extremes

or

$$b \times c = a \times d$$

Example 2.3.1

Confirm that the proportion 3:4 equals the proportion 15:20.

$$3{:}4 = 15{:}20$$
$$4 \times 15 = 3 \times 20$$
$$60 = 60$$

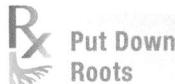

Put Down Roots

The word *ratio* comes from the Latin term *ratio* meaning "to reason or calculate." The word *proportion* also has its roots in Latin, with the phrase *pro portione* meaning "for or according to the relation of parts." Thus, a ratio-proportion calculation is based on determining the relationship of parts to each other.

The **ratio-proportion method** is one of the most frequently used methods for calculating medication doses in the pharmacy. You can use this method any time one ratio is complete and the other ratio has a missing component. In other words, if you know three of the four values in a proportion, you can solve for the missing value. When setting up ratios in the proportion, it is important that the numbers remain in the correct ratio and that the numbers have the correct units of measurement in both the numerator and the denominator. Table 2.2 lists the rules for using the ratio-proportion method. Table 2.3 lists the steps for solving for an unknown quantity, typically designated by the letter *x*.

TABLE 2.2   Rules for Using the Ratio-Proportion Method

Rule 1. Three of the four amounts must be known.
Rule 2. The numerators must have the same unit of measurement.
Rule 3. The denominators must have the same unit of measurement.

TABLE 2.3   Steps for Solving for *x* in the Ratio-Proportion Method

Step 1. Create a proportion by placing the ratios in fraction form and use a variable to represent the unknown (*x* is often used).
Step 2. Check that the unit of measurement in the numerators is the same and the unit of measurement in the denominators is the same.
Step 3. Use the means-extremes property of proportions to cross multiply and solve for the unknown variable.
Step 4. Check your answer by seeing if the product of the means equals the product of the extremes.

Example 2.3.2

A medication is available as 250 mg/5 mL. How many milliliters represent a dose of 375 mg?

In this case, set the ordered dose ratio equal to the pharmacy-stocked medication ratio. In setting up a proportion, the ratios on the two sides of the equal sign may be flipped over as long as *both* ratios are reversed.

$$\text{prescription order ratio} = \text{pharmacy shelf ratio}$$

$$\frac{375 \text{ mg}}{x \text{ mL}} = \frac{250 \text{ mg}}{5 \text{ mL}}$$

Be sure to check that the unit of measurement in the numerators is the same (both are milligrams) and that the unit of measurement in the denominators is the same (both are milliliters).

Using the ratio-proportion method:

$$x \text{ mL } (250 \text{ mg}) = 5 \text{ mL } (375 \text{ mg})$$

$$\frac{x \text{ mL } (250 \text{ mg})}{250 \text{ mg}} = \frac{5 \text{ mL } (375 \text{ mg})}{250 \text{ mg}}$$

$$x = 7.5 \text{ mL}$$

Check your answer by checking that the product of the means equals the product of the extremes.

$$\frac{375 \text{ mg}}{7.5 \text{ mL}} = \frac{250 \text{ mg}}{5 \text{ mL}}$$

$$375 : 7.5 = 250 : 5$$

$$375 \times 5 = 7.5 \times 250$$

$$1{,}875 = 1{,}875$$

Using the dimensional analysis method:

$$\frac{375 \text{ mg}}{1} \times \frac{5 \text{ mL}}{250 \text{ mg}} = 7.5 \text{ mL}$$

Example 2.3.3

The label shown below is the stock your pharmacy has available for gentamicin. How many milliliters will need to be prepared if the patient is prescribed 50 mg?

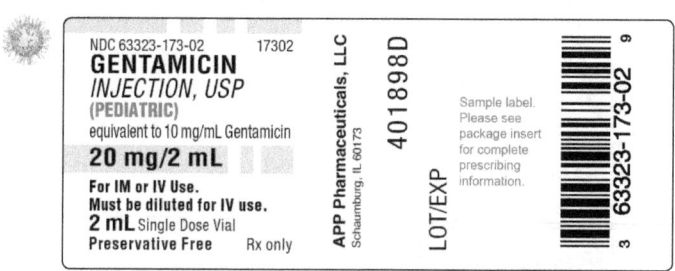

$$\frac{50 \text{ mg}}{x \text{ mL}} = \frac{20 \text{ mg}}{2 \text{ mL}}$$

Be sure to check that the unit of measurement in the numerators is the same (both are milligrams) and that the unit of measurement in the denominators is the same (both are milliliters).

Using the ratio-proportion method:

$$x \text{ mL} (20 \text{ mg}) = 2 \text{ mL} (50 \text{ mg})$$

$$\frac{x \text{ mL} (20 \text{ mg})}{20 \text{ mg}} = \frac{2 \text{ mL} (50 \text{ mg})}{20 \text{ mg}}$$

$$x = 5 \text{ mL}$$

Check your answer by checking that the product of the means equals the product of the extremes.

$$\frac{50 \text{ mg}}{5 \text{ mL}} = \frac{20 \text{ mg}}{2 \text{ mL}}$$

$$50{:}5 = 20{:}2$$

$$50 \times 2 = 5 \times 20$$

$$100 = 100$$

Using the dimensional analysis method:

$$\frac{50 \text{ mg}}{1} \times \frac{2 \text{ mL}}{20 \text{ mg}} = 5 \text{ mL}$$

Example 2.3.4

The label shown below is the stock available at your pharmacy. How many milligrams of diazepam will need to be dispensed to the patient if the prescription is for 4 mL?

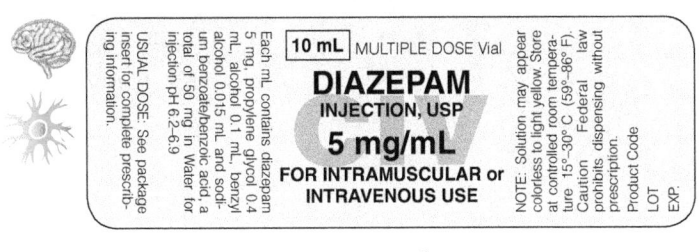

$$\frac{x \text{ mg}}{4 \text{ mL}} = \frac{5 \text{ mg}}{1 \text{ mL}}$$

Be sure to check that the unit of measurement in the numerators is the same (both are milligrams) and that the unit of measurement in the denominators is the same (both are milliliters).

Using the ratio-proportion method:

$$x \text{ mg} (1 \text{ mL}) = 5 \text{ mg} (4 \text{ mL})$$

$$\frac{x \text{ mg} (1 \text{ mL})}{1 \text{ mL}} = \frac{5 \text{ mg} (4 \text{ mL})}{1 \text{ mL}}$$

$$x = 20 \text{ mg}$$

Check your answer by checking that the product of the means equals the product of the extremes.

$$\frac{20 \text{ mg}}{4 \text{ mL}} = \frac{5 \text{ mg}}{1 \text{ mL}}$$

$$20:4 = 5:1$$

$$20 \times 1 = 4 \times 5$$

$$20 = 20$$

Using the dimensional analysis method:

$$\frac{4 \text{ mL}}{1} \times \frac{5 \text{ mg}}{1 \text{ mL}} = 20 \text{ mg}$$

In addition to being useful for calculating drug doses in the pharmacy, the ratio-proportion method can be used for converting between units of measure. To solve a conversion problem, use a conversion factor as one of the proportions. A **conversion factor** is an equivalency equal to 1. For example, since 1 g = 1,000 mg, an example of a conversion factor is 1 g/1,000 mg or 1,000 mg/1 g. Additional conversion factors are presented in Appendix C.

☑ TAKE NOTE

Conversion factors are extremely helpful in pharmacy calculations. While it is not necessary to memorize all the conversion factors in Appendix C, you may find it helpful to memorize the ones commonly used in your practice setting. Most practice settings use the following conversion factors: 1 kg/2.2 lb, 1 in/2.54 cm, and 1 oz/30 mL.

For Good Measure

When setting up a proportion to solve a conversion, the units in the numerators must match, and the units in the denominators must match.

Example 2.3.5

How many milligrams are equivalent to 3 g?

$$\frac{x \text{ mg}}{3 \text{ g}} = \frac{1,000 \text{ mg}}{1 \text{ g}}$$

Be sure to check that the unit of measurement in the numerators is the same (both are milligrams) and that the unit of measurement in the denominators is the same (both are grams).

Using the ratio-proportion method:

$$x \text{ mg } (1 \text{ g}) = 1,000 \text{ mg } (3 \text{ g})$$

$$\frac{x \text{ mg } (1 \text{ g})}{1 \text{ g}} = \frac{1,000 \text{ mg } (3 \text{ g})}{1 \text{ g}}$$

$$x = 3,000 \text{ mg}$$

Check your answer by checking that the product of the means equals the product of the extremes.

$$\frac{3{,}000 \text{ mg}}{3 \text{ g}} = \frac{1{,}000 \text{ mg}}{1 \text{ g}}$$

$$3{,}000{:}3 = 1{,}000{:}1$$

$$3{,}000 \times 1 = 3 \times 1{,}000$$

$$3{,}000 = 3{,}000$$

Using the dimensional analysis method:

$$\frac{3 \cancel{\text{g}}}{1} \times \frac{1{,}000 \text{ mg}}{1 \cancel{\text{g}}} = 3{,}000 \text{ mg}$$

Example 2.3.6

Change 44 lb to kilograms. The conversion chart in Appendix C states that 1 kg = 2.2 lb.

$$\frac{x \text{ kg}}{44 \text{ lb}} = \frac{1 \text{ kg}}{2.2 \text{ lb}}$$

Be sure to check that the unit of measurement in the numerators is the same (both are kilograms) and that the unit of measurement in the denominators is the same (both are pounds).

Using the ratio-proportional method:

$$x \text{ kg } (2.2 \text{ lb}) = 1 \text{ kg } (44 \text{ lb})$$

$$\frac{x \text{ kg } (\cancel{2.2 \text{ lb}})}{\cancel{2.2 \text{ lb}}} = \frac{1 \text{ kg } (44 \cancel{\text{ lb}})}{2.2 \cancel{\text{ lb}}}$$

$$x = 20 \text{ kg}$$

Check your answer by checking that the product of the means equals the product of the extremes.

$$\frac{20 \text{ kg}}{44 \text{ lb}} = \frac{1 \text{ kg}}{2.2 \text{ lb}}$$

$$20{:}44 = 1{:}2.2$$

$$20 \times 2.2 = 44 \times 1$$

$$44 = 44$$

Using the dimensional analysis method:

$$\frac{44 \cancel{\text{ lb}}}{1} \times \frac{1 \text{ kg}}{2.2 \cancel{\text{ lb}}} = 20 \text{ lb}$$

The ratio-proportion method can also be used to solve many types of percentage problems. When setting up the ratios, remember that a percentage may be written in fraction form, with the percent value over 100. For example, 95% is equivalent to $^{95}/_{100}$.

Example 2.3.7

A patient needs to take 75% of a recommended dose before it may be discontinued. The recommended dose is 650 mg. How much must the patient take before it is discontinued?

Write the percentage (75%) as a fraction ($^{75}/_{100}$) and solve for x.

$$\frac{x \text{ mg}}{650 \text{ mg}} = \frac{75 \text{ mg}}{100 \text{ mg}}$$

Be sure to check that the unit of measurement in the numerators is the same (both are milligrams) and that the unit of measurement in the denominators is the same (both are milligrams).

Using the ratio-proportional method:

$$x \text{ mg} (100 \text{ mg}) = 650 \text{ mg} (75 \text{ mg})$$

$$\frac{x \text{ mg} (\cancel{100 \text{ mg}})}{\cancel{100 \text{ mg}}} = \frac{650 \cancel{\text{ mg}} (75 \text{ mg})}{100 \cancel{\text{ mg}}}$$

$$x = 487.5 \text{ mg}$$

Check your answer by checking that the product of the means equals the product of the extremes.

$$\frac{487.5 \text{ mg}}{650 \text{ mg}} = \frac{75}{100 \text{ mg}}$$

$$487.5{:}650 = 75{:}100$$

$$487.5 \times 100 = 650 \times 75$$

$$48{,}750 = 48{,}750$$

Using the dimensional analysis method:

$$\frac{650 \cancel{\text{ mg}} \text{ (total amount)}}{1} \times \frac{75 \text{ mg (portion of total)}}{100 \cancel{\text{ mg}} \text{ (total amount)}} = 487.5 \text{ mg}$$

Example 2.3.8

A patient has taken 85% of a recommended dose. If the amount taken is 320 mg, what was the recommended dose?

Another way of phrasing this question is "320 mg is 85% of what amount?"

$$\frac{320 \text{ mg}}{x \text{ mg}} = \frac{85 \text{ mg}}{100 \text{ mg}}$$

Be sure to check that the unit of measurement in the numerators is the same (both are milligrams of the portion of the whole) and that the unit of measurement in the denominators is the same (both are milligrams of the total amount).

Using the ratio-proportion method:

$$x \text{ mg } (85 \text{ mg}) = 320 \text{ mg } (100 \text{ mg})$$

$$\frac{x \text{ mg } (\cancel{85 \text{ mg}})}{\cancel{85 \text{ mg}}} = \frac{320 \cancel{\text{ mg}} (100 \text{ mg})}{85 \cancel{\text{ mg}}}$$

$$x = 376.5 \text{ mg}$$

Check your answer by checking that the product of the means equals the product of the extremes.

$$\frac{320 \text{ mg}}{376.5 \text{ mg}} = \frac{85 \text{ mg}}{100 \text{ mg}}$$

$$320{:}376.5 = 85{:}100$$

$$320 \times 100 = 376.5 \times 85$$

$$32{,}000 = 32{,}000$$

Using the dimensional analysis method:

$$\frac{320 \cancel{\text{ mg}} \text{ (portion of total)}}{1} \times \frac{100 \text{ mg (total amount)}}{85 \cancel{\text{ mg}} \text{ (portion of total)}} = 376.5 \text{ mg}$$

2.3 Problem Set

Solve for x for each of the following ratios. Round your answers to the nearest hundredth when necessary.

1. $\dfrac{x}{10} = \dfrac{20}{40}$

2. $\dfrac{x}{0.6} = \dfrac{0.8}{6.12}$

3. $\dfrac{x}{9} = \dfrac{5}{10}$

4. $\dfrac{x}{1} = \dfrac{0.5}{5}$

5. $\dfrac{x}{50} = \dfrac{0.4}{125}$

6. $\dfrac{13}{15} = \dfrac{5}{x}$

7. $\dfrac{x}{68} = \dfrac{72}{90}$

8. $\dfrac{14}{3} = \dfrac{x}{52}$

9. $\dfrac{x}{27} = \dfrac{49}{51}$

10. $\dfrac{13}{x} = \dfrac{52}{64}$

11. $\dfrac{14}{23} = \dfrac{27}{x}$

12. $\dfrac{31}{13} = \dfrac{51}{x}$

13. $\dfrac{47}{9} = \dfrac{x}{15}$

14. $\dfrac{9}{26} = \dfrac{x}{31}$

15. $\dfrac{37}{x} = \dfrac{11}{23}$

Set up proportions and solve for x to answer the following questions. Round your answers to the nearest hundredth.

16. 72 is what percent of 254?

17. 90% of what number is 44?

18. 44% of what number is 100?

19. 28% of what number is 34?

20. 24.5 is what percent of 45?

Change the following weights using the conversion factor 1 g = 1,000 mg.

21. 100 mg = _____ g

22. 247 mg = _____ g

23. 1420 mg = _____ g

24. 495 mg = _____ g

25. 3781 mg = _____ g

26. 0.349 g = _____ mg

27. 1.5 g = _____ mg

28. 0.083 g = _____ mg

29. 0.01 g = _____ mg

30. 2.1 g = _____ mg

Change the following weights using the conversion factor 1 kg = 2.2 lb. Round your answer to the tenths place.

31. 6.3 lb = _____ kg

32. 15 lb = _____ kg

33. 97 lb = _____ kg

34. 115 lb = _____ kg

35. 186 lb = _____ kg

36. 7.5 kg = _____ lb

37. 3.6 kg = _____ lb

38. 79.2 kg = _____ lb

39. 90 kg = _____ lb

40. 0.5 kg = _____ lb

Applications

Set up a proportion using x as the unknown and solve the following. Explain in your own words how you set up the proportion.

41. Progesterone is available as 50 mg/mL. The order calls for 100 mg of progesterone. How many milliliters will you prepare?

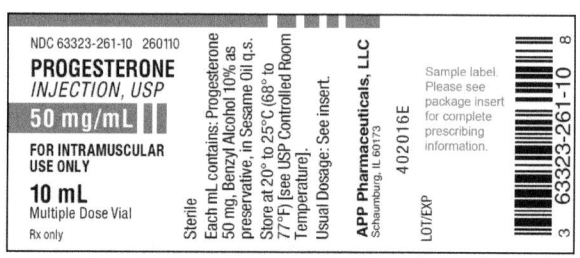

NDC 63323-261-10 260110
PROGESTERONE
INJECTION, USP
50 mg/mL
FOR INTRAMUSCULAR USE ONLY
10 mL
Multiple Dose Vial
Rx only

Sterile
Each mL contains: Progesterone 50 mg, Benzyl Alcohol 10% as preservative, in Sesame Oil q.s.
Store at 20° to 25°C (68° to 77°F) [see USP Controlled Room Temperature].
Usual Dosage: See insert.

APP Pharmaceuticals, LLC
Schaumburg, IL 60173

402016E

Sample label. Please see package insert for complete prescribing information.

LOT/EXP

63323-261-10

42. Capicillin is available as a 125 mg tablet. How many tablets are needed to give a dose of 375 mg?

43. Soakamycin is available as a concentration of 20 mg/mL. How many milliliters are needed to prepare a foot soak that contains 300 mg?

44. You are going to buy some folders to file your orders. After doing research, you find that the most cost-effective price is $7.40 per box of 100 folders. You have $15 to spend. How many 100 count boxes can you buy?

45. The patient is to get an intramuscular injection of 10,000 units of Musclesporin. You have a bottle containing 250,000 units per 15 mL. How many milliliters must be prepared to administer this dose?

48. A prescriber ordered a dose of 300 mg. The medication is available as a 500 mg/10 mL solution. How many milliliters are needed to provide the ordered dose?

46. A prescriber ordered a dose of 60 mg gentamicin. The medication is available as a 20 mg/2 mL solution. How many milliliters are needed to provide the ordered dose?

49. A prescriber ordered a dose of 30 mg lamivudine oral solution. The medication is available in a 5 mg/mL oral solution. How many milliliters are needed to provide the ordered dose?

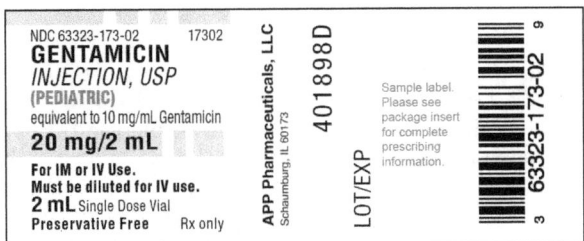

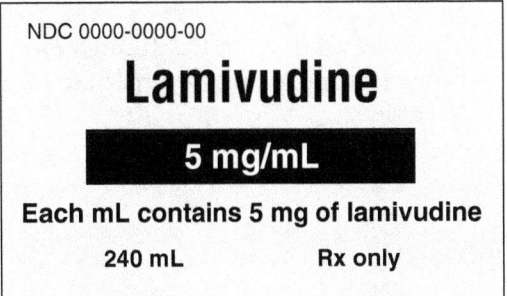

47. A prescriber ordered a dose of 60 mg famotidine. The medication is available as a 40 mg/4 mL solution. How many milliliters are needed to provide the ordered dose?

50. A prescriber ordered a dose of 30 mg. The medication is available as a 20 mg/mL solution. How many milliliters are needed to provide the ordered dose?

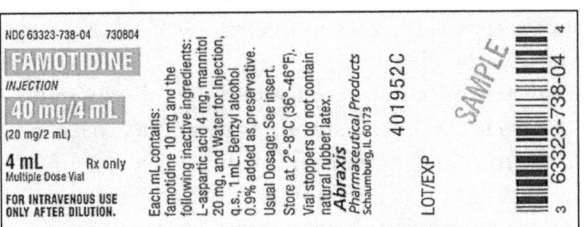

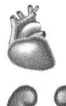 Use the following medication label to determine the doses needed for questions 51–55.

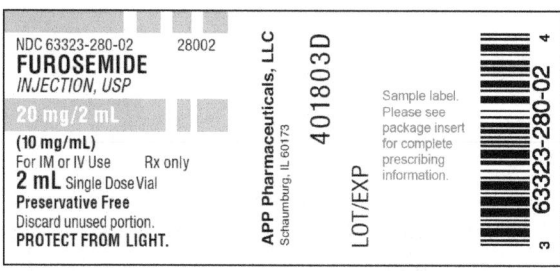

NDC 63323-280-02   28002
FUROSEMIDE
INJECTION, USP

20 mg/2 mL

(10 mg/mL)
For IM or IV Use   Rx only
2 mL Single Dose Vial
Preservative Free
Discard unused portion.
PROTECT FROM LIGHT.

APP Pharmaceuticals, LLC
Schaumburg, IL 60173

401803D

LOT/EXP

63323-280-02

Sample label.
Please see
package insert
for complete
prescribing
information.

51. The order calls for 5 mL of furosemide. How many milligrams are needed to fulfill the order?

52. The order calls for 80 mg of furosemide. How many milliliters are needed to fill the order?

53. The order calls for 50 mg of furosemide. How many milliliters are needed to fill the order?

54. The order calls for 12.5 mg of furosemide. How many milliliters are needed to fill the order?

55. The order calls for 3.5 mL furosemide. How many milligrams are needed to fill the order?

Self-check your work in Appendix A.

2.4 Percentage of Error

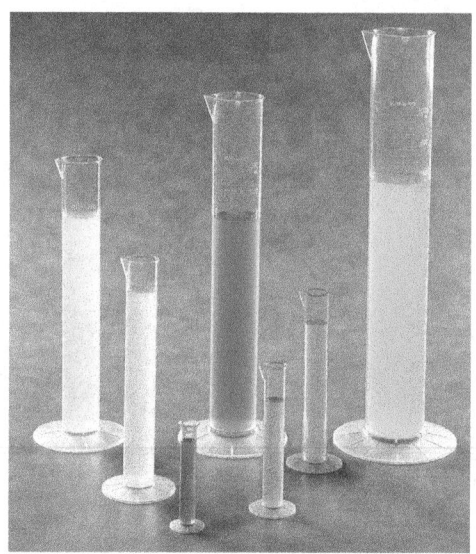

Graduated cylinders are used to accurately measure liquids in the pharmacy.

Percentages are used in a variety of ways when preparing medication doses. In the compounding pharmacy, percentages are used to determine the possible percentage of error and the least weighable quantity of a substance for safe preparation. Percentages are also used when doing the business of the pharmacy, such as calculating the percentage of sales, percentage of discount, and percentage of markup. These applications will be covered in Chapter 9, "Using Business Math in the Pharmacy."

When measuring a liquid or weighing a solid ingredient in the pharmacy, a certain amount of error is expected. Not all graduated cylinders used in the pharmacy are equally accurate, although they are usually much more accurate than the measuring devices found in patients' homes. Graduated cylinders used in pharmacies may be conical or cylindrical, with the cylindrical shape being more accurate. Similarly, pharmacy balances, though generally very accurate when compared with other small scales, may exhibit slight variations. A Class III prescription balance is a type of balance commonly used to weigh very small quantities in the pharmacy. Regardless of the measuring tool being used, it is important to know the margin of error of a particular balance or graduated cylinder. Margin of error can be expressed as a percentage, called **percentage of error**.

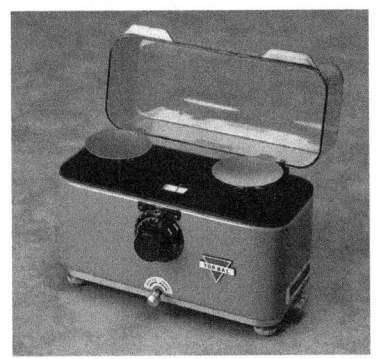

A Class III prescription balance can accurately weigh small quantities.

When weighing a substance, the balance will approximate the actual weight to a certain degree of accuracy. Pharmacy balances are generally marked with their degree of accuracy. This degree has been determined by comparing quantities weighed on the balance with the weights obtained from another balance whose accuracy is known. This determination of accuracy is performed in the factory and typically is not done in the pharmacy.

If a substance was weighed or measured incorrectly, and you have something that will allow you to more accurately measure the amount in question, then you can determine the percentage of error by using the following formula:

$$\frac{\text{amount of error}}{\text{quantity desired}} \times 100 = \text{percentage of error}$$

In this equation, the amount of error is the difference between the actual amount and the quantity desired, or

$$\text{actual amount} - \text{quantity desired} = \text{amount of error*}$$

*Use the absolute value or positive integer.

The percentage of error is a range both above and below the target measurement. It is inconsequential whether the result is over or under the target (i.e., whether it is positive or negative). Percentage of error is always expressed as a positive value.

Example 2.4.1

 You are to dispense 50 mL of cetirizine solution. The original measurement shows 50 mL. When you double-check the amount using a more accurate graduated cylinder, the actual amount is 52 mL. What is the amount of error in the first measurement?

Calculate the difference in the two measurements to determine the amount of error.

$$\text{actual amount} - \text{quantity desired} = \text{amount of error}$$
$$52 \text{ mL} - 50 \text{ mL} = 2 \text{ mL}$$

The amount of error is 2 mL.

Example 2.4.2

You are to dispense 120 mL of a liquid. The original measurement is 120 mL. When you double-check the amount using a more accurate graduated cylinder, the actual amount is 126 mL. What is the percentage of error of the first measurement?

Calculate the difference in the two measurements to determine the amount of error.

$$\text{actual amount} - \text{quantity desired} = \text{amount of error}$$
$$126 \text{ mL} - 120 \text{ mL} = 6 \text{ mL}$$

Use the percentage of error equation to determine the percentage of error of the measurement.

$$\frac{\text{amount of error}}{\text{quantity desired}} \times 100 = \frac{6 \text{ mL}}{120 \text{ mL}} \times 100 = 5\%$$

The percentage of error is 5%.

Example 2.4.3

You are to dispense 30 g of a powder. The original measurement is 30 g. When you double-check the amount using a more accurate balance, the actual amount is 31.8 g. What is the percentage of error of the first measurement?

Calculate the difference in the two amounts to determine the amount of error.

$$31.8 \text{ g} - 30 \text{ g} = 1.8 \text{ g}$$

Use the percentage of error equation to determine the percentage of error of the measurement.

$$\frac{\text{amount of error}}{\text{quantity desired}} \times 100 = \frac{1.8 \text{ g}}{30 \text{ g}} \times 100 = 6\%$$

The percentage of error is 6%.

Example 2.4.4

You are to dispense 453 mg of a powder. The original measurement is 453 mg. When you double-check the amount using a more accurate balance, the actual amount is 438 mg. What is the percentage of error of the first measurement?

Calculate the difference in the two measurements to determine the amount of error.

$$438 \text{ mg} - 453 = -15 \text{ mg and we take the absolute value of } -15 \text{ which is } 15.$$

Use the percentage of error equation to determine the percentage of error of the measurement.

$$\frac{\text{amount of error}}{\text{quantity desired}} \times 100 = \frac{15 \text{ mg}}{453 \text{ mg}} \times 100 = 3.3\%$$

The percentage of error is 3.3%.

Example 2.4.5

You are to weigh 60 g of a cream base for a topical compound. Your error range is 3%. What will be the least amount and the largest amount acceptable?

Multiply the percentage (in decimal form) by the target weight.

$$60 \text{ g} \times 0.03 = 1.8 \text{ g}$$

Determine the range.

$$60 \text{ g} - 1.8 \text{ g} = 58.2 \text{ g} \qquad 60 \text{ g} + 1.8 \text{ g} = 61.8 \text{ g}$$

Therefore, the acceptable range is 58.2 g to 61.8 g.

Example 2.4.6

You are preparing an order by measuring 800 mL from a 1 L normal saline IV bag. When you check the volume of the fluid in a graduated cylinder, the amount measured is actually 820 mL. You have an acceptable range of 2%. What is the percentage of error in this measurement? Did you meet your target?

Determine the difference in the two measurements to determine the amount of error.

$$820 \text{ mL} - 800 \text{ mL} = 20 \text{ mL}$$

Use the percentage of error equation to determine the percentage of error of the measurement.

$$\frac{\text{amount of error}}{\text{quantity desired}} \times 100 = \frac{20 \text{ mL}}{800 \text{ mL}} \times 100 = 2.5\%$$

Because 2.5% is larger than the acceptable percentage of error, the target range was not met.

2.4 Problem Set

Calculate the percentage of error for the following measurements. Then, round to the nearest hundredths place. Assume that the measured amount is equal to the quantity desired.

1. The measured weight was 185 mg, but the actual weight is 189 mg.

2. The measured weight was 500 mg, but the actual weight is 476 mg.

3. The measured weight was 1,200 mg, but the actual weight is 1,507 mg.

4. The measured weight was 15 mg, but the actual weight is 12.5 mg.

5. The measured weight was 400 mcg, but the actual weight is 415 mcg.

6. The measured volume was 5 mL, but the actual volume is 6.3 mL.

7. The measured volume was 15 mL, but the actual volume is 13 mL.

8. The measured volume was 15 mL, but the actual volume is 20 mL.

9. The measured volume was 1.5 L, but the actual volume is 1.45 L.

10. The measured volume was 700 mL, but the actual volume is 726 mL.

Determine the percentage of error for the following measurements, and identify those within a percentage of error of 3%.

11. The measured volume was 3 mL, but the actual volume is 2.6 mL.

12. The measured volume was 12.5 mL, but the actual volume is 12.1 mL.

13. The measured volume was 1.8 mL, but the actual volume is 1.5 mL.

14. The measured volume was 3.2 mL, but the actual volume is 3.29 mL.

Determine the percentage of error for the following measurements, and identify those within a percentage of error of 6%.

15. The measured weight was 150 mg, but the actual weight is 149 mg.

16. The measured weight was 200 mg, but the actual weight is 192 mg.

17. The measured weight was 30 mg, but the actual weight is 31.5 mg.

18. The measured weight was 454 mg, but the actual weight is 450 mg.

State the acceptable range of error for each of the following. Round to the nearest hundredths place.

19. The desired volume is 200 mL, and the percentage of error is 0.5%.

20. The desired volume is 10.3 mL, and the percentage of error is 0.75%.

21. The desired volume is 830 mL, and the percentage of error is 2%.

22. The desired weight is 18 g, and the percentage of error is 0.15%.

23. The desired weight is 750 mg, and the percentage of error is 0.4%.

Applications

24. If a generic drug manufacturer meets a bioavailability (the degree to which a drug becomes available to the target tissue after administration) comparison to within 20%, and a drug normally has a bioavailability of 100 mg, what is the range of accuracy?

25. A new brand of vitamins claims to have bioavailability within 12% of a national brand of vitamin C. The national brand has 500 mg of vitamin C per tablet. What is the range of vitamin C contained in the tablet?

Self-check your work in Appendix A.

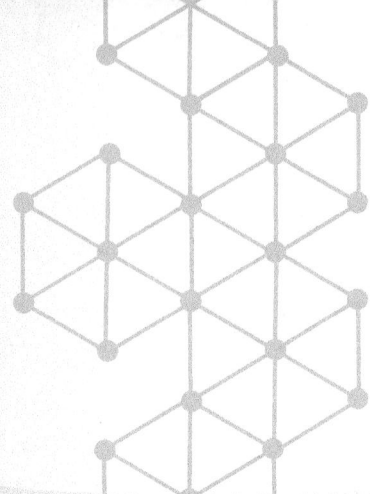

- Ratios are used to describe the amount of medication per dose or unit.

- Ratios may also be written as fractions.

- Ratios may be written in reverse order (1:100 or 100:1) or may be written flipped upside down (1/100 or 100/1).

- Ratios may be multiplied when a larger dose is desired or divided when a smaller dose is desired.

- Percent is the number of parts per 100 parts.

- Ratios, percents, fractions, and decimals may all be used to express the same value.

- When converting a percent to a numerical value, divide by 100, or move the decimal point two places to the left.

- When converting a numerical value to a percent, multiply by 100, or move the decimal point two places to the right.

- Proportions are an expression of equivalency between two ratios (or fractions).

- A proportion with one missing value may be solved if three of the four values are known.

- When using the ratio-proportion method to solve for a missing value, the numerators must have the same unit of measure, and the denominators must have the same unit of measure.

- The ratio-proportion method may be used to convert between units of measure by setting the ratio desired to be converted equal to a unit of 1.

- Percentage of error is calculated by dividing the amount of error by the quantity desired, and multiplying by 100.

- Error range is the amount above or below the target.

KEY TERMS

conversion factor an equivalency equal to 1 that can be used when converting units of measure using the ratio-proportion method

percent the number of parts per 100; can be written as a fraction, a decimal, or a ratio

percentage of error the percentage by which a measurement is inaccurate

proportion an expression of equality between two ratios

ratio a numerical representation of the relationship between two parts of the whole or between one part and the whole

ratio-proportion method a conversion method based on comparing a complete ratio to a ratio with a missing component

solution liquid mixture in which the minor component, the solute, is uniformly distributed within the major component, the solvent

suspension mixture in which solute particles are mixed with, but not dissolved, in a fluid

CHAPTER REVIEW

Finding Solutions

To gain practice in handling challenging situations in the workplace, consider the following real-world scenarios, and then use the guiding questions to help you formulate your responses.

Note: *To indicate your answer for Scenario A, Question 1, ask your instructor for the handout depicting measuring devices.*

Scenario A: A patient with poison ivy has been taking over-the-counter (OTC) Benadryl for itching. The doctor has told him to take 50 mg every six hours. The medication is available in a 12.5 mg/5 mL solution.

1. On the handout that you obtained from your instructor, indicate how many milliliters the patient will need for each dose.

2. If the patient uses three doses per day, how many milliliters will he need to last three days?

3. How many 4 fluid ounce bottles (120 mL) will the patient need to purchase?

 Scenario B: A patient has brought her newborn infant into the pharmacy. She said the baby weighs 9½ pounds.

4. What is the infant's weight in kilograms?

Scenario C: You have been asked to reorder and restock a special-order lip balm that your pharmacy carries. A carton of 24 tubes costs the pharmacy $21.50. You know that you may not spend more than $100.00 and that you may not purchase a partial carton.

5. How many cartons can you buy?

6. What will the cost be for this quantity of cartons?

7. How many tubes of lip balm will this provide?

8. How much money will be left over after the cost of the lip balm?

9. The company charges an additional 4% of the cost of the product for shipping. How much is this?

Scenario D: You receive a prescription for the antibiotic amoxicillin 125 mg/5 mL suspension. This medication is for a pediatric patient weighing 20 kg, and it is determined that each dose should be 25 mg.

10. How many milliliters are needed for each 25 mg dose?

11. The patient needs to take 2 doses per day for a total of 50 mg. How many milliliters are needed for 50 mg of medication?

12. The total prescription requires that 500 mg of medication be dispensed. How many milliliters are needed to equal 500 mg of amoxicillin?

13. How would you express the concentration of amoxicillin in mg/10 ml?

Scenario E: You study hard for your pharmacy calculations exam and do very well. The exam had 50 questions, and you missed only 2 questions.

14. What percent of the questions did you get correct?

15. You classmate got a score of 80%. How many questions did he miss?

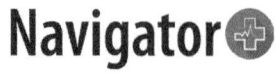

Navigator

Access interactive chapter review exercises, practice activities, flash cards, and study games.

3

Developing Prescription Literacy Skills

Learning Objectives

1 Identify the elements of a complete prescription order.

2 Apply calculation operations in handling prescription orders.

3 Recognize the elements of a medication label.

4 Apply calculation operations to information on medication labels.

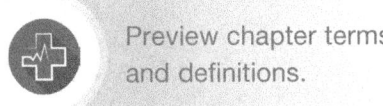
Preview chapter terms and definitions.

3.1 Elements of a Prescription Order

Put Down Roots

The word *prescription* is derived from the Latin word *praescriptio*, meaning "order, direction, a writing before." Therefore, a prescription is an order for a medication that is written before the medication is given or dispensed to the patient.

A **prescription** is an order for a medication or mixture of medications written (or otherwise recorded and/or transmitted) by a practitioner to be filled by a pharmacist or technician. Prescriptions may be received in the pharmacy by several means: a handwritten order, a digital or computerized order, or a phone order. The pharmacy technician needs to interpret the prescription to determine which calculations will be necessary to fill this order correctly and appropriately. Although the legal requirements for information necessary on a prescription are regulated by state law and vary from one state to another, the following elements appear on every prescription: patient information, prescriber information, and drug designation. Figure 3.1 illustrates the parts of a prescription written for a community pharmacy, and Figure 3.2 illustrates the parts of a medication order written for a hospital pharmacy. (These figures are shown on the following pages.)

Patient Information

Every prescription order must have enough information to uniquely identify the patient. In addition to the patient's full name (first and last), most states also require outpatient prescriptions (prescriptions for patients that are not in hospitals or other medical institutions) to include the patient's address (street, city, state). It is also good practice to include the patient's age or date of birth on every prescription, and some states and most insurers require this information.

FIGURE 3.1
Elements of a Prescription for a Community Pharmacy

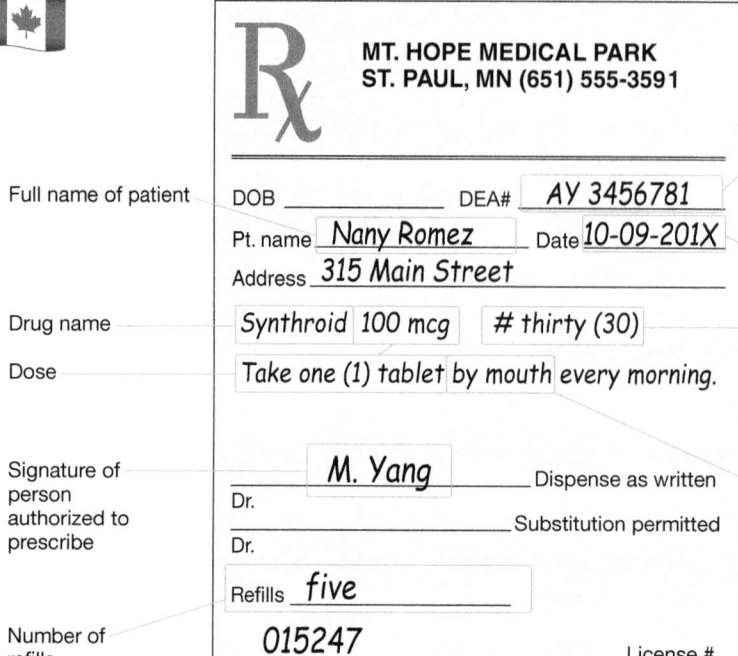

Full name of patient

Drug name

Dose

Signature of person authorized to prescribe

Number of refills

DEA number for controlled drug and insurance

Date of prescription

Amount of drug to be dispensed
Note: Amounts should be written out to prevent alterations.

Route of administration

Prescriptions for inpatients (patients admitted to a hospital or other medical institution), often referred to as "orders," usually substitute the patient's hospital identification number and room number for the patient's address. Inpatient prescription orders are typically submitted electronically or written on a form pre-stamped with the patient's admission date, the admitting physician's name, and the patient's date of birth, in addition to the patient's name and hospital number. Hospital medication order forms frequently require a notation of the patient's allergy information as well.

Many pharmacies require that the patient's height and weight be available, either on the prescription itself or in the patient's file. If height and weight are included, it is important to include the units for each. Patient weights may be measured in either kilograms (kg) or pounds (# or lb). Heights are generally measured in centimeters (cm) or inches (″ or in.). These measurements are quite different from one another: A 100 kg patient is more than twice the size of a 100 lb patient; a 76 cm patient is most likely a child under three years of age, whereas a 76″ patient is a very tall adult! (Conversions of height and weight units are covered in Chapters 4 and 5.)

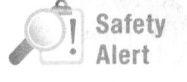
Safety Alert

Every number should always be followed by the appropriate unit.

Prescriber Information

In most states, outpatient prescription orders must include the name, authority (medical doctor, doctor of osteopathy, etc.), and address of the prescribing practitioner. Frequently, the prescription order includes the prescriber's telephone number. Prescriptions for controlled substances must also bear a registration code known as a **DEA number**. DEA numbers are issued by the Drug Enforcement Administration (DEA), an agency of the federal government, and signify the authority of the holder to prescribe or handle controlled substances. A DEA number is *always* two letters followed by seven digits. The last of the seven digits is a **check digit**, calculated by following the steps in Table 3.1.

FIGURE 3.2
**Elements of
a Hospital
Medication
Order**

Patient identification
(name, identification number)

Room number
or bed location

Name and dose
of medication

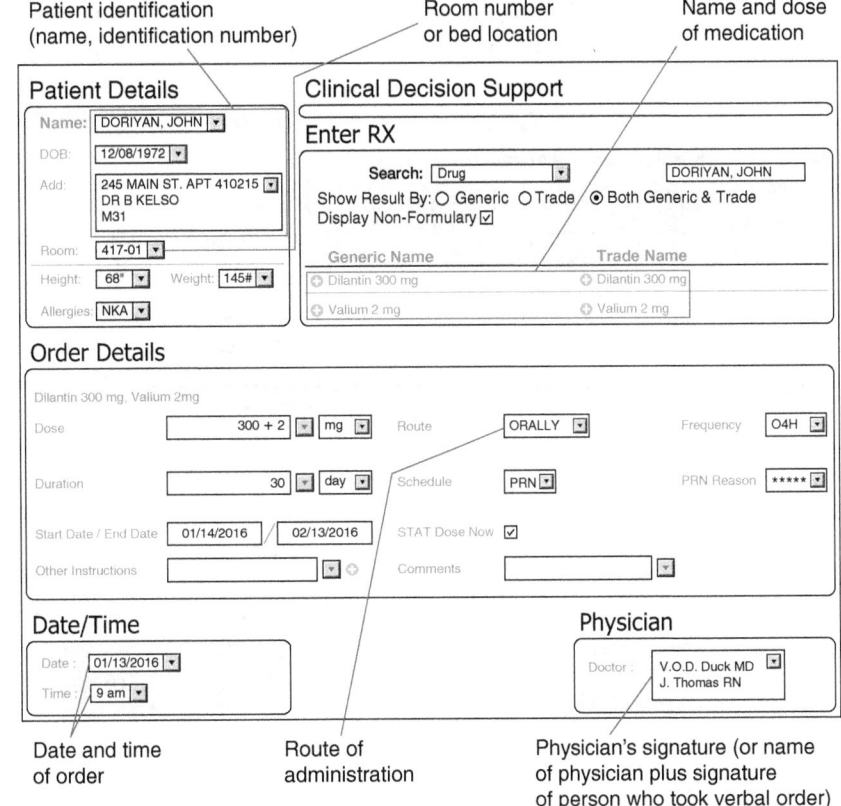

Patient Details

Name: DORIYAN, JOHN

DOB: 12/08/1972

Add: 245 MAIN ST. APT 410215
DR B KELSO
M31

Room: 417-01

Height: 68" Weight: 145#

Allergies: NKA

Clinical Decision Support

Enter RX

Search: Drug   DORIYAN, JOHN

Show Result By: ○ Generic ○ Trade ◉ Both Generic & Trade
Display Non-Formulary ☑

Generic Name	Trade Name
Dilantin 300 mg	Dilantin 300 mg
Valium 2 mg	Valium 2 mg

Order Details

Dilantin 300 mg, Valium 2mg

Dose: 300 + 2 mg   Route: ORALLY   Frequency: O4H

Duration: 30 day   Schedule: PRN   PRN Reason: *****

Start Date / End Date: 01/14/2016 / 02/13/2016   STAT Dose Now ☑

Other Instructions: Comments:

Date/Time

Date: 01/13/2016

Time: 9 am

Physician

Doctor: V.O.D. Duck MD
J. Thomas RN

Date and time
of order

Route of
administration

Physician's signature (or name
of physician plus signature
of person who took verbal order)

The first two letters of the DEA number provide information about the prescriber. The first letter usually (but not always) designates the level of authority of the holder. For example, A, B, and F are used for primary-level practitioners such as physicians and dentists, and M is used to indicate mid-level practitioners such as nurse practitioners, nurse midwives, nurse anesthetists, clinical nurse specialists, and physician assistants. The second letter in the DEA number is the first letter of the prescriber's last name. Therefore, the first two letters of the DEA number for Dr. Mary Smith might be AS, BS, or FS, whereas the first two letters for nurse practitioner David Jones might be MJ.

DEA numbers are carefully regulated, and a DEA number that does not have a correct check digit (as determined by the steps in Table 3.1) is invalid. The check digit gives pharmacists and pharmacy technicians one way to check whether a DEA number was falsified. Note that passing the check test does not necessarily mean that a DEA number is valid. Many unethical or criminally minded people know the formula and are able to compose DEA numbers that *appear* to be valid but were not issued by the DEA. If a pharmacy technician discovers an invalid DEA number or suspects a problem with the authenticity of a prescription, he or she should notify a pharmacist immediately.

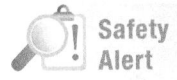

Safety Alert

The check digit calculation is necessary, but it is not sufficient for verifying the validity of a DEA number.

TABLE 3.1 DEA Check Digit Formula

Step 1. Add the first, third, and fifth digits of the DEA number.

Step 2. Add the second, fourth, and sixth digits of the DEA number.

Step 3. Double the sum obtained in Step 2 (i.e., multiply it by 2).

Step 4. Add the results of Steps 1 and 3. The last digit of this sum should match the check digit, the last digit of the DEA number.

The following examples demonstrate how the steps in Table 3.1 can be used to check for false DEA numbers.

Example 3.1.1

 A patient brings a prescription for methylphenidate tablets to the pharmacy, signed by Dr. Johnson and bearing a DEA number of BJ 2345678. Could this be a valid DEA number?

Begin by reviewing the letters of the DEA number. The first letter is consistent with the prescriber's level of authority (A, B, or F for a primary practitioner), and the second letter matches the last name of the physician (J).

Now, check the validity of the check digit.

Step 1. Add the first, third, and fifth digits of the DEA number.

$$2 + 4 + 6 = 12$$

Step 2. Add the second, fourth, and sixth digits of the DEA number.

$$3 + 5 + 7 = 15$$

Step 3. Multiply the sum obtained in Step 2 by 2.

$$15 \times 2 = 30$$

Step 4. Add the results of Steps 1 and 3. The last digit of this sum should match the check digit, the last digit of the DEA number.

$$12 + 30 = 42$$

Because the check digit is 8, not 2, this DEA number is invalid.

Example 3

 A patient brings a prescription for oxycodone to the pharmacy, signed by nurse-midwife Ann Johnson and bearing a DEA number of MJ 3456781. (In the state where the prescription is received, advanced practice nurses are authorized to prescribe narcotic analgesics.) Could this be a valid DEA number?

Begin by reviewing the letters of the DEA number. The first letter is consistent with the prescriber's level of authority (M for a nurse practitioner), and the second letter matches the last name of the prescriber (J).

Now, check the validity of the check digit.

Step 1. Add the first, third, and fifth digits of the DEA number.

$$3 + 5 + 7 = 15$$

Step 2. Add the second, fourth, and sixth digits of the DEA number.

$$4 + 6 + 8 = 18$$

Step 3. Multiply the sum obtained in Step 2 by 2.

$$18 \times 2 = 36$$

Step 4. Add the results of Steps 1 and 3. The last digit of this sum should match the check digit, the last digit of the DEA number.

$$15 + 36 = 51$$

Because the check digit is 1, this DEA number meets the criteria for a valid registration.

Inpatient prescriptions are most often ordered on the premises where the patient is located and where the medication will be administered. Such prescriptions may be ordered only by practitioners with privileges within that institution. Physician addresses and DEA numbers are generally not required on the actual medication orders because the institutional pharmacy that will fill the orders usually has this information on file for each authorized practitioner.

Drug Designation

A prescription order must always designate the medication that is intended for the patient. Medications may have three names: a chemical name, a generic name, and a brand name. These various names are referred to as *nomenclature*. Sometimes, the drug will be identified by its **generic name**, the name by which it was approved by the Food and Drug Administration (FDA) as a unique chemical product safe and effective for use in its approved indication or use. The generic name of a drug is the same, regardless of the company that manufactures it or the dosage form or packaging in which it is supplied. Other times, a physician will specify a brand name. The **brand name** is a registered trademark of the manufacturer and may indicate the dose form or packaging of the drug as well. State law and (in the case of inpatients) institutional policy

Put Down Roots

The word *nomenclature*—a term used in pharmacy to indicate naming guidelines for medications—has its beginnings in the Roman Empire. The word means the "calling or assigning of names" and comes from the Latin roots *nomen* meaning "name" and *calare* meaning "to call out."

☑ TAKE NOTE

Patients may be curious about the difference between generic and brand name drugs. As a pharmacy technician, it is important that you understand how generic and brand name drugs are similar and how they are different. Generic drugs are required to have the same active ingredient(s), strength, dosage form, and route of administration as brand name drugs. Generic drug manufacturers must also prove that their drug works equivalently to the brand name product. However, the inactive ingredients do not have to be the same between products. A small amount of variability may be present, which is permitted and monitored by the Food and Drug Administration.

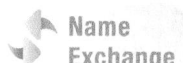
govern the extent to which generic products can be substituted for brand name drugs. In some instances, the pharmacy can automatically substitute an equivalent product with the same generic name (but a different brand name) for cost savings or convenience. In other situations, the pharmacy must supply the exact brand prescribed, unless the pharmacist has discussed a substitution with the prescriber.

Figure 3.3 identifies the standard parts of a drug label for Cleocin Phosphate. As shown in this example, the label of a brand name drug will indicate both the brand and generic names. Medications with a given name (brand or generic) are frequently available in a variety of strengths, doses, or dosage forms, and information about the particular strength, dose, and dosage form is clearly stated on the drug label. Digoxin, for instance, is available as a generic product and as several branded preparations. It is available as a tablet in two different strengths (0.125 mg and 0.25 mg), an oral solution of 0.05 mg/mL, and injections of 0.1 mg/mL and 0.25 mg/mL. Many other drugs present a similar array of choices (brand names, dosage forms, strengths, or concentrations), and the proper product to select must be clear in the prescription order. Figure 3.4 shows labels for the same drug in different dosage forms. Note how the labels use color to help distinguish the unique information.

FIGURE 3.3
Parts of a Drug Label

Although medication labels from different manufacturers vary slightly in format, the labels' components remain the same. Pharmacy technicians must be able to identify and interpret all parts of a drug label.

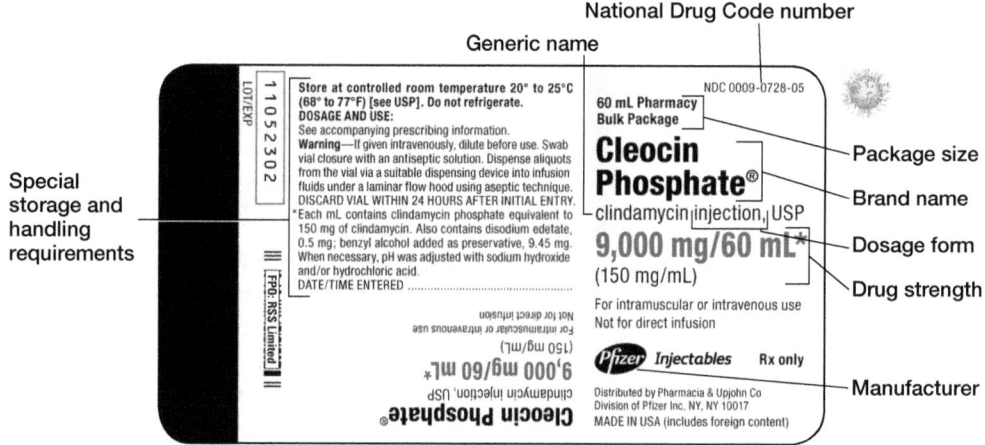

FIGURE 3.4
Comparison of Dosage Forms

(a) 20 mg tablet
(b) 40 mg tablet
(c) 40 mg/4 mL solution

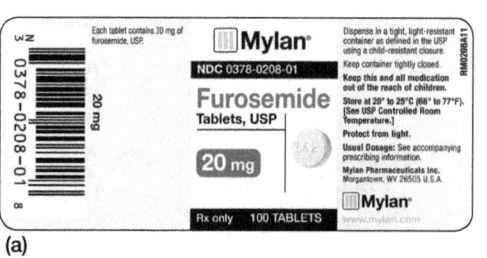

(a)

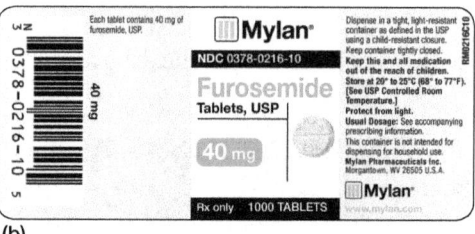

(b)

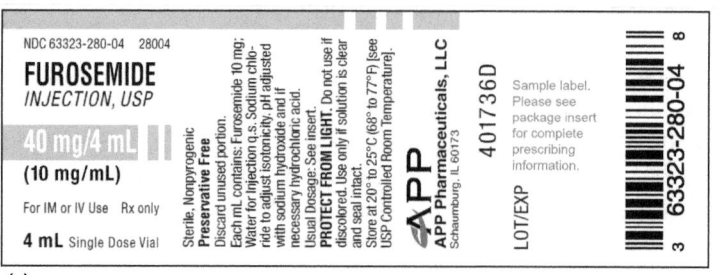

(c)

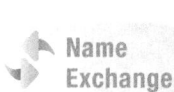

It is important to correctly match a prescription order with the appropriate medication available in the pharmacy. The following example demonstrates this procedure.

Example 3.1.3

The pharmacy receives an order for epinephrine 1 mg/mL. The computer system lists epinephrine 1:10,000, 1:2,000, and 1:1,000 injections are available in stock. Which one matches the order?

As discussed in Chapter 2, ratios can be written as fractions. The available drug concentrations are 1:10,000, or 1 g/10,000 mL; 1:2,000, or 1 g/2,000 mL; and 1:1,000, or 1 g/1,000 mL.

Convert the strength of 1 mg/mL into a concentration ratio of g/mL. Use the conversion factor 1,000 mg = 1 g or 1 mg = 1/1,000 g (because both sides of the equation were divided by 1,000).

$$\frac{1 \text{ mg}}{1 \text{ mL}} \text{ is the concentration of epinephrine ordered.}$$

From above, we know that 1 mg = 1/1,000 g. Substitute this into the concentration ratio.

$$\frac{1 \text{ mg}}{1 \text{ mL}} = \frac{\frac{1}{1,000} \text{ g}}{1 \text{ mL}} = \frac{1 \text{ g}}{1,000 \text{ mL}}$$

1 g/1,000 mL is equivalent to 1:1,000. Therefore, the 1:1,000 injection matches the order. The label appears below.

You can also use dimensional analysis to solve this problem.

$$\frac{1 \text{ mg}}{\text{mL}} \times \frac{1 \text{ g}}{1,000 \text{ mg}} = \frac{1 \text{ g}}{1,000 \text{ mL}}$$

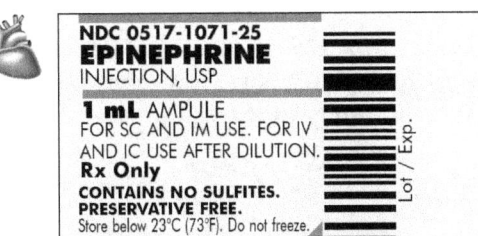

NDC 0517-1071-25
EPINEPHRINE
INJECTION, USP
1 mL AMPULE
FOR SC AND IM USE. FOR IV
AND IC USE AFTER DILUTION.
Rx Only
CONTAINS NO SULFITES.
PRESERVATIVE FREE.
Store below 23°C (73°F). Do not freeze.
AMERICAN REGENT, INC.
SHIRLEY, NY 11967 Rev. 5/05
Lot / Exp.

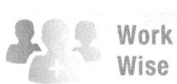

Work Wise

While calculating quantity dispensed may seem tedious, it is important when dispensing medication. If you miscalculate, a patient may receive too much or too little of a medication, and both scenarios may be harmful.

Quantity to Dispense

Every outpatient prescription order must indicate to the pharmacist what quantity to dispense. Sometimes, the indication is straightforward, as in Figure 3.1, where the physician has written the number of tablets to dispense next to "#" (used as a number symbol). This number is often written as a Roman numeral or spelled out ("thirty" for #30) to make it more difficult to alter the number to obtain a greater number of tablets. Other times, the physician will indicate the number of doses the patient is to take or the number of days the therapy is to last, and the pharmacy staff will calculate the quantity to dispense from the information on the prescription.

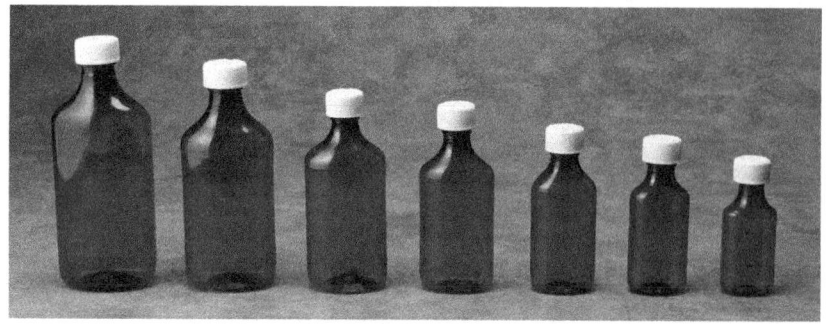

When the quantity to dispense has been determined, the pharmacy technician selects the proper dispensing container. Commonly, amber bottles (ovals) are used for liquids and amber vials for tablets or capsules. Amber bottles are often marked with both fluid ounce and milliliter lines. Common practice uses the metric system, so the quantity indicated on the prescription drug label will usually be indicated in milliliters. When preparing tablets or capsules to fill a prescription, the tablets or capsules are generally counted out by fives, using a specially designed tray and plastic or metal spatula, and placed in amber vials.

Amber medication bottles come in many sizes. The pharmacy technician must select the appropriate size to match the dispensed volume.

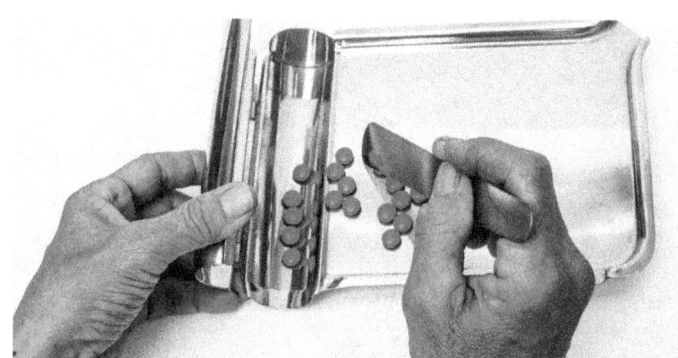

Tablets are frequently counted out by fives on a tray with a spatula and then placed in the dispensing container.

The following examples show how to calculate the quantity to dispense.

Example 3.1.4

 A prescription for amoxicillin 125 mg chewable tablets twice daily is written for a patient in your pharmacy. How many chewable tablets should be dispensed for a 10-day supply?

$$\frac{1 \text{ tablet}}{\text{dose}} \times \frac{2 \text{ doses}}{\text{day}} \times \frac{10 \text{ days}}{1} = 20 \text{ tablets}$$

Therefore 20 tablets should be dispensed for a 10-day supply.

Example 3.1.5

A prescription for an antacid reads, "Take one ounce three times a day," and instructs the pharmacy to dispense a five-day supply. What volume is to be dispensed?

The patient takes one ounce three times a day. First determine the number of ounces taken in one day. Note that the units cancel out, as shown below.

$$\frac{x \text{ oz}}{1 \text{ day}} = \frac{1 \text{ oz}}{1 \text{ dose}} \times \frac{3 \text{ doses}}{1 \text{ day}} = \frac{3 \text{ oz}}{1 \text{ day}}$$

You can determine the amount to dispense by multiplying the daily dose by the number of days.

$$x \text{ oz} = \frac{3 \text{ oz}}{1 \text{ day}} \times 5 \text{ days} = 15 \text{ oz}$$

This can also be calculated in one step.

$$\frac{1 \text{ oz}}{\text{day}} \times \frac{3 \text{ doses}}{\text{day}} \times \frac{5 \text{ days}}{1} = 15 \text{ oz}$$

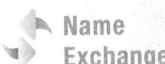

Name Exchange

Dificid is a brand name medication for the generic drug fidaxomicin. Both names appear on a medication label.

Example 3.1.6

A prescription for Dificid reads, "Take 200 mg every 12 hours," and instructs the pharmacy to dispense a one-week supply. The pharmacy has the following product in stock. How many tablets are dispensed?

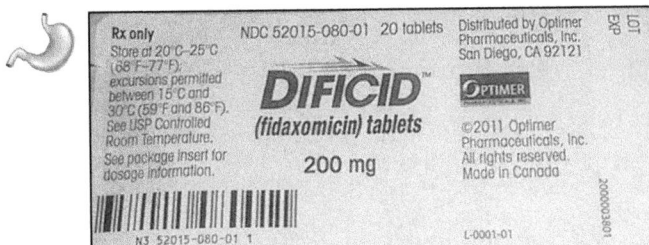

Because 1 tablet contains 200 mg, the patient will take 1 tablet every 12 hours, and there are 24 hours in a day. You can determine the number of tablets the patient will need in a single 24-hour period (a day) by setting up a ratio.

$$\frac{1 \text{ tablet}}{12 \text{ hours}} \times \frac{24 \text{ hours}}{1 \text{ day}} \times \frac{7 \text{ days}}{1} = 14 \text{ tablets}$$

Therefore 14 tablets are needed for a 7-day supply.

Calculating Days' Supply

As each prescription is received in the pharmacy, personnel scan the prescription for completeness and validity, interpret the order, and then enter the information into the computer system. The electronic information becomes a part of the patient's permanent health record. Some information that must be entered into the computer is not always written on the prescription but must be calculated by the pharmacy technician or pharmacist. The pharmacist must verify the accuracy of the calculations and the data that is entered into the computer. Any calculation that the technician performs that requires written work should be available to the pharmacist when he or she verifies the accuracy of the prescription entry and calculations.

Whether prescriptions are written for a specified number of doses or a specified duration of time, the technician needs to calculate the **days' supply** (the number of days that a prescription or medication order will last a patient when taken as directed by the prescriber). A prescription that is written for a specified number of doses such as #30 and with a dosing schedule of TID (three times daily) will last 10 days. Another prescription may be written for a patient to use a medication TID for 10 days, and the physician has indicated the quantity as QS (a sufficient quantity). You would calculate that the patient needs 30 doses to complete the therapy prescribed by the physician.

The most common information that requires a calculation is verifying that the days' supply and the quantity dispensed will meet the needs of the patient according to what the prescriber has indicated.

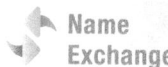

Example 3.1.7

Calculate the days' supply for the following prescription.

 Ibuprofen 800 mg

Take one tablet by mouth two times daily with food

Dispense 60 tablets

$$\frac{x \text{ days}}{60 \text{ tablets}} = \frac{1 \text{ day}}{2 \text{ tablets}}$$

Recall the means-extreme proportion property to cross multiply and solve for x (see Chapter 2 for more details).

$$x \text{ days} (2 \text{ tablets}) = 1 \text{ day} (60 \text{ tablets})$$

$$x \text{ days} = 30 \text{ days}$$

You can check your answer by ensuring that the product of the means equals the product of the extremes (detailed in Chapter 2).

You can also use dimensional analysis to solve this problem.

$$\frac{60 \text{ tablets}}{1} \times \frac{1 \text{ day}}{2 \text{ tablets}} = 30 \text{ days}$$

Example 3.1.8

Calculate the days' supply for the following prescription.

 Acetaminophen 120 mg/codeine 12 mg per 5 mL elixir

Take 15 mL by mouth three times daily

Dispense 270 mL

Since the patient takes the medication three times daily, multiply 15 mL by 3. The patient takes 45 mL each day.

$$\frac{x \text{ days}}{270 \text{ mL}} = \frac{1 \text{ day}}{45 \text{ mL}}$$

$$x \text{ days} (45 \text{ mL}) = 1 \text{ day} (270 \text{ mL})$$

$$x \text{ days} = 6 \text{ days}$$

Therefore the prescription is for a 6 days' supply.

You can also use dimensional analysis to solve this problem.

$$\frac{270 \text{ mL}}{1} \times \frac{1 \text{ day}}{45 \text{ mL}} = 6 \text{ days}$$

3.1 Problem Set

Which of the following DEA numbers meet the standard validity test? Justify your answer.

1. DEA number JC 2169870 for Dr. James Cardillo

2. DEA number MG 3081659 for nurse-midwife Laura Gonzales

3. DEA number BH 9998070 for Dr. Blanche McKennon

4. DEA number AL 6230618 for Dr. George Lewis

5. DEA number AD 7638224 for Dr. Anita Chan

6. DEA number BN 4412209 for Dr. Srisha Narayana

7. DEA number AK 3051492 for Dr. Satoru Kudaishi

8. DEA number MS 2864228 for clinical nurse specialist Katherine Schultz

Choose a drug product to fill the following orders.

9. acetic acid 1:400 irrigation

   a. glacial acetic acid
   b. 0.25% acetic acid
   c. 25% acetic acid
   d. 4% acetic acid

10. isoproterenol 5 mg/mL solution
    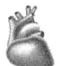
    a. isoproterenol 5% solution
    b. isoproterenol 0.05% solution
    c. isoproterenol 1:200 solution
    d. isoproterenol 1:2 solution

Identify the information indicated for each drug label.

11. Brand name: _____

    Generic name: _____

    Dosage form: _____

    Strength: _____

    Total quantity: _____

    Storage requirement(s): _____

    Manufacturer: _____

    NDC number: _____

NDC 52427-285-01   Rx Only

100 mg

Macrobid®
(nitrofurantoin monohydrate/ macrocrystals)

URINARY TRACT ANTIBACTERIAL
100 Capsules

Almatica ⚕ Pharma

Store at controlled room temperature (59° to 86°F or 15° to 30°C).
THIS IS A BULK CONTAINER AND NOT INTENDED FOR DISPENSING.
Dispense in a tight container.
DOSAGE: Adults: One 100-mg capsule every 12 hours with food. See package outsert for full prescribing information.

Mfg. by:
Norwich Pharmaceuticals, Inc.
Norwich, NY 13815 USA
Dist. by:
Almatica Pharma, Inc.
Pine Brook, NJ 07058 USA
Rev 03/12 285-01-04   PKG01455

12. Brand name: _____

    Generic name: _____

    Dosage form: _____

    Strength: _____

    Total quantity: _____

    Storage requirement(s): _____

    Manufacturer: _____

    NDC number: _____

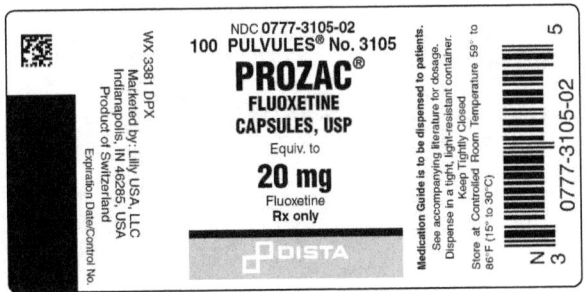

13.　Brand name: _____

　　　Generic name: _____

　　　Dosage form: _____

　　　Strength: _____

　　　Total quantity: _____

　　　Storage requirement(s): _____

　　　Manufacturer: _____

　　　NDC number: _____

15.　Brand name: _____

　　　Generic name: _____

　　　Dosage form: _____

　　　Strength: _____

　　　Total quantity: _____

　　　Storage requirement(s): _____

　　　Manufacturer: _____

　　　NDC number: _____

30 Capsules　NDC 0002-3238-30
PU 3238

strattera®
atomoxetine HCl

Rx only

18 mg

Each capsule equivalent
to 18 mg atomoxetine

Do not use if Lilly inner seal
is missing or broken.

www.strattera.com　Lilly

Store at 25°C (77°F); excursions permitted to 15° to 30°C (59° to 86°F) [see USP Controlled Room Temperature].

Eli Lilly and Company
Indianapolis, IN 46285, USA
Product of Ireland

Expiration Date/Control No.

WW 8715 AMX

Medication Guide is to be dispensed to patients.
Keep tightly closed.
Keep out of the reach of children.
See accompanying literature for dosage information.

0002-3238-30

Store below 86°F (30°C).
Dispense in tight, light-resistant containers (USP).
TARTRAZINE DYE FREE.

DOSAGE AND USE
Adults: 25 mg t.i.d. to 100 mg q.i.d.
Children: Under 6 years— 50 mg daily in divided doses. Over 6 years– 50 to 100 mg daily in divided doses. See accompanying prescribing information.
*Each capsule contains hydroxyzine pamoate equivalent to 50 mg hydroxyzine hydrochloride.

Rx only

NDC 0069-5420-66

100 Capsules

Vistaril®　50
(hydroxyzine pamoate)

50 mg*

Distributed by
Pfizer　Pfizer Labs
Division of Pfizer Inc, NY, NY 10017

4375
MADE IN USA

FPO UPC: 80% x 5.5 mm
0069-5420-66

05-2186-32-9

LOT
&
EXP
AREA

14.　Brand name: _____

　　　Generic name: _____

　　　Dosage form: _____

　　　Strength: _____

　　　Total quantity: _____

　　　Storage requirement(s): _____

　　　Manufacturer: _____

　　　NDC number: _____

16.　Brand name: _____

　　　Generic name: _____

　　　Dosage form: _____

　　　Strength: _____

　　　Total quantity: _____

　　　Storage requirement(s): _____

　　　Manufacturer: _____

　　　NDC number: _____

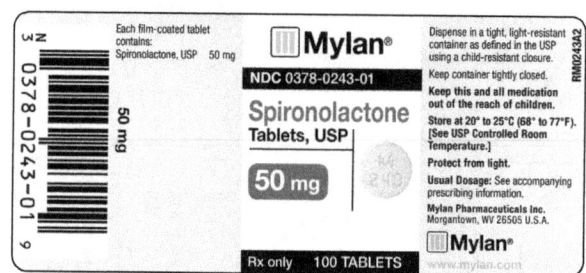

Each film-coated tablet contains:
Spironolactone, USP　50 mg

Mylan®

NDC 0378-0243-01

Spironolactone
Tablets, USP

50 mg

Dispense in a tight, light-resistant container as defined in the USP using a child-resistant closure.
Keep container tightly closed.
Keep this and all medication out of the reach of children.
Store at 20° to 25°C (68° to 77°F). [See USP Controlled Room Temperature.]
Protect from light.
Usual Dosage: See accompanying prescribing information.
Mylan Pharmaceuticals Inc.
Morgantown, WV 26505 U.S.A.

Mylan®

Rx only　100 TABLETS
www.mylan.com

0378-0243-01

50 mg

NDC 0406-9915-01　100 Capsules

Restoril™　C IV
(temazepam)
Capsules USP
7.5 mg　Rx only

Each capsule contains:
Temazepam USP........7.5 mg
PHARMACIST: PLEASE DISPENSE WITH
MEDICATION GUIDE PROVIDED WITH PRODUCT
Mallinckrodt

USUAL ADULT DOSAGE:
See package insert.
STORAGE: Store at 20° to 25°C (68° to 77°F) [see USP Controlled Room Temperature].
Dispense in a well-closed, light-resistant container with a child-resistant closure.
Do not accept if seal over bottle opening is broken or missing.
Mallinckrodt Inc.
Hazelwood, MO 63042 USA

COVIDIEN™

Lot No.:

Exp.:

Applications

How much medication should be dispensed for the following prescriptions?

17.

℞ Ibuprofen 400 mg tablet #XX

Take one tablet by mouth four times daily with food.

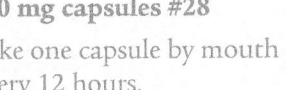

18.

℞ Amoxicillin capsule 500 mg

Take one capsule three times daily for 10 days.

19.

℞ Prednisone 5 mg tablet

Take four tablets twice daily for two days,
then three tablets twice daily for two days,
then four tablets once daily for two days,
then three tablets once daily for two days,
then two tablets once daily for two days,
then one tablet once daily for two days.

20.

℞ Milk of Magnesia

Take one ounce every night at bedtime for one week.

21.

℞ Phenytoin 100 mg capsule #CL

Take three capsules every morning.

What is the days' supply for each of these prescriptions?

22.

℞ Cephalexin 500 mg capsules #28

Take one capsule by mouth every 12 hours.

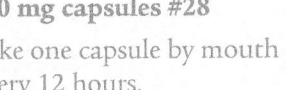

23.

℞ Bactrim DS Tablets #90

Take one tablet by mouth each morning.

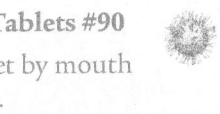

24.

℞ Norpace Capsules 100 mg #120

Take one capsule by mouth every 6 hours.

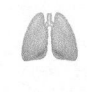

25.

℞ Advair HFA 45/21

Dispense one inhaler with 120 doses.
Use inhaler two times daily.

Self-check your work in Appendix A.

3.2 Prescription Directions

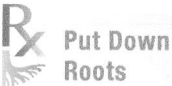

Rx Put Down Roots

The word *signa* comes from the Latin word *signāre*, meaning "to write, mark, or label." The signa, or sig, refers to the prescriber's instructions for the proper use of a medication.

A very important part of each prescription is the **signa (sig)**, a term that comes from the Latin word for "to write." It consists of the prescriber's instructions for proper use of the medication and usually includes the following information:

- **Dose:** how much medication the patient will take at each administration. It is generally expressed as a number of units (e.g., tablets, capsules), an amount of drug (e.g., weight in milligrams or grains), or a volume of medication (e.g., ounces, teaspoonfuls).

- **Route of administration:** how the drug is to be administered. Routes of administration include oral (by mouth), injection (into veins, into muscles, under the skin), rectal, or topical (to the eye, ear, skin, or mucous membranes), among others.

- **Dosing schedule:** how often the drug is to be taken and, in some cases, how long therapy is to be continued.

Work Wise

If you are not familiar with a medical abbreviation ask for clarification: an abbreviation mistake can have serious consequences. There are also many resources available that you can consult. Medical dictionaries often have an abbreviations index. An online source is Stedman's Online (http://stedmansonline.com/reference).

Abbreviations

Healthcare professionals have developed their own shorthand for many aspects of patient care, and it is reflected in the abbreviations used in prescription directions. Many of the abbreviations used in prescriptions are derived from the initials of Latin or Greek words or phrases. Others come from medical terminology in English, and some even combine terms from multiple languages. Table 3.2 on the following page lists some of the most common abbreviations used in prescriptions. Appendix B provides a more complete listing of abbreviations.

When abbreviations are standardized (to have only one meaning) and are clearly written, they are useful because they save space and time. Abbreviations can cause serious problems, however, if they are misinterpreted. Sometimes confusion occurs when the same set of letters can have two different meanings. For example, "IVP" means "IV Push" or "administer by injection into the vein from a syringe" when used on a hospital medication order for an intravenous (IV) medication. In another context, however, "IVP" designates "intravenous pyelogram," an X-ray examination of the urinary tract.

Abbreviations are also problematic when they are not written clearly. The abbreviation "q6 pm," for example, means "every evening at 6 p.m.," but if written hastily or printed using a fax machine low in toner, it may appear to say "q6 h," meaning every six hours. The abbreviation "qhs" means "nightly at bedtime" but could be misread as "qhr," meaning "every hour." Some abbreviations are so error-prone that the Joint Commission—an independent organization that evaluates and accredits practices in hospital systems—has declared that they are absolutely unacceptable for use in accredited institutions. To that end, the Joint Commission has published the Official "Do Not Use" List containing abbreviations that may lead to confusion among healthcare personnel and, consequently, may result in medication errors. This list can be found at http://PharmCalc6e.ParadigmEducation.com/JointCommission. Another organization, the Institute for Safe Medication Practices (ISMP), has published an extensive list of dangerous abbreviations and symbols to avoid in the healthcare setting. This document, called the ISMP's Error-Prone Abbreviations, Symbols, and Dose Designations, can be found at http://PharmCalc6e.ParadigmEducation.com/ISMP.

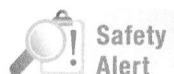

Safety Alert

Pharmacy personnel must exercise care when interpreting abbreviations on prescriptions.

You should commit the common abbreviations to memory because they are a part of the pharmacy technician's everyday language. The easiest ones to start with are the ones that indicate how many times per day a patient should take a medication: BID (twice daily), TID (three times daily), and QID (four times daily). The abbreviations are sometimes written in lowercase letters and sometimes written in uppercase letters. The letter "q" means "every" and is sometimes placed in front of other abbreviations.

TABLE 3.2 Common Prescription Abbreviations

Abbreviation	Translation	Abbreviation	Translation
ac	before meals	mL	milliliter
AD	right ear	NKA	no known allergy
AS	left ear	NKDA	no known drug allergy
AU	both ears	npo	nothing by mouth
am	morning	OD	right eye
bid	twice daily	OS	left eye
c̄	with	OU	both eyes
cap	capsule	pc	after meals
DAW	dispense as written	po	by mouth
D/C	discontinue	prn	as needed
g	gram	q	every
gr	grain	qh	every hour
gtt	drop	q2 h	every 2 hours
h or hr	hour	qid	four times a day
hs	bedtime	qs	a sufficient quantity
IM	intramuscular	stat	immediately
IV	intravenous	tab	tablet
L	liter	tid	three times daily
mcg	microgram	ud	as directed
mEq	milliequivalent	wk	week

Note: Some prescribers may write abbreviations using capital letters or periods. However, periods should not be used with metric units or medical abbreviations as they can be a source of medication errors.

Safety Alert

Instructions to patients on dispensed medications must be clear and should not include abbreviations.

Directions for Patients

Because most patients are not familiar with the abbreviations and shorthand used on prescriptions, directions must be "translated" from the sig and written on the label placed on the dispensing packaging so that the patient can understand the directions. Sometimes, descriptive terms are added if appropriate. For example, a prescription for a fentanyl transdermal patch may have the sig "ī q 3d." The pharmacy label on the patient's package, however, must read, "Apply one patch every 72 hours." Similarly, a prescription for hydrochlorothiazide 25 mg tablets may bear a sig of "12.5 mg po qam," but the patient's label must read, "Take one-half tablet by mouth every morning." It is important that directions for patients be set forth in clear and unambiguous terms on the label, even if the doctor and the pharmacist explain verbally in great detail how the medication is to be used. It is easy for patients to misunderstand or forget what they were told days or weeks earlier, and having the label available for instructions at every dose is necessary for safe medication use.

Even with appropriate prescription instruction translation, patients may still require additional assistance. For example, when patients are receiving liquid medicines, doses are often given in mLs. Most patients are not familiar with measuring volumes in mLs. Special dosing devices – such as syringes, spoons, and cups – are often used to help patients.

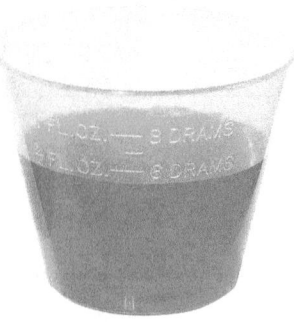

One fluid ounce is the size of most plastic dispensing cups.

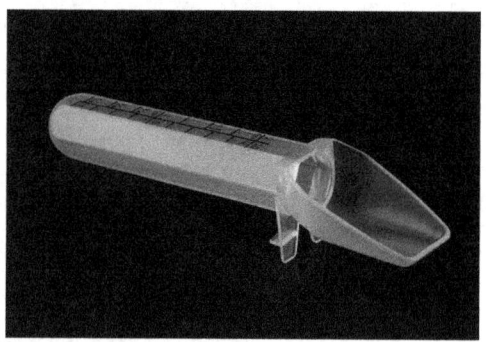

Dosing spoons are a way to accurately measure liquid medicines.

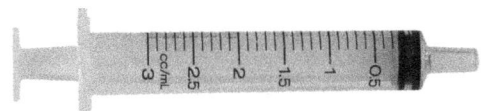

Oral dosing syringes are used for liquid medicines that are ingested by mouth. These syringes should not be confused for syringes for parenteral use.

3.2 Problem Set

Write out the meanings of these common abbreviations used in prescriptions.

1. bid

2. DAW

3. IM

4. IV

5. mL

6. NKA

7. npo

8. q3 h

9. qid

10. tid

Answer the following questions.

11. What is a route of administration?

12. Name four routes of administration.

13. Give one abbreviation for a route of administration and write out its meaning.

14. Give one abbreviation for a dosing schedule and write out its meaning.

15. Explain the difference between an IM administration and an IV administration of a medication.

Applications

Translate the following directions from a prescription order into wording that would be appropriate on a label for the patient's use.

16.

℞ **Diphenhydramine capsules**
ii cap po four times daily prn itching
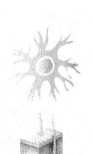

17.

℞ **Nitroglycerin Transdermal Systems**
ī on qhs off qam

18.

℞ **Nitroglycerin ointment**
½ in q6 h

19.

℞ **Nateglinide 60 mg tablets**
120 mg po tid ac

20.

℞ **Potassium Chloride 20 mEq tablets**
10 mEq po bid
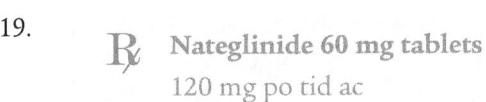

21.

℞ **Tobramycin eyedrops**
ii gtt q4 h OD

22.

℞ **Alendronate tablets**
i po q wk 30 minutes ac breakfast c̄ H_2O
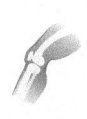

Determine the days' supply and quantity to dispense for the following prescriptions:

23.

℞ **Dyazide capsules**
Take one capsule each morning for 6 weeks.
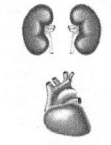

24.

℞ **Amoxicillin 500 mg capsules**
Take one capsule tid for 10 days and then one daily until gone.
Dispense #40.

25.

℞ **Promethazine 25 mg**
Take one tablet three times daily.
Dispense #63.
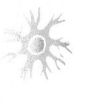

Self-check your work in Appendix A.

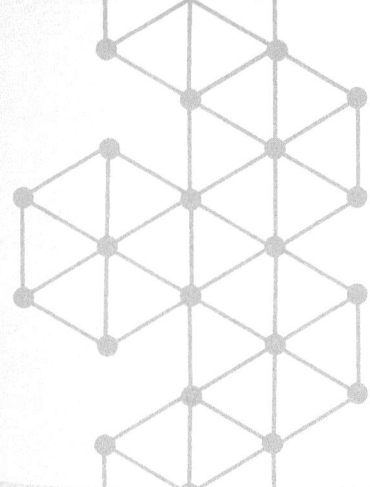

- Prescriptions can arrive at the pharmacy in many forms: electronically, handwritten, typed, faxed, or via telephone or voice mail.

- Prescriptions must be checked for validity before being filled.

- Patient information should be complete on the prescription to meet safety, legal, and insurance requirements.

- DEA numbers can be checked for validity by using a formula and performing a calculation.

- Drugs are identified on prescriptions using a brand and/or generic name.

- Drug labels contain standard information, including:

  — generic name of the drug (and brand name, when there is one)

  — strength per unit

  — dosage form

  — quantity enclosed

  — manufacturer

  — special handling or storage requirements

  — National Drug Code (NDC)

- Some drug labels will display the strength per unit in several different manners.

- Quantity to dispense may need to be calculated if the prescriber does not indicate the amount to be dispensed on the prescription.

- Days' supply should be calculated to meet the need of the patient according to the duration of therapy indicated by the physician.

- Days' supply must be entered into the patient's record and submitted to insurance for every prescription.

- Prescriptions are written using shorthand that consists mainly of abbreviations derived from the initials of Latin or Greek phrases.

- Prescription instructions for the patient are called the signa (or sig).

- Route of administration for medications should always be specified on the prescription or medication order.

- "Do Not Use" abbreviations should be avoided.

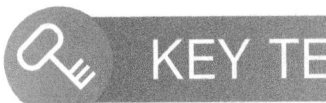

KEY TERMS

brand name the name under which the manufacturer markets a drug; a registered trademark of the manufacturer; also known as the *trade name*

check digit the last digit of a DEA number that is used to check validity

days' supply the number of days that a prescription or medication order will last a patient when taken as directed by the prescriber

DEA number a number issued by the Drug Enforcement Administration (DEA) to signify the authority of the holder to prescribe or handle controlled substances; made up of two letters followed by seven digits, the last of which is a check digit used to check the validity of the DEA number

dose on a prescription, the indication of how much medication the patient will take at each administration

dosing schedule on a prescription, the indication of how often the drug is to be taken

generic name the name under which a drug is approved by the Food and Drug Administration; sometimes denotes a drug that is not protected by a trademark; also referred to as a *USAN (United States Adopted Name)*

prescription an order for medication for a patient that is written by a physician or a qualified licensed practitioner to be filled by a pharmacist or technician

route of administration on a prescription, the indication of how the medication is to be given

signa (sig) the part of the prescription that provides instructions for proper use of the medication, including the dose, route of administration, and dosing schedule

Finding Solutions

To gain practice in handling challenging situations in the workplace, consider the following real-world scenarios, and then use the guiding questions to help you formulate your responses.

Note: *To indicate your answers for Scenario C, Questions 9 and 10, ask your instructor for the handout depicting a dosing spoon and oral syringe and the handout depicting a dosing spoon and medicine cup.*

Scenario A: A prescription for a large quantity of narcotic pain medication has come into the pharmacy. Although the order is written on a hospital prescription blank, you are suspicious that the prescription may not be valid. The written directive is oddly worded, and the dose is not what is typically associated with the medication prescribed. A DEA number is hand-written at the bottom of the prescription.

1. Perform a check on the DEA number: AB 4423921. Is it valid?

2. The sig indicates that the patient should take 3 tabs q.i.d. or prn. What does this mean?

3. The drug name written is "Norco Hydrocodone APAP." What part of the drug name indicates the brand name, and what part indicates the generic name?

Scenario B: An older adult patient with significant vision loss has asked you to write out instructions for his medication in very large print so that he can read them more easily. Write out the instructions (sig) for the following medications:

4. Lasix 20 mg; take 1 tab PO QDay in AM for edema

5. ranitidine 150 mg; take 1 tab PO BID for stomach

6. acyclovir 800 mg; take 1 tab PO four times daily for 5 days for shingles
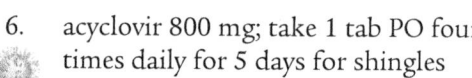

7. verapamil 80 mg; take 1 tab PO TID for angina
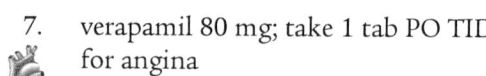

8. diazepam 2 mg; take 1 tab PO HS for sleep
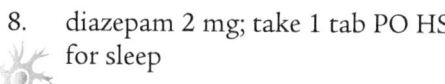

Scenario C: Mrs. Zapata has three children with chicken pox, and the pediatrician's office has advised her to purchase OTC Benadryl for itching. Her oldest child can take capsules, but the two younger ones need liquid.
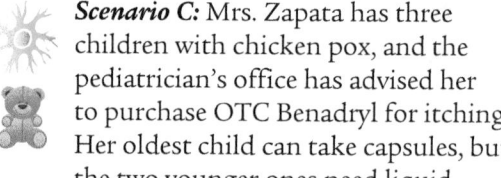

9. On the handout that you obtained from your instructor, select the most accurate measuring device (either the dosing spoon or the oral syringe) to administer a ½ tsp dose to a child. Fill in the correct volume on the measuring device.

10. On the handout that you obtained from your instructor, select the most accurate measuring device (either the dosing spoon or the medicine cup) to administer a 2 tsp dose to a child. Fill in the correct volume on the measuring device.

Scenario D:

℞ **MT. HOPE MEDICAL PARK**
ST. PAUL, MN (651) 555-3591

DOB _____ DEA# __AY 3456781__

Pt. name _Nany Romez___ Date _10-09-201X_

Address _315 Main Street_

Synthroid 100 mcg   # thirty (30)

Take one (1) tablet by mouth every morning.

_____M. Yang_____ ___ Dispense as written
Dr.
_____ ___ Substitution permitted
Dr.

Refills _five_____

___015247_____ ___ License #

Mrs. Romez brings this prescription to the pharmacy.

11. Perform a checksum on the DEA number. Is it valid?

12. How would you abbreviate the signa?

13. What is the days' supply for this prescription?

14. If Mrs. Romez wanted a 90-day supply of this medication, how many tablets would need to be dispensed?

15. Mrs. Romez tells you she weighs 164 lbs. How many kilograms is this?

Scenario E: Use the following prescription to answer the next two questions.

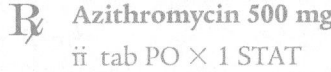 ℞ **Azithromycin 500 mg**
ii tab PO × 1 STAT

16. Translate the directions from the prescription into wording that would be appropriate on a patient label.

17. If the instructions included "ac" how would that change your translation?

Navigator ✚

Access interactive chapter review exercises, practice activities, flash cards, and study games.

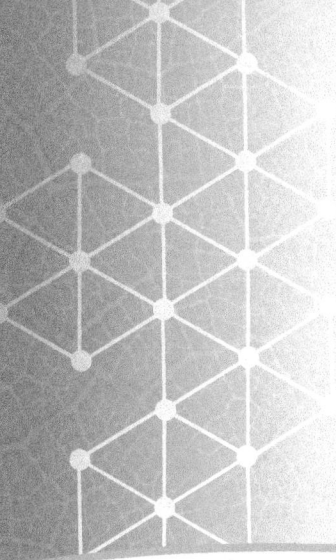

4 Applying Metric Measurements and Calculating Doses

Learning Objectives

1 Identify the basic units and prefixes of the metric system.

2 Convert units within the metric system by moving the decimal point, using the ratio-proportion method, and using the dimensional analysis method.

3 Calculate drug doses using the ratio-proportion and dimensional analysis methods.

4 Calculate doses based on weight and body surface area.

5 Calculate a pediatric dose using the patient's weight or age and the appropriate adult dose.

Preview chapter terms and definitions.

4.1 Basic Metric Units

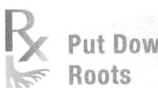
Put Down Roots

Three units of measure in the metric system have their roots in the Greek language. The word *meter* is from the Greek term *metron*, meaning "measure"; the word *gram* is from the Greek term *gramma*, meaning "small weight"; and the word *liter* is from the Greek term *litra*, meaning "pound."

Chapter 1 presented a brief overview of the decimal number system. Because of its accuracy, the decimal system is used in pharmacy measurements. Based on subdivisions and multiples of 10, the **metric system** uses decimals to indicate tenths, hundredths, and thousandths.

Identifying Metric Units of Measure

The metric system's three basic units of measure are the meter, the gram, and the liter (see Table 4.1). The **meter**, the unit for measuring length, has limited use in the pharmacy. A patient's height is often measured in feet and inches but could be measured in meters or centimeters. One meter is approximately three feet (approximately 39.37 inches). The **gram**, the unit for measuring weight (mass), is used in the pharmacy for measuring the amount of medication in solid form and for indicating the amount of solid medication in a solution. One gram is the weight of one cubic centimeter of water at 4 °C. The **liter** is the unit used for measuring the volume of liquid medications and liquids for solutions. One liter equals 1,000 milliliters, and one milliliter equals the volume in one cubic centimeter.

TABLE 4.1 Metric Units of Measure

Metric Unit	Measurement
meter (m)	length
gram (g)	weight (mass)*
liter (L)	volume

* Mass is a measurement of how much matter is in an object; weight is a measurement of how hard gravity is pulling on that object. Your mass is the same no matter where you are (Earth, the moon, another planet), but your weight differs based on where you are. To prevent confusion, we will use gram as the unit of measurement for weight.

Using Metric Prefixes and Abbreviations

The set of prefixes shown in Table 4.2 is used to designate multiples of the basic metric units. The three prefixes most widely used in pharmaceutical calculations are kilo-, milli-, and micro-. The abbreviations shown in Table 4.3 are commonly used for metric measurements.

Metric units are commonly used in pharmacy practice. Therefore, it is important to memorize the basic metric units along with their prefixes. All units in the metric system use the same prefixes. An example is the gram: the larger unit is the kilogram, whereas two of the smaller units are the milligram and microgram.

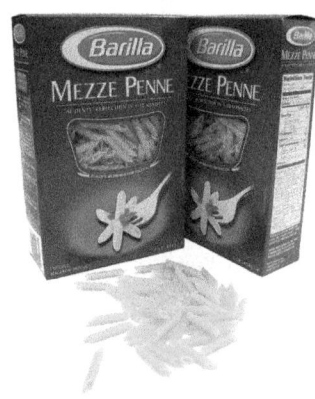

One kilogram is equivalent to a little more than two 1-lb boxes of pasta.

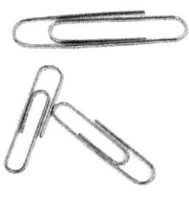

A single large paper clip, or two small paper clips, weighs about 1 g.

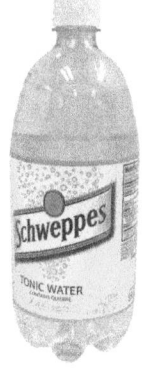

Remembering the amount of liquid that is contained in a standard, 1-L bottle will help you visualize the amount of liquid in 1 liter.

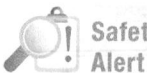
Safety Alert

Pharmacy technicians should use the medication labels, not the color or shape of the pills, to confirm the amount of drug contained in a tablet or capsule.

Most people can visualize an object that weighs a kilogram or a gram, and many can create a mental picture of a container that can hold a liter or a milliliter of a liquid. However, it is harder to see something that weighs only a microgram. Medications that contain micrograms, or even milligrams, of an active ingredient will almost always contain an inactive filler so that the dosage form becomes measurable. For example, a tablet with a weight of 300 micrograms would be hard to see and too small to handle. The tablets shown in Figure 4.1 contain different amounts of levothyroxine, but they are all the same size. Even though levothyroxine is available in a variety of doses, the tablet sizes remain the same. The colors of the tablets and the package labeling differentiate the amount of active ingredient.

TABLE 4.2 Metric System Prefixes

Prefix	Value
nano (n)	$\frac{1}{1,000,000,000}$ (one-billionth of the basic unit, or 0.000000001 or 10^{-9})
micro (mc)	$\frac{1}{1,000,000}$ (one-millionth of the basic unit, or 0.000001 or 10^{-6})
milli (m)	$\frac{1}{1,000}$ (one-thousandth of the basic unit, or 0.001 or 10^{-3})
centi (c)	$\frac{1}{100}$ (one-hundredth of the basic unit, or 0.01 or 10^{-2})
deci (d)	$\frac{1}{10}$ (one-tenth of the basic unit, or 0.1 or 10^{-1})
kilo (k)	1,000 (one thousand times the basic unit or 10^{3})

TABLE 4.3 Metric Abbreviations

Measurement	Metric Unit	Abbreviation
Weight	kilogram	kg
	gram	g
	milligram	mg
	microgram	mcg
Volume	kiloliter	kL
	liter	L
	milliliter	mL*
	microliter	mcL
Length	kilometer	km
	meter	m
	millimeter	mm
	micrometer	mcm†

* equivalent to cc, which stands for cubic centimeters, but cc is considered a dangerous abbreviation because it can be mistaken for "u"

† sometimes abbreviated as μm, but μm is considered a dangerous abbreviation because it can be mistaken for mg

FIGURE 4.1 Levothyroxine

       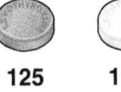 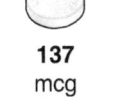 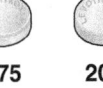

| **25** mcg orange | **50** mcg white | **75** mcg violet | **88** mcg olive | **100** mcg yellow | **112** mcg rose | **125** mcg brown | **137** mcg turquoise | **150** mcg blue | **175** mcg lilac | **200** mcg pink | **300** mcg green |

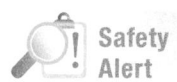 **Safety Alert**

For a decimal value less than 1, use a leading zero to prevent errors.

Writing Parts of a Unit

Parts of a unit are written as a decimal number. For example, two and one-half milligrams is written as 2.5 mg. A leading zero is used if there is no whole number preceding the decimal point. For example, one-half liter is written as 0.5 L, and one-quarter gram is written as 0.25 g. These leading zeros help prevent medication errors.

When writing dosage strengths, unnecessary zeros after the decimal point are generally left off to reduce the chance of misreading the value. For example, 0.25 mL, 5 L, and 15.6 mL should not be written as 0.250 mL, 5.0 L, and 15.60 mL.

4.1 Problem Set

State the abbreviation for each of the following metric units.

1. microgram

2. milligram

3. liter

4. gram

5. kilogram

6. meter

7. centimeter

8. milliliter

9. cubic centimeter

10. deciliter

Write the following numbers using an Arabic number with a decimal value and the appropriate abbreviation.

11. six-tenths of a gram

12. fifty kilograms

13. four-tenths of a milligram

14. four-hundredths of a liter

15. four and two-tenths of a gram

16. five-thousandths of a gram

17. six-hundredths of a gram

18. two and six-tenths liters

19. three-hundredths of a liter

20. two-hundredths of a milliliter

Applications

21. The Taro Pharmaceutical Company has donated a container labeled 5 kg of bulk Genocillin granules. The standard dose is 375 mg. How many single dose units can be obtained from the container?

22. The pharmacy receives the following prescription.

> ℞ **Metformin tablets**
> **500 mg**
> ii q am
> i with lunch
> ii 8 pm
> 30 days' supply

a. How many tablets will be dispensed?

b. How many milligrams will the patient take over the course of one month (30 days)?

23. If the total daily dose of a drug is 0.9 g and it is given tid, what is the amount of each dose in grams?

24. A patient is to receive 1.2 g of cimetidine per day in four divided doses.

    a. How many grams will be in each dose?

    b. If the available dosage forms are shown in the following labels, which will be chosen?

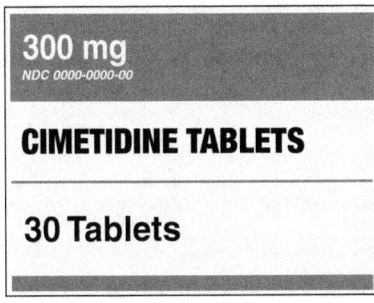

300 mg
NDC 0000-0000-00

CIMETIDINE TABLETS

30 Tablets

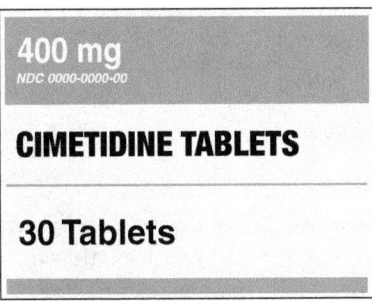

400 mg
NDC 0000-0000-00

CIMETIDINE TABLETS

30 Tablets

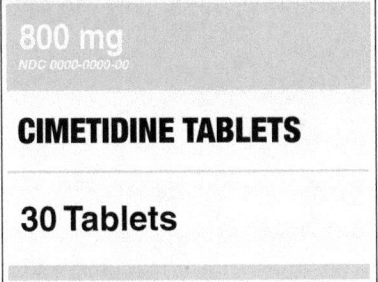

800 mg
NDC 0000-0000-00

CIMETIDINE TABLETS

30 Tablets

25. The following prescription for potassium permanganate has been brought into the compounding pharmacy.

 Potassium permanganate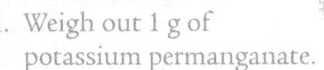

1. Weigh out 1 g of potassium permanganate.
2. Add to a 1-L bottle of sterile water for irrigation. (Be sure to wear gloves, as this chemical stains.)
3. Replace cap on bottle and swirl to dissolve potassium permanganate.

The solution expires 30 days after mixing.

a. What is the percentage of potassium permanganate in this solution?

b. If today is August 1, 2017, what expiration date will you place on the bottle?

Self-check your work in Appendix A.

4.2 Conversions within the Metric System

In this section, you will learn three ways to convert units within the metric system: moving the decimal point, using the ratio-proportion method, and using the dimensional analysis method. Once you learn the three methods of conversion, select the method you are most comfortable with and use only that method when making conversions. Before calculating a needed dose, you should be confident that the number you are working with is accurate and that the correct conversion has been made.

Moving the Decimal Point

To change the metric units of a number to smaller or larger units, you can multiply or divide by an appropriate multiple of 1,000. (See Table 4.4.) For instance, to convert 5 g to milligrams, multiply 5 by 1,000 to get 5,000 mg. One way to multiply by 1,000 is to move the decimal point three places to the right. Multiplying 17 L by 1,000,000 yields 17,000,000 mcL. (Move the decimal point six places to the right.) Conversely, changing to a larger unit requires division. Therefore, to convert 25 m to kilometers, divide by 1,000 to get 0.025 km. One way to divide by 1,000 is to move the decimal point three places to the left. Similarly, 3 mcL divided by 1,000 yields 0.003 mL, and 22 mL divided by 1,000 yields 0.022 L. In each case, move the decimal point three places to the left.

TABLE 4.4 Metric Unit Equivalents

Kilo	Base	Milli	Micro
0.001 kg	1 g	1,000 mg	1,000,000 mcg
0.001 kL	1 L	1,000 mL	1,000,000 mcL
0.001 km	1 m	1,000 mm	1,000,000 mcm

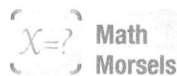 **Math Morsels**

Moving the decimal point three spaces to the right is the same as multiplying by 1,000. Moving the decimal point three places to the left is the same as dividing by 1,000.

The key to understanding the relationships of "kilo," "base," "milli," and "micro" in the metric system is to remember that the decimal point must be moved three places when converting from one unit to the next. Moving the decimal point three places is a quick way to multiply or divide the number by 1,000. The three places are representative of the three zeros in 1,000.

$$1 \text{ kg} = 1,000 \text{ g}$$
$$1 \text{ g} = 1,000 \text{ mg}$$
$$1 \text{ mg} = 1,000 \text{ mcg}$$
$$1 \text{ L} = 1,000 \text{ mL}$$

When converting from a smaller to a larger unit of measure, move the decimal point three places to the left.

$$4,500 \text{ mL} = 4.500 \text{ L}$$
$$1,287 \text{ mg} = 1.287 \text{ g}$$
$$480 \text{ mL} = 0.480 \text{ L}$$

When converting from a larger to a smaller unit of measure, move the decimal point three places to the right.

$$0.954 \text{ g} = 954 \text{ mg}$$
$$1.5 \text{ g} = 1500 \text{ mg}$$
$$0.238 \text{ g} = 238 \text{ mg}$$
$$0.621 \text{ mg} = 621 \text{ mcg}$$

At first, it may be difficult to conceptualize conversions from smaller to larger units. It can be helpful to think about this in terms of more familiar units. Suppose you have $1,000,000 all in one dollar bills (a smaller unit). In other words, you have 1,000,000 one dollar bills. Say you wanted larger units and exchanged your dollar bills for $100 bills. You would then have 10,000 one hundred dollar bills (move the decimal point two places to the left). Now say you exchange all your $100 bills for $1,000 dollar bills (assume that one thousand dollar bills are still printed). You would have 1,000 one thousand dollar bills (move the decimal point one place to the left). In the end, you have the same amount of total dollars ($1,000,000), but you changed the units from smaller (one dollar bills) to larger (one hundred and then one thousand dollar bills).

For Good Measure

When setting up proportions, units in the numerators must match, and units in the denominators must match.

Using the Ratio-Proportion Method

If you have difficulty remembering which way to move the decimal point when converting between units of measure in the metric system, the ratio-proportion method introduced in Chapter 2 is an effective alternative. This method is a foolproof way to convert metric units. Set up the conversion by placing the unknown and the value to be converted on one side of the equation and the conversion factor (the ratio of the desired unit to the given unit) on the other side.

When setting up proportions to solve for an unknown, remember that the units in the numerators must match and the units in the denominators must match. Checking to make sure the units match before completing the calculation will ensure accuracy in the conversion. The next examples demonstrate conversions by moving the decimal point, followed by the same conversions using the ratio-proportion method.

Safety Alert

Always remember to check your answer by multiplying the two means and the two extremes in the ratio. The products of the means and extremes must be equal.

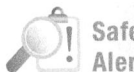

Example 4.2.1

Convert 2,300 mg to grams.

Moving the decimal point:

One method is to divide by 1,000 by moving the decimal point three places to the left.

$$2{,}300 \text{ mg} = 2.\underset{\sim}{300} \text{ g} = 2.3 \text{ g}$$

Using the ratio-proportion method:

$$\frac{x \text{ g}}{2{,}300 \text{ mg}} = \frac{1 \text{ g}}{1{,}000 \text{ mg}}$$

$$x \text{ g} \,(1{,}000 \text{ mg}) = 1\text{g} \,(2{,}300 \text{ mg})$$

$$\frac{x \text{ g} \,(\cancel{1{,}000 \text{ mg}})}{\cancel{1{,}000 \text{ mg}}} = \frac{1 \text{ g} \,(2{,}300 \,\cancel{\text{mg}})}{1{,}000 \,\cancel{\text{mg}}}$$

$$x = 2.3 \text{ g}$$

You can check your answer by verifying that the product of the means equals the product of the extremes (see Chapter 2 for more details).

Example 4.2.2

Convert 3.2 mg to micrograms.

Moving the decimal point:

You can multiply by 1,000 by moving the decimal point three places to the right.

$$3.2 \text{ mg} = 3200 \text{ mcg} = 3,200 \text{ mcg}$$

Using the ratio-proportion method:

$$\frac{x \text{ mcg}}{3.2 \text{ mg}} = \frac{1,000 \text{ mcg}}{1 \text{ mg}}$$

$$x \text{ mcg } (1 \text{ mg}) = 1,000 \text{ mcg } (3.2 \text{ mg})$$

$$x = 3,200 \text{ mcg}$$

Example 4.2.3

Convert 3.785 L to milliliters.

Moving the decimal point:

Multiply by 1,000 by moving the decimal point three places to the right.

$$3.785 \text{ L} = 3785 \text{ mL} = 3,785 \text{ mL}$$

Using the ratio-proportion method:

$$\frac{x \text{ mL}}{3.785 \text{ L}} = \frac{1,000 \text{ mL}}{1 \text{ L}}$$

$$x \text{ mL } (1 \text{ L}) = 1,000 \text{ mL}(3.785 \text{ L})$$

$$x = 3,785 \text{ mL}$$

Example 4.2.4

Convert 454 g to kilograms.

Moving the decimal point:

Divide by 1,000 by moving the decimal point three places to the left.

$$454 \text{ g} = 0.454 \text{ kg} = 0.454 \text{ kg}$$

Using the ratio-proportion method:

$$\frac{x \text{ kg}}{454 \text{ g}} = \frac{1 \text{ kg}}{1,000 \text{ g}}$$

$$x \text{ kg } (1,000 \text{ g}) = 1 \text{ kg } (454 \text{ g})$$

$$x = 0.454 \text{ kg}$$

Using the Dimensional Analysis Method

The **dimensional analysis method** (also known as the factor-label method or unit factor method) is a problem-solving method that uses the fact that any number or expression can be multiplied by one without changing its value. In this method, the given number and unit are multiplied by the ratio of the desired unit to the given unit. The unit in the denominator will match the given unit, so the units will cancel each other out, and the unit remaining in the numerator will be the unit to which you are converting. Chapter 1 includes a more thorough explanation of the mathematics and rationale behind the dimensional analysis method, as well as examples of converting seconds, minutes, and hours.

Example 4.2.5

Convert **486 mg to grams.**

$$486 \text{ mg} \times \frac{1 \text{ g}}{1,000 \text{ mg}} = 0.486 \text{ g}$$

Example 4.2.6

Convert **4.5 L to milliliters.**

$$4.5 \text{ L} \times \frac{1,000 \text{ mL}}{1 \text{ L}} = 4,500 \text{ mL}$$

Example 4.2.7

Convert **240 mL to liters.**

$$240 \text{ mL} \times \frac{1 \text{ L}}{1,000 \text{ mL}} = 0.24 \text{ L}$$

Example 4.2.8

Convert **0.725 mg to micrograms.**

$$0.725 \text{ mg} \times \frac{1,000 \text{ mcg}}{1 \text{ mg}} = 725 \text{ mcg}$$

Example 4.2.9

Convert **0.519 g to micrograms.**

This conversion requires two steps. The first step is to convert grams to milligrams, and the second step is to convert milligrams to micrograms.

$$0.519 \text{ g} \times \frac{1,000 \text{ mg}}{1 \text{ g}} \times \frac{1,000 \text{ mcg}}{1 \text{ mg}} = 519,000 \text{ mcg}$$

4.2 Problem Set

Convert the following units within the metric system by using the ratio-proportion method. Retain all significant figures and do not round the answers.

1. 1,964 mcg = _____ mg

2. 418 mg = _____ g

3. 651 mg = _____ mcg

4. 0.84 mg = _____ mcg

5. 0.012 g = _____ mcg

6. 9,213,406 mcg = _____ g

7. 284 mg = _____ g

8. 9,382.5 mcg = _____ mg

9. 12,321 mcg = _____ g

10. 184 g = _____ kg

Convert the following units within the metric system by using the dimensional analysis method. Retain all significant figures and do not round the answers.

11. 52 mL = _____ L

12. 2.06 g = _____ mg

13. 16 mg = _____ mcg

14. 256 mg = _____ g

15. 2,703,000 mcg = _____ g

16. 6.9 L = _____ mL

17. 62.5 mg = _____ g

18. 15 kg = _____ g

19. 2,785,000 mcg = _____ g

20. 8.234 mg = _____ mcg

Convert the following units by moving the decimal point, or by using the method that you prefer. Show all work. Retain all significant figures and do not round the answers.

21. 2 kg = _____ mg

22. 21 L = _____ mL

23. 576 mL = _____ L

24. 823 kg = _____ mg

25. 27 mcg = _____ mg

26. 5,000 mcg = _____ mg

27. 20 mcg = _____ mg

28. 4.624 mg = _____ mcg

29. 3.19 g = _____ mg

30. 8,736 mcg = _____ mg

31. 830 mL = _____ L

32. 0.94 L = _____ mL

33. 1.84 g = _____ mg

34. 560 mg = _____ g

35. 1,200 mcg = _____ mg

36. 125 mcg = _____ mg

37. 0.275 mg = _____ mcg

38. 480 mL = _____ L

39. 239 mg = _____ g

40. 1,500 mg = _____ g

41. The following prescription has come into the pharmacy.

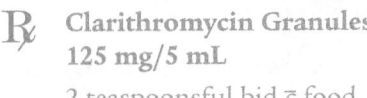

℞ **Clarithromycin Granules**
    125 mg/5 mL

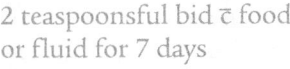

2 teaspoonsful bid c̄ food
or fluid for 7 days

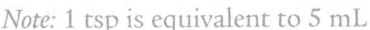

Note: 1 tsp is equivalent to 5 mL

a. How many milliliters will the patient take daily?

b. How many milliliters should be dispensed for the patient?

c. How many grams will the patient take daily?

d. Using the following drug label, how many bottles of clarithromycin will be needed to fill this prescription?

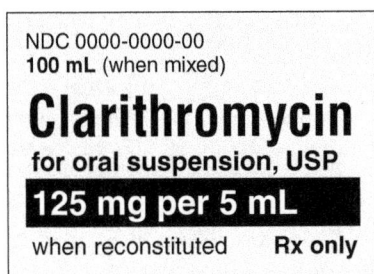

NDC 0000-0000-00
100 mL (when mixed)

Clarithromycin
for oral suspension, USP

125 mg per 5 mL

when reconstituted   **Rx only**

42. A patient is to take 1.5 g of amoxicillin before a dental procedure. The capsules available are shown in the following label. How many capsules will be dispensed to this patient?

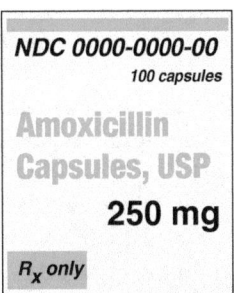

NDC 0000-0000-00

100 capsules

Amoxicillin Capsules, USP

250 mg

R_x only

43. A patient is to receive 1,000 mg of vancomycin two times daily, diluted in IV solution. The following label shows the stock available.

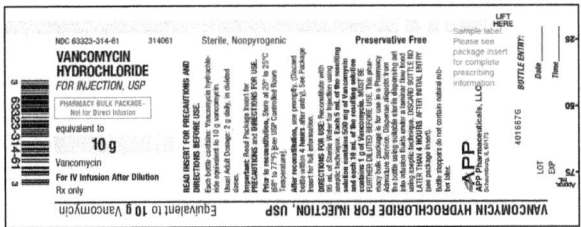

a. How many doses are available in one vial?

b. How many days will one unopened vial last?

Self-check your work in Appendix A.

4.3 Problem Solving in the Pharmacy

Many pharmacy calculations require problem solving. Real life situations in the pharmacy are similar to mathematical story problems, or problems presented as text, usually in a scenario. When faced with a story problem or other problem in which the calculation needed is not absolutely clear, it is important to begin by asking the question, "What am I looking for?" In dose calculations, this is usually a weight, expressed in milligrams, or a volume, expressed in milliliters.

Using the Ratio-Proportion Method to Solve Story Problems

In Chapter 2, you learned some basic calculations using the ratio-proportion method and applied that method to converting between units of measure in the metric system. Now you will use ratios and proportions mathematically to compare a readily available product, consisting of an active ingredient and a **vehicle**, to a desired (prescribed) dosage. A vehicle is an inert (chemically inactive) medium, such as syrup, in which a medication is administered. Like the available product, the desired dosage will consist of an active ingredient and a vehicle.

$$\frac{\text{active ingredient (desired)}}{\text{vehicle (desired)}} = \frac{\text{active ingredient (on hand)}}{\text{vehicle (on hand)}}$$

Keep in mind that the ratios on the two sides of the equation may be inverted (that is, the vehicle may be in the numerator and the active ingredient may be in the denominator). However, the same units must appear in both numerators, and the same units must appear in both denominators.

You can use the steps outlined in Table 4.5 as a basis for solving story problems or dose calculations using the ratio-proportion method. Usually, you can use the following equation to solve a story problem.

$$\frac{\text{desired amount of medication}}{\text{prescriber's order}} = \text{ratio of pharmacy stock}$$

TABLE 4.5 Steps for Using the Ratio-Proportion Method for Solving Story Problems

Step 1. Read through the entire problem and identify what the question is asking for. This unknown amount becomes the variable x, labeled with the unit you are looking for such as x mg or x mL.

Step 2. Identify the prescriber's order. Circle the dose ordered by the physician.

Step 3. Identify the appropriate stock available in the pharmacy. The ratio of pharmacy stock, such as 1 mg/tablet or 125 mg/5 mL, should be found on the labels of the drugs used in the pharmacy. Underline this information.

Step 4. Identify extraneous information. It is often helpful to draw a single line through any information you identify as not needed. This prevents you from using that information in your setup. Use a pencil in case you need that information again.

Step 5. Estimate what your answer should be. Compare the ordered dose to what is on hand. Will the dose be larger or smaller than the dosage unit given?

Step 6. Use the ratio-proportion method to solve for x. When using the ratio-proportion method to solve the problem, place the prescriber-ordered dosage on the left side of the proportion and the pharmacy on-hand ratio on the right side.

Step 7. Round your answer appropriately. Weights are typically rounded to the nearest whole milligram, and volumes are typically rounded to the nearest tenth of a milliliter.

Example 4.3.1

A physician has ordered 370 mg of a medication, and you have a 10-mL vial of solution containing 250 mg/3 mL on hand. How many milliliters will you measure out?

Step 1. Identify the question being asked. You need to find the number of milliliters, so x mL is the unknown.

Step 2. Identify the prescribed amount and circle it. In this problem, the physician has ordered 370 mg.

Step 3. Identify the product available in the pharmacy and underline it. In this problem, the pharmacy has 250 mg/3 mL of the medication.

Step 4. Identify extraneous information and draw a line through it. In this problem, it is not important to know that the medication comes in a 10-mL vial.

Step 5. Estimate the answer. The ordered dose of 370 mg is greater than the dosage strength of 250 mg, so the dose volume should be greater than 3 mL.

Step 6. Use the ratio-proportion method to solve for x mL.

$$\frac{x \text{ mL}}{370 \text{ mg}} = \frac{3 \text{ mL}}{250 \text{ mg}}$$

$$x \text{ mL} = 4.44 \text{ mL}$$

Step 7. Because this is a liquid, and volumes are typically rounded to the nearest tenth of a milliliter, round to 4.4 mL.

Example 4.3.2

A physician has ordered 100 mg of amoxicillin to be given to a child 3 times a day for 10 days. Amoxicillin is available in a 150-mL bottle with a dose strength of 125 mg/5 mL. How many milliliters will the child need at each dose?

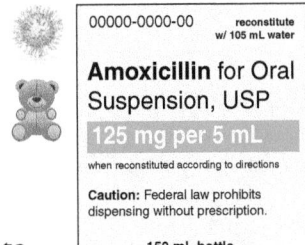

00000-0000-00   reconstitute
                     w/ 105 mL water

Amoxicillin for Oral
Suspension, USP

125 mg per 5 mL

when reconstituted according to directions

Caution: Federal law prohibits
dispensing without prescription.

150 mL bottle

Step 1. Identify the question being asked. You need to find the number of milliliters, so x mL is the unknown.

Step 2. Identify the prescribed amount and circle it. In this problem, the physician has ordered 100 mg at each dose.

Step 3. Identify the product available in the pharmacy and underline it. In this problem, the pharmacy has 125 mg/5 mL of amoxicillin.

Step 4. Identify extraneous information and draw a line through it. In this problem, it is not important to know "three times a day for 10 days" and that the size of the amoxicillin bottle is 150 mL.

Step 5. Estimate the answer. The ordered dose of 100 mg is less than the dose strength of 125 mg, so the dose volume should be less than 5 mL.

Step 6. Use the ratio-proportion method to solve for x mL:

$$\frac{\text{desired amount of medication}}{\text{prescriber's order}} = \text{ratio of pharmacy stock}$$

$$\frac{x \text{ mL}}{100 \text{ mg}} = \frac{5 \text{ mL}}{125 \text{ mg}}$$

$$\text{mL} = 4 \text{ mL}$$

Step 7. No rounding is needed because the answer for this liquid measure does not extend beyond a tenth of a milliliter.

Some medications are ordered by a certain volume rather than by milligrams or or other units of weight. For example, a cough syrup may be ordered as 10 mL every 4 hours, and it may be necessary to calculate how much of the active ingredient is in this dose. The steps presented in Table 4.5 can also be used to solve this type of problem. In this case, however, the unknown will be the amount of the active ingredient instead of the overall volume.

Example 4.3.3

A physician has ordered 10 mL of amoxicillin to be given to a child three times daily for seven days. Amoxicillin is available in a 150-mL bottle with a dosage strength of 250 mg/5 mL. How many milligrams will the child get at each dose?

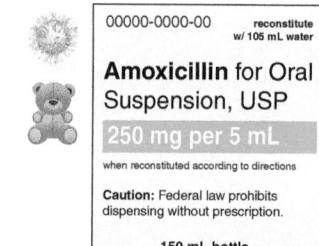

Step 1. The unknown is x mg.

Step 2. The prescribed amount is 10 mL of amoxicillin.

Step 3. The pharmacy has 250 mg/5 mL of amoxicillin.

Step 4. The extraneous information includes "three times daily for 7 days" and that the size of the amoxicillin bottle is 150 mL.

Step 5. The answer will be greater than 250 mg because 10 mL is greater than 5 mL.

Step 6. Use the ratio-proportion method to solve for x mg.

$$\frac{x\ \text{mg}}{10\ \text{mL}} = \frac{250\ \text{mg}}{5\ \text{mL}}$$

$$x\ \text{mg} = 500\ \text{mg}$$

Step 7. No rounding is needed because the answer for this weight does not have a decimal point and the significant figures are correct.

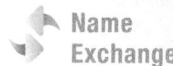 **Name Exchange**

Cefaclor is a generic drug name and is marketed under several brand names, including Ceclor. Cefaclor is a cephalosporin antibiotic used to treat bacterial infections.

Example 4.3.4

A physician has ordered cefaclor 375 mg/5 mL oral suspension. A 100-mL bottle is prepared and is labeled to administer 7.5 mL twice daily for five days. How many milligrams is the patient receiving at each dose?

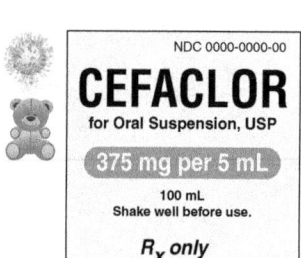

Step 1. The unknown is x mg.

Step 2. The prescribed amount is 7.5 mL suspension.

Step 3. Once the suspension is prepared, it contains 375 mg cefaclor/5 mL of suspension.

Step 4. The extraneous information includes "twice daily for five days" and that the size of the cefaclor bottle is 100 mL.

Step 5. The answer will be greater than 375 mg because 7.5 mL is greater than 5 mL.

Step 6. Use the ratio-proportion method to solve for *x* mg.

$$\frac{x \text{ mg}}{7.5 \text{ mL}} = \frac{375 \text{ mg}}{5 \text{ mL}}$$

$$x \text{ mg} = 562.5 \text{ mg}$$

Step 7. The answer of 562.5 mg is rounded to the nearest whole milligram, or 563 mg.

Using Dimensional Analysis to Calculate a Medication Dose

Just as you used the dimensional analysis method to convert metric units earlier in this chapter, you can now use it to solve medication dose problems by "converting" a dose from milligrams to tablets, or from milligrams to milliliters. You accomplish this by multiplying the dose ordered by the ratio for the on-hand product. As in the metric conversions practiced earlier in the chapter, you set up the ratio so that the units of the given dose and the units in the denominator cancel out. When using the dimensional analysis method to solve drug dosage problems, you can still use the steps in Table 4.5 to analyze the information. The only difference is in the setup in Step 6.

The dimensional analysis method tends to be used most frequently for simple dosage calculations such as the number of tablets. For example, if a doctor has prescribed 100 mg of a medication, and you have that medication on hand in 50 mg tablets, you can quickly determine that the patient will need two 50 mg tablets for the prescribed 100 mg dose. Although you may be able to do the calculations in the following exercises mentally, it is important to work through the steps to be sure you understand each step in the calculation.

Example 4.3.5

A physician has ordered a 25 mg dose of hydrochlorothiazide. You have a 100-count bottle of 50 mg tablets. What will you prepare to fill the order?

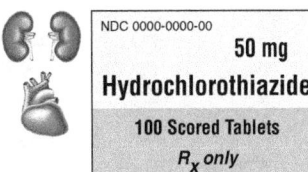

NDC 0000-0000-00
50 mg
Hydrochlorothiazide
100 Scored Tablets
R$_x$ only

Step 1. The unknown is x tablets.

Step 2. The prescribed amount is 25 mg.

Step 3. The pharmacy has 50 mg tablets.

Step 4. The extraneous information includes "100-count bottle."

Step 5. The answer will be less than 1 tablet, as the requested dose is less than the number of milligrams in 1 tablet.

Step 6. Use the dimensional analysis method to convert the units.

$$25 \text{ mg} \times \frac{1 \text{ tablet}}{50 \text{ mg}} = 0.5 \text{ tablet}$$

Step 7. No rounding is required.

Example 4.3.6

A physician has ordered a 750 mg dose of amoxicillin. You have 150 mL of a 250 mg/5 mL suspension. What will you prepare to fill the order?

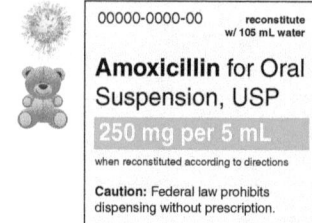

00000-0000-00   reconstitute w/ 105 mL water

Amoxicillin for Oral Suspension, USP

250 mg per 5 mL

when reconstituted according to directions

Caution: Federal law prohibits dispensing without prescription.

150 mL bottle

Step 1. The unknown is x mL.

Step 2. The prescribed amount is 750 mg of amoxicillin.

Step 3. The pharmacy has 250 mg/5 mL.

Step 4. The extraneous information includes "150 mL suspension."

Step 5. The answer will be approximately three times as large as the unit given.

Step 6. Use dimensional analysis to convert the units.

$$750 \;\cancel{mg} \times \frac{5 \text{ mL}}{250 \;\cancel{mg}} = 15 \text{ mL}$$

Step 7. No rounding is required.

Example 4.3.7

A prescriber has ordered that a patient use 250 mg of amoxicillin twice daily for 10 days. You have 150 mL of 250 mg/5 mL amoxicillin suspension in stock. How many milliliters are needed for a one-day supply?

Step 1. The unknown is x mL.

Step 2. The prescriber ordered 250 mg twice daily.

Step 3. The extraneous information includes "10 days" and "150 mL".

Step 4. The answer will be greater than 5 mL (the volume of 250 mg of amoxicillin).

Step 5. Use dimensional analysis to convert the units.

$$\frac{250 \;\cancel{mg}}{\cancel{dose}} \times \frac{2 \;\cancel{doses}}{\text{day}} \times \frac{5 \text{ mL}}{\cancel{mg}} = \frac{10 \text{ mL}}{\text{day}}$$

Step 6. No rounding is required.

Example 4.3.8

Using the same prescription and amoxicillin suspension from Example 4.3.7, calculate how many milliliters of amoxicillin 250 mg/5 mL suspension are needed for a 10-day supply. The patient weighs 25 kg.

Step 1. The unknown is x mL.

Step 2. The prescriber ordered 250 mg twice daily for 10 days.

Step 3. The extraneous information includes the patient's weight.

Step 4. The answer will be greater than 10 L.

Step 5. Use dimensional analysis to convert the units.

$$\frac{10 \text{ days}}{1} \times \frac{10 \text{ mL}}{\text{day}} = 100 \text{ mL}$$

Step 6. No rounding is required.

You solved for a 10-day supply volume in two steps: first converting mg/dose to mL/day in Example 4.3.7, and then converting mL/day to mL for a 10-day supply. You can alternately solve this problem using one longer equation.

$$\frac{10 \text{ days}}{1} \times \frac{2 \text{ doses}}{\text{day}} \times \frac{250 \text{ mg}}{\text{dose}} \times \frac{5 \text{ mL}}{250 \text{ mg}} = 100 \text{ mL}$$

4.3 Problem Set

Calculate the following doses using the ratio-proportion method.

1. A patient has a prescription order for 30 mg of a medication. The pharmacy has a partial container of 7.5 mg tablets. How many tablets will the patient need?

2. A prescription order is written for 20 mg of medication. The pharmacy has on hand a 10-mL vial of 25 mg/2 mL solution. How many milliliters will be prepared for this patient?

3. A patient is prescribed 125 mg of carbamazepine suspension. The label provided shows the medication that the pharmacy has in stock. How many milliliters will be prepared for this patient?

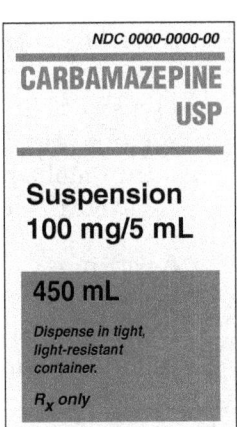

NDC 0000-0000-00

CARBAMAZEPINE USP

Suspension 100 mg/5 mL

450 mL

Dispense in tight, light-resistant container.

R$_x$ only

4. A patient is to receive 4 mg of haloperidol. The pharmacy has on hand a 1-mL vial of 5 mg/1 mL solution. How many milliliters are needed to fill this prescription?

5. A loading dose of 1750 mg is needed. The pharmacy has on hand a 500-count bottle of 250 mg capsules. How many capsules will be needed to fill this prescription?

6. A patient is to receive 40 mg of morphine sulfate. The pharmacy has the following medication available. How many milliliters will be prepared for this patient?

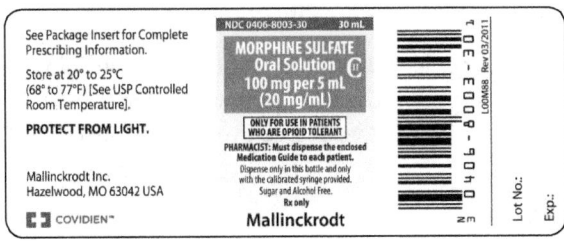

See Package Insert for Complete Prescribing Information.

Store at 20° to 25°C (68° to 77°F) [See USP Controlled Room Temperature].

PROTECT FROM LIGHT.

Mallinckrodt Inc.
Hazelwood, MO 63042 USA

COVIDIEN™

NDC 0406-8003-30   30 mL

MORPHINE SULFATE Oral Solution
100 mg per 5 mL (20 mg/mL)

ONLY FOR USE IN PATIENTS WHO ARE OPIOID TOLERANT

PHARMACIST: Must dispense the enclosed Medication Guide to each patient. Dispense only in this bottle and only with the calibrated syringe provided. Sugar and Alcohol Free.
Rx only

Mallinckrodt

Lot No.:
Exp.:

7. A patient is to receive 400 mg of erythromycin ethylsuccinate three times daily. The label provided shows the available medication. How many milliliters will be prepared for the morning dose?

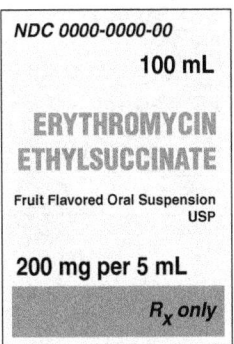

NDC 0000-0000-00

100 mL

ERYTHROMYCIN ETHYLSUCCINATE

Fruit Flavored Oral Suspension
USP

200 mg per 5 mL

R$_x$ only

8. The pharmacy receives the following order.

℞ **Amoxicillin**
1 g bid

Zantac (ranitidine hydrochloride)
75 mg bid

Carafate (sucralfate)
500 mg tid ac and at bedtime

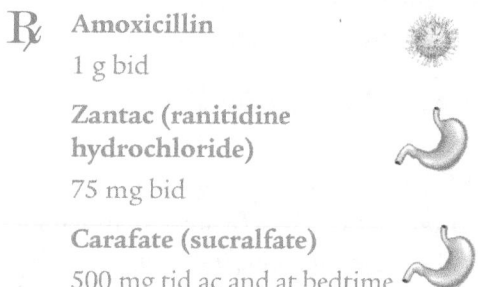

a. Amoxicillin is available as a 250 mg/5 mL suspension. How many milliliters of medication would you draw up in each oral syringe for the patient?

b. Zantac is available as 15 mg/mL. How many milliliters will you draw up in each oral syringe for the patient?

c. Carafate is available as 1 g tablets. How many tablets will be needed for one day?

9. A total regimen of therapy calls for 10 mg of a medication to be given to a patient over several days. In the pharmacy, a solution is available with 40 mcg/mL. How many milliliters must be dispensed to complete the regimen?

10. A patient was given 2 mL of gentamicin, shown in the label below. How many milligrams were given to the patient?

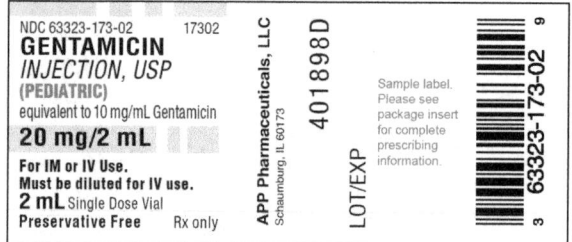

11. A patient receives 1 mg of atropine, shown in the label. How many milliliters is this?

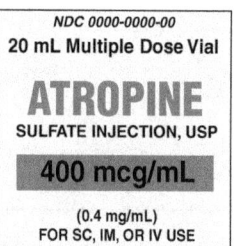

12. A patient receives 1.2 mL of the atropine solution shown in the preceding problem. How many micrograms is this?

13. A prescriber orders a 0.63 mL dose of medication. The pharmacy stock solution contains 80 mg/15 mL. How many micrograms are in the dose?

14. A capsule contains 35 mg of an active ingredient. How many capsules would you need to accumulate 1.05 kg of the ingredient?

15. A total regimen of a drug calls for 880 mg to be given. If two doses provide 80 mg, how many doses will have to be given?

16. You have 560 mL of a solution that contains 1,600 mg. How many micrograms are in 4 mL of solution? (Round your answer to the nearest tenth.)

17. A total regimen of therapy calls for 10 mg of a medication to be given to a patient over several days. In the pharmacy, a solution is available with 40 mcg/mL. How many milliliters must be dispensed to complete the regimen?

18. A patient is to receive 2,000 units of heparin. Use the following label to determine how many milliliters of heparin you will prepare.

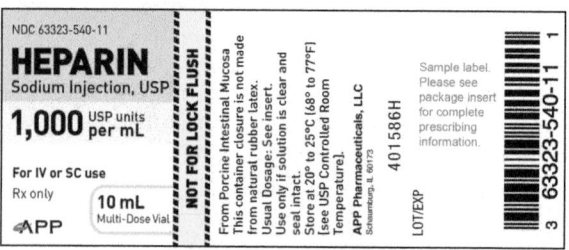

Use the following label to answer questions 19 and 20:

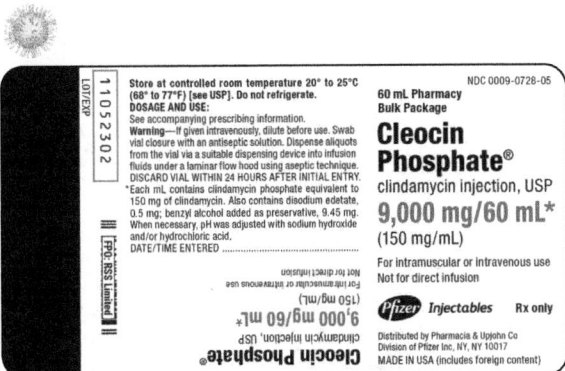

19. A medication order states that the patient is to take 900 mg of Cleocin. Use the medication label above to determine how many milliliters this will be.

20. A patient receives 4 mL of Cleocin. Use the medication label above to determine how many milligrams this will be.

Use the following label to answer questions 21 and 22:

Each 5 mL (1 teaspoonful) contains zidovudine 50 mg and sodium benzoate 0.2% added as a preservative.

See package insert for dosage and administration.

Store at 15° to 25°C (59° to 77°F).

NDC 0000-0000-00
Zidovudine Syrup
240 mL   Rx only

21. A patient is to take 12.5 mL of zidovudine syrup as shown. How many milligrams is this?

22. A patient is prescribed 100 mg of zidovudine syrup as shown. How many milliliters is this?

Use the following label to answer questions 23 and 24:

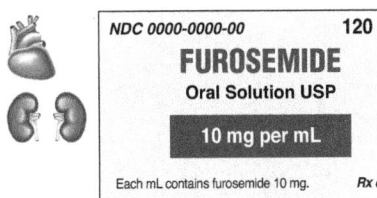

NDC 0000-0000-00   120 mL
FUROSEMIDE
Oral Solution USP
10 mg per mL
Each mL contains furosemide 10 mg.   Rx only

23. A pediatric patient is to take 0.5 mL of furosemide oral solution, and the medication shown in the label is to be used to fill the order. How many milligrams will the child take with each dose?

24. A pediatric patient is to take 0.8 mL of furosemide oral solution, and the medication shown in the label is to be used to fill the order. How many milligrams will the child take with each dose?

Use the adjacent label to answer questions 25 and 26:

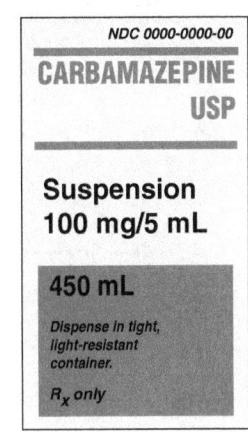

NDC 0000-0000-00
CARBAMAZEPINE USP
Suspension 100 mg/5 mL
450 mL
Dispense in tight, light-resistant container.
R$_x$ only

25. A patient is to take 150 mg of carbamazepine every 12 hours, and the medication is available as presented in the label. How many milliliters will the patient take at each dose?

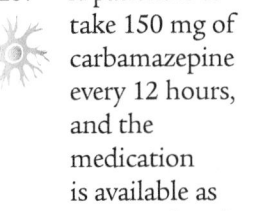

26. A patient is to take 0.5 g of carbamazepine. How many milliliters will be prepared?

Use the following label to answer questions 27 and 28:

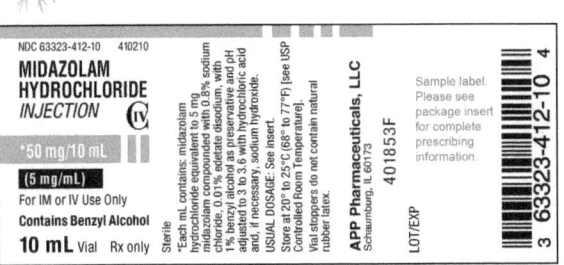

NDC 63323-412-10   410210
MIDAZOLAM HYDROCHLORIDE INJECTION (IV)
*50 mg/10 mL
(5 mg/mL)
For IM or IV Use Only
Contains Benzyl Alcohol
10 mL Vial   Rx only

APP Pharmaceuticals, LLC
Schaumburg, IL 60173
401853F
LOT/EXP

27. A patient is to receive 50 mg of midazolam intramuscularly (IM) every 4 to 6 hours as needed, and the medication shown in the label is to be used to fill the order. How many milliliters will the patient need for one dose?

28. A patient is to receive 0.8 mL of midazolam solution IM stat. How many milligrams is this?

Use the following label to answer questions 29 and 30:

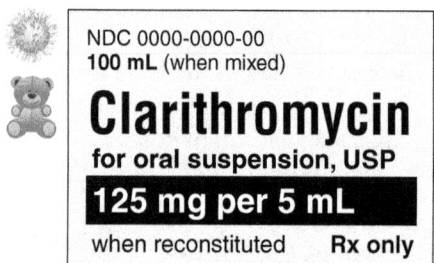

NDC 0000-0000-00
100 mL (when mixed)

Clarithromycin
for oral suspension, USP
125 mg per 5 mL
when reconstituted   **Rx only**

29. A patient is to take 100 mg of clarithromycin. How many milliliters will this be?

30. A patient is to take 7.5 mL of clarithromycin. How many milligrams will this be?

Use the following label to answer questions 31 and 32:

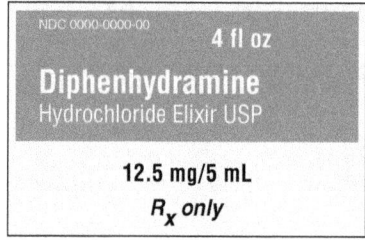

NDC 0000-0000-00   4 fl oz

Diphenhydramine
Hydrochloride Elixir USP

12.5 mg/5 mL
R_x only

31. A pediatric patient is to receive 20 mg of diphenhydramine hydrochloride. How many milliliters of elixir will be administered?

32. An adult patient who has been stung by a wasp is to receive 50 mg of diphenhydramine hydrochloride immediately. How many milliliters of elixir will be administered?

33. A patient is to take 150 mg of nortriptyline per day. The pharmacy has on hand 25 mg, 50 mg, and 75 mg capsules.

   a. Select the product that will result in the patient taking the fewest number of capsules daily.

   b. How many capsules will need to be dispensed for a week's supply?

34. The pharmacy receives the following order.

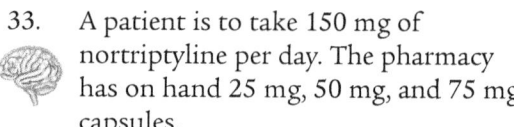

℞   **Cephalexin Suspension**
    500 mg po qid

    Hydrochlorothiazide
    50 mg po qam

    Phenytoin
    480 mg PO qday

    Carbamazepine
    200 mg tid

   a. Cephalexin is available in a 200-mL bottle of 250 mg/5 mL suspension. How many milliliters will the patient need for the first day?

   b. Hydrochlorothiazide is available from the pharmacy in a 1,000-count bottle of 25 mg tablets. How many tablets will be needed for the first day of hospitalization?

   c. Phenytoin is available as 125 mg/5 mL. How many milliliters will be measured out for the patient's daily dose?

   d. The pharmacy has a 450-mL bottle of 100 mg/5 mL carbamazepine solution. How many milliliters will be prepared for this patient for the first day?

Self-check your work in Appendix A.

4.4 Customized Doses

Most manufacturers offer dose ranges as prescribing guidelines. In some cases, the suggested dose may be based on the patient's weight or the patient's weight and height. In these cases, it is necessary to calculate patient-specific doses.

Calculating Doses Based on Weight

The patient's weight may be especially important when calculating a customized dose of a medication. Medications that have a small margin of safety should have a customized dose. More commonly, pediatric (aged birth to 18 years) and older adults (aged 65 and above) often need customized doses because their weight differs from that of the typical adult patients the medications are designed for. Also, the body systems of pediatric and older adult patients may not metabolize or eliminate the medication as an adult's body might. In these cases, manufacturers will often offer prescribing guidelines for medications based upon a therapeutic amount or range per unit of body weight. The most common unit used is milligram of a medication per kilogram of body weight (or mg/kg).

The following examples demonstrate calculations used to customize a dose. When calculating weights and doses associated with a patient's weight, round to the tenth, unless greater accuracy can be measured, as indicated in the example or question provided.

Example 4.4.1

A patient weighs 60 kg, and she is to receive a medication of 15 mg/kg. If the medication is available in a 300 mg capsule, how many capsules will be dispensed for one dose?

This problem has two parts. The first part asks for the dose, and the second part asks for the number of capsules to be dispensed for one dose. You can solve both parts of this problem using either the ratio-proportion method or the dimensional analysis method.

Using the ratio-proportion method:

Step 1: Determine the dose.

$$\frac{x \text{ mg}}{60 \text{ kg}} = \frac{15 \text{ mg}}{1 \text{ kg}}$$

$$x = 900 \text{ mg}$$

Step 2: Determine the number of capsules to be dispensed for one dose.

$$\frac{x \text{ capsules}}{900 \text{ mg}} = \frac{1 \text{ capsule}}{300 \text{ mg}}$$

$$x = 3 \text{ capsules}$$

Using the dimensional analysis method:

You can also use dimensional analysis to solve this problem in either one or two steps.

Two-Step Method

Step 1: Determine the dose.

$$\frac{60 \ \cancel{kg}}{1} \times \frac{15 \ mg}{\cancel{kg}} = 900 \ mg$$

Step 2: Determine the number of capsules to be dispensed for one dose.

$$\frac{900 \ \cancel{mg}}{1} \times \frac{1 \ capsule}{300 \ \cancel{mg}} = \frac{3 \ capsules}{dose} = 3 \ capsules$$

One-Step Method

$$\frac{60 \ \cancel{kg}}{1} \times \frac{15 \ \cancel{mg}}{\cancel{kg}} \times \frac{1 \ capsules}{300 \ \cancel{mg}} = 3 \ capsules$$

Example 4.4.2

A patient weighs 74 kg, and he is to receive a medication of 0.4 mg/kg. What will his dose be? If the medication is available in a 15 mg/10 mL solution, how many milliliters of medication will the patient receive in a dose?

This problem has two parts. The first part asks for the dose, and the second part asks for the number of milliliters to be dispensed. You can solve both parts of this problem using either the ratio-proportion method or the dimensional analysis method.

Using the ratio-proportion method:

Step 1: Determine the dose.

$$\frac{x \ mg}{74 \ kg} = \frac{0.4 \ mg}{1 \ kg}$$

$$x \ mg \ (1 \ kg) = 0.4 \ mg \ (74 \ kg)$$

$$x = 29.6 \ mg$$

Step 2: Determine the number of milliliters to be dispensed for one dose.

$$\frac{x \ mL}{29.6 \ mg} = \frac{10 \ mL}{15 \ mg}$$

$$x \ mL \ (15 \ mg) = 10 \ mL \ (29.6 \ mg)$$

$$x = 19.73 \ mL, \ rounded \ to \ 19.7 \ mL$$

Using the dimensional analysis method:

You can also use dimensional analysis to solve this problem in either one or two steps.

Two-Step Method

Step 1: Determine the dose.

$$\frac{74 \text{ kg}}{1} \times \frac{0.4 \text{ mg}}{\text{kg}} = 29.6 \text{ mg}$$

Step 2: Determine the number of milliliters to be dispensed for one dose.

$$\frac{29.6 \text{ mg}}{1} \times \frac{10 \text{ mL}}{15 \text{ mg}} = 19.73 \text{ mL, rounded to } 19.7 \text{ mL}$$

One-Step Method

$$\frac{74 \text{ kg}}{1} \times \frac{0.4 \text{ mg}}{\text{kg}} \times \frac{10 \text{ mL}}{15 \text{ mg}} = 19.73 \text{ mL, rounded to } 19.7 \text{ mL}$$

Calculating Doses Based on Body Surface Area

Body surface area (BSA) is a measurement that is based on weight and height variables and expressed as meters squared (m^2). BSA can be estimated using a nomogram (a graph used to show the relation between to or more values). Table 4.6 outlines the steps for using a BSA nomogram, and Figures 4.2 and 4.3 are nomograms used for estimating BSA for children and adults. Some medications, such as chemotherapy medications, require BSA to calculate a patient-specific dose.

TABLE 4.6 Steps for Reading a Nomogram for Estimating BSA

Step 1. Mark the patient's height on the left column.
Step 2. Mark the patient's weight on the right column.
Step 3. Draw a line or place a straight-edge on the two marks.
Step 4. Determine the BSA by noting where the straight edge crosses the center column. When the straight edge crosses between two numbers, the BSA should be estimated to the nearest one-half unit.

BSA can also be calculated using an equation. A popular equation to calculate BSA is the Mosteller Method. This formula takes the patient's height and weight into account. The Mosteller Method formula is shown below.

$$\text{BSA (in meters squared or } m^2) = \sqrt{\frac{\text{height (cm)} \times \text{weight (kg)}}{3,600}}$$

FIGURE 4.2 Nomogram for Estimating Body Surface Area of Children

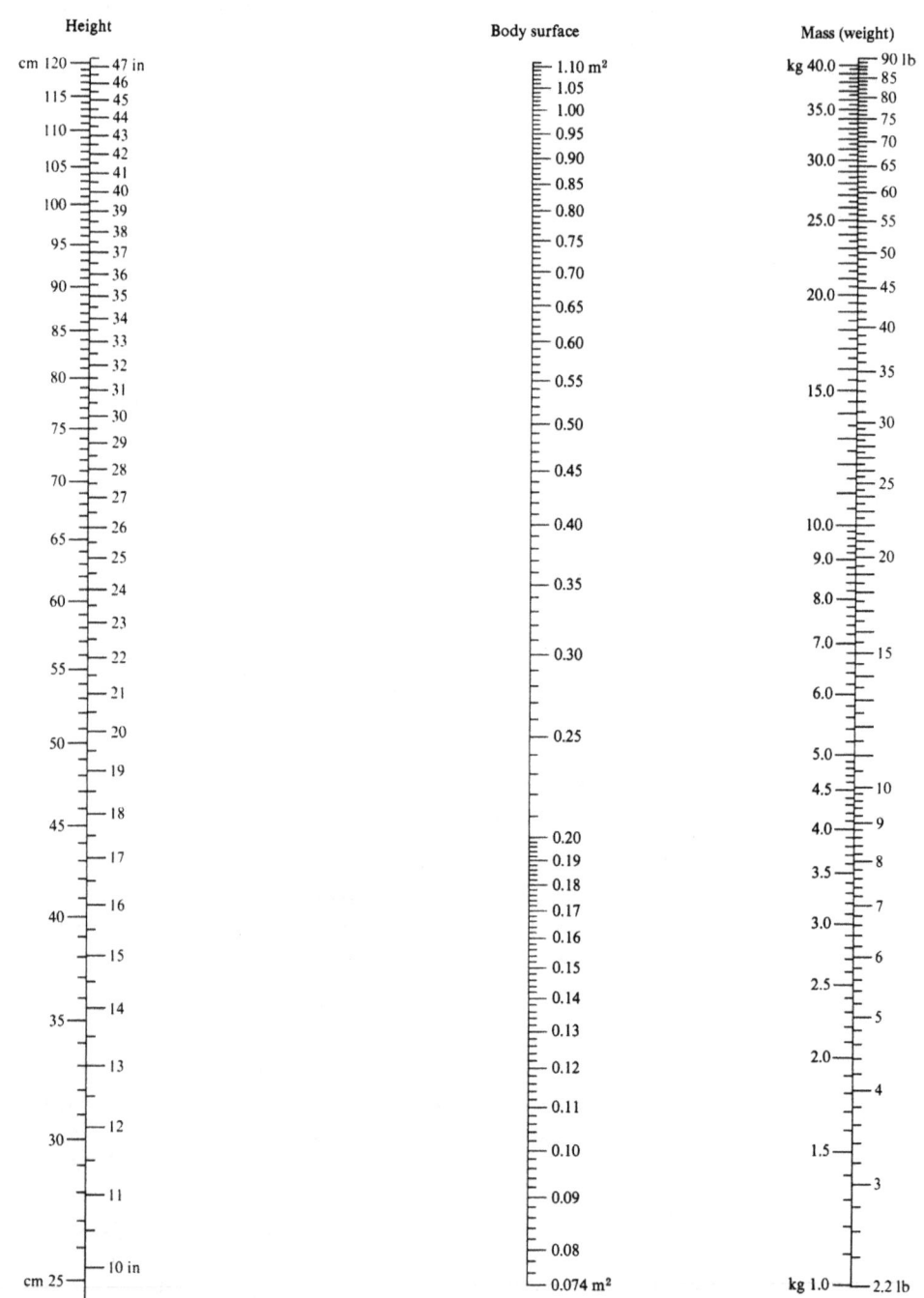

Copyright © Novartis and used with permission.

FIGURE 4.3 Nomogram for Estimating Body Surface Area of Adults

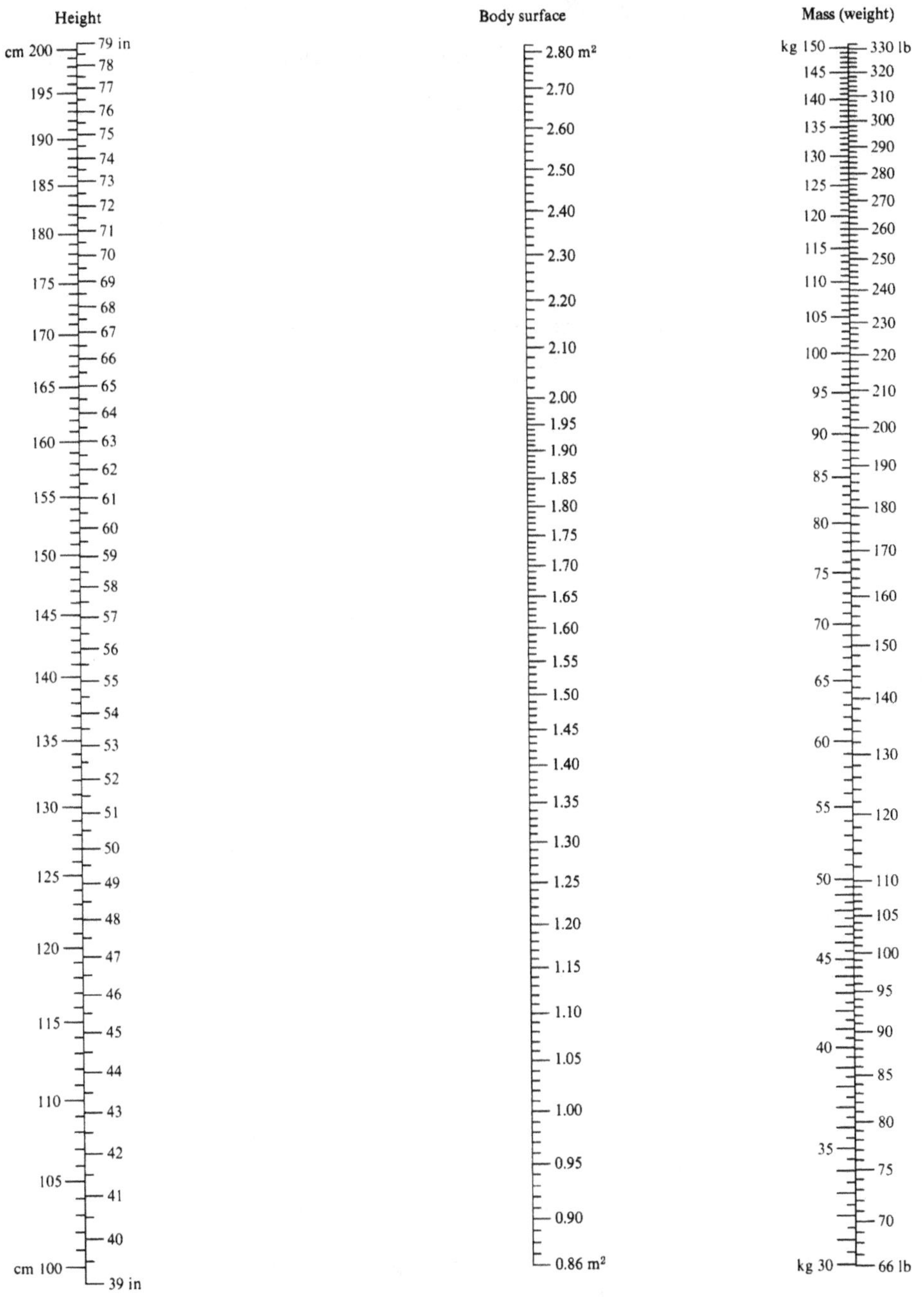

Height	Body surface	Mass (weight)
cm 200 — 79 in	2.80 m²	kg 150 — 330 lb
78	2.70	145 — 320
195 — 77		140 — 310
76	2.60	135 — 300
190 — 75	2.50	130 — 290
74		125 — 280
185 — 73	2.40	— 270
72		120 — 260
180 — 71	2.30	115 — 250
70	2.20	110 — 240
175 — 69		105 — 230
68	2.10	100 — 220
170 — 67		
66	2.00	95 — 210
165 — 65	1.95	90 — 200
64	1.90	
160 — 63	1.85	— 190
62	1.80	85 — 180
155 — 61	1.75	80 —
60	1.70	— 170
150 — 59	1.65	75 — 160
58	1.60	
145 — 57	1.55	70 — 150
56	1.50	
140 — 55	1.45	65 — 140
54	1.40	
135 — 53	1.35	60 — 130
52	1.30	
130 — 51	1.25	55 — 120
50	1.20	
125 — 49	1.15	50 — 110
48	1.10	— 105
120 — 47		45 — 100
46	1.05	— 95
115 — 45	1.00	— 90
44		40 — 85
110 — 43	0.95	— 80
42	0.90	35 — 75
105 — 41		— 70
40	0.86 m²	
cm 100 — 39 in		kg 30 — 66 lb

Copyright © Novartis and used with permission.

4.4 *Customized Doses*   **117**

Example 4.4.3

A patient is 180 cm tall and weighs 110 kg. What is the patient's BSA?

Use the Mosteller Method formula to calculate BSA:

$$BSA = \sqrt{\frac{180 \text{ cm} \times 110 \text{ kg}}{3,600}}$$

$$BSA = 2.35 \text{ m}^2$$

The patient's BSA is 2.35 m². The BSA could also be estimated using the nomogram in Figure 4.3.

Example 4.4.4

A pediatric patient is 40 inches tall and weighs 50 lbs. What is the patient's BSA?

Step 1. Convert the patient's height and weight to centimeters and kilograms.

Using dimensional analysis:

$$\frac{40 \text{ in}}{1} \times \frac{2.54 \text{ cm}}{1 \text{ in}} = 101.6 \text{ cm}$$

$$\frac{50 \text{ lb}}{1} \times \frac{1 \text{ kg}}{2.2 \text{ lb}} = 22.7 \text{ kg}$$

Step 2. Use the Mosteller Method formula to calculate BSA.

$$BSA = \sqrt{\frac{101.6 \text{ cm} \times 22.7 \text{ kg}}{3,600}}$$

$$BSA = 0.80 \text{ m}^2$$

The patient's BSA is 0.80 m². The BSA could also be estimated using the nomogram in Figure 4.2.

The following examples use the dimensional analysis method of solving pharmacy calculations. Please note that the ratio-proportion method could be used instead.

Example 4.4.5

A patient is to receive a medication with the dose based on 50 mg/m². If the patient has a BSA of 0.90 m², what will the dose be? If the medication is available only in 15 mg tablets, how many will be dispensed for one dose?

Two-Step Method

Step 1. Because the dose is to be based on 50 mg/m², multiply by the number of square meters of the BSA, in this case 0.90.

$$0.90 \, \cancel{m^2} \times \frac{50 \text{ mg}}{\cancel{m^2}} = 45 \text{ mg}$$

Step 2. Use the dose to determine the number of tablets to dispense.

$$45 \, \cancel{mg} \times \frac{1 \text{ tablet}}{15 \, \cancel{mg}} = 3 \text{ tablets}$$

One-Step Method

$$\frac{0.90 \text{ m}^2}{1} \times \frac{50 \text{ mg}}{m^2} \times \frac{1 \text{ tablet}}{15 \text{ mg}} = 3 \text{ tablets}$$

Example 4.4.6

A patient with a BSA of 1.30 m² is to receive a medication with the dose based on 0.80 mg/m². The prescription is to be divided into three equal doses. How much will each dose be? If the medication is available only as 50 mcg tablets, how many tablets will be dispensed?

Two-Step Method

Step 1. Multiply the number of mg/m² by the number of m², which is the BSA.

$$1.30 \, \cancel{m^2} \times \frac{0.80 \text{ mg}}{\cancel{m^2}} = 1.04 \text{ mg}$$

$$1.04 \text{ mg} \div 3 \text{ doses} = 0.35 \text{ mg/dose}$$

Step 2. Convert the dose in milligrams to micrograms, the units of the tablets, by using the equivalency 1 mg 5 1,000 mcg.

$$0.35 \, \cancel{mg} \times \frac{1,000 \text{ mcg}}{1 \, \cancel{mg}} = 350 \text{ mcg}$$

Therefore, a dose is 350 mcg. Since the tablets are 50 mcg each,

$$350 \, \cancel{mcg} \times \frac{1 \text{ tablet}}{50 \, \cancel{mcg}} = 7 \text{ tablets}$$

One-Step Method

$$\frac{1.30 \, \cancel{m^2}}{1 \, \cancel{day}} \times \frac{0.80 \, \cancel{mg}}{\cancel{m^2}} \times \frac{1 \, \cancel{day}}{3 \text{ doses}} \times \frac{1000 \, \cancel{mcg}}{1 \, \cancel{mg}} \times \frac{1 \text{ tablet}}{50 \, \cancel{mcg}} = 6.93 \text{ tablets/dose, which rounds to 7 tablets}$$

Calculating Pediatric Doses

If a manufacturer does not suggest an exact pediatric dose for a medication, such as a dose based on body weight or BSA, an appropriate dose may be calculated using the normal adult dose and one of several formulas. **Young's Rule** bases the suggested dose on a child's age in years, and **Clark's Rule** bases the suggested dose on a child's weight. Both formulas include the usual adult dose, but because the manufacturer often provides this as a range (such as 20–30 mg), the physician or pharmacist must determine the "usual dose" for purposes of the formula.

Young's Rule

$$\frac{\text{age (in years)}}{\text{age} + 12 \text{ years}} \times \text{adult dose} = \text{pediatric dose}$$

Clark's Rule

$$\frac{\text{weight (in lb)}}{150 \text{ lb}} \times \text{adult dose} = \text{pediatric dose}$$

Many medications have a broad dose range, and the patient's response and adverse reactions can vary widely, even in adults. For this reason, many physicians prefer to prescribe to children only those medications that have a known suggested pediatric dose. Consequently, Young's and Clark's Rules are used infrequently. A more common method for determining pediatric doses, using dosing tables, will be presented in Chapter 5. In addition, for pediatric doses, it is also common practice to round down to the nearest whole number or down to the most accurate, measurable amount. The pharmacy technician should verify the common practice used in his or her pharmacy workplace.

Example 4.4.7

A 6-year-old child needs a dose of a medication that has a suggested adult dose of 500 mg. Using Young's Rule, what is the appropriate pediatric dose? Round to the nearest milligram.

$$\frac{6 \text{ years}}{6 \text{ years} + 12 \text{ years}} \times 500 \text{ mg} = 166.66 \text{ mg, rounded down to } 166 \text{ mg}$$

Example 4.4.8

An 80 lb child needs a dose of a medication that has a suggested adult dose of 250 mg. Using Clark's Rule, what is the appropriate pediatric dose? Round to the nearest milligram.

$$\frac{80 \text{ lb}}{150 \text{ lb}} \times 250 \text{ mg} = 133.33 \text{ mg, rounded down to } 133 \text{ mg}$$

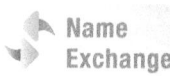

Example 4.4.9

Calculate the dose of acetaminophen for a 5-year-old child who weighs 44 lb (20 kg). The normal adult dose is 650 mg every 4 to 6 hours as needed. Determine the child's dose based on Young's Rule and Clark's Rule. Round to the nearest milligram.

Young's Rule: $\dfrac{5\ \text{years}}{5\ \text{years} + 12\ \text{years}} \times 650\ \text{mg} = 191.18\ \text{mg}$, rounded down to 191 mg

Clark's Rule: $\dfrac{44\ \text{lb}}{150\ \text{lb}} \times 650\ \text{mg} = 190.67\ \text{mg}$, rounded down to 190 mg

---

Example 4.4.10

The manufacturer in Example 4.4.9 recommends a dosage range of 10–15 mg/kg for a child age 4–5 years. What is the dosage range for the 5-year-old child who weighs 20 kg? Round to the nearest milligram.

$$20\ \cancel{kg} \times \frac{10\ \text{mg}}{\cancel{kg}} = 200\ \text{mg}$$

$$20\ \cancel{kg} \times \frac{15\ \text{mg}}{\cancel{kg}} = 300\ \text{mg}$$

Thus, the manufacturer's suggested dosage range for this child is 200–300 mg. This is a little more than the dose determined by the formulas in Example 4.4.9. For this medication, in fact, the manufacturer specifically recommends a dose of 240 mg per dose for a child between the ages of 4 and 5 years.

4.4 Problem Set

Determine the BSA for each patient described using the Mosteller method. Then use the BSA nomogram to determine the following BSA values. (For homework purposes, round to the hundredths place.)

1. Child of normal height and weight: 28 in., 20 lb

2. Child of normal height and weight: 34 in., 32 lb

3. Child of normal height and weight: 48 in., 51 lb (approximate your answer)

4. Child of normal height and weight: 95 cm, 21 kg

5. Young adult of normal height and weight: 141 cm, 42.5 kg

6. Adult: 60 in., 78 kg

7. Adult: 66 in., 64 kg

8. Adult: 71 in., 76 kg

9. Adult: 58 in., 57 kg

10. Adult: 200 cm, 80 kg

Applications

Calculate the following weight-based doses based on the provided recommended dose. (For homework purposes, round to the hundredths place.)

11. 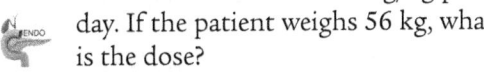 Cortisone is dosed at 0.5 mg/kg per day. If the patient weighs 56 kg, what is the dose?

12. 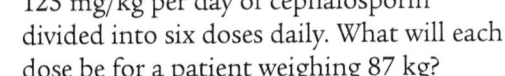 A postsurgical patient is to receive 125 mg/kg per day of cephalosporin divided into six doses daily. What will each dose be for a patient weighing 87 kg?

13. A premature infant is to receive 4 mL/kg of a medication. If the infant weighs 1.4 kg, how much medication will be administered?

14. A drug is to be given at a dose of 0.625 mg/kg.

    a. If a patient weighs 80 kg, what is the proper dose?

    b. The dose determined above is to be divided and given three times over the course of 24 hours. What is the size of each dose, to the nearest hundredth of a milligram?

15. A newborn weighs 6 kg and is to be given medication at 5 mg/kg per day in two divided doses. How much will each dose be?

16. A patient weighs 68.64 kg and is to be dosed at 125 mg/kg per day. How many milligrams is this?

17. A child weighs 10 kg and is to be dosed at 10 mg/kg per day. The medication should be administered in equal doses every 12 hours. How many milligrams are in each dose?

Calculate the following BSA-based doses based on the provided recommended dose.

18. A patient is to receive medication with the dose based on 25 mg/m² per day, divided into two equal doses. This patient has a BSA of 1.1 m². How much will each dose be?

19. A patient is to receive medication with the dose based on 0.75 mg/m². This patient has a BSA of 0.67 m². How much of the medication will you prepare? (Round to the nearest tenth.)

20. The medication order for a patient says that the dose is to be based on 100 mg/m². If this patient has a BSA of 0.85 m², how much will be prepared?

21. A child is to receive acyclovir at 250 mg/m². The child's BSA is 0.71 m². What will the dose be?

22. Methotrexate is to be given at 3.3 mg/m². The patient has a BSA of 0.83 m². What will the dose be?

Determine if the following doses are safe according to the manufacturer's recommended doses.

23. A pediatric patient weighs 40 lb and is 43 in. in height. The manufacturer of vincristine has a recommended dose of 2 mg/m². The physician has ordered 1.9 mg of vincristine. Is the physician's order safe according to the recommended dose?

24. A pediatric patient weighs 27 lb and is 30 in. in height. The manufacturer of methotrexate has a recommended dose of 3.3 mg/m². The physician has ordered 2.5 mg of methotrexate. Is the physician's order safe according to the recommended dose?

25. A pediatric patient weighs 23 lb and is 32 in. in height. The manufacturer of acyclovir has a recommended dose of 250 mg/m² every 8 hours. The physician has ordered 200 mg of acyclovir tid. Is the physician's order safe according to the recommended dose?

26. A patient weighs 40.9 kg and is 58 in. in height. The manufacturer of erythromycin has a recommended dose of 50 mg/kg per day. The physician has ordered 300 mg of erythromycin tid. Is the physician's order safe according to the recommended dose?

Calculate dosage ranges for the following and determine whether the prescribed dose is in the recommended safe range.

27. A pediatric patient weighs 36.4 kg and is 48 in. in height. The manufacturer of cefazolin has a recommended dose of 50 to 100 mg/kg per day. The physician has prescribed 250 mg tid.

   a. Calculate the minimum daily dose for this pediatric patient.

   b. Calculate the maximum daily dose for this pediatric patient.

   c. Is the physician's dose within the recommended safe range?

   d. How many milliliters will be prepared for one prescribed dose if the product is available as a 500 mg/50 mL solution?

28. A pediatric patient weighs 5.45 kg and has a length of 21 in. The manufacturer of amoxicillin has a recommended dose of 20 to 40 mg/kg per day. The physician has ordered 125 mg tid.

   a. Calculate the minimum daily dose for this pediatric patient.

   b. Calculate the maximum daily dose for this pediatric patient.

   c. Is the physician's dose within the recommended safe range?

   d. How many milliliters will be prepared for one prescribed dose if the product is available as a 125 mg/5 mL suspension?

29. A pediatric patient weighs 11.8 kg and is 31 in. in height. The physician has ordered acetaminophen with codeine, and safe dosing of acetaminophen with codeine is based on the amount of codeine. The manufacturer of codeine has a recommended dose of 0.5 to 1 mg/kg per dose. The physician has ordered 10 mL of 12 mg codeine/5 mL oral elixir.

   a. Calculate the minimum daily dose for this pediatric patient.

   b. Calculate the maximum daily dose for this pediatric patient.

   c. How many milligrams of codeine are in the 10 mL of oral elixir?

   d. Is the physician's dose within the recommended safe range?

30. A pediatric patient weighs 9.32 kg and is 28 in. in length. The manufacturer of ibuprofen has a recommended dose of 5 to 10 mg/kg every 6 to 8 hours. The physician has ordered 125 mg q8 h.

   a. Calculate the minimum daily dose for this pediatric patient.

   b. Calculate the maximum daily dose for this pediatric patient.

   c. Is the physician's dose within the recommended safe range?

   d. How many milliliters will be prepared for one prescribed dose if the product is available as a 100 mg/5 mL suspension?

31. A pediatric patient weighs 50 kg and is 65 in. in height. The manufacturer of cephalexin has a recommended dose of 25 to 50 mg/kg per day in two or four equal doses. The physician has ordered 500 mg bid.

   a. Calculate the minimum daily dose for this pediatric patient.

   b. Calculate the maximum daily dose for this pediatric patient.

   c. Is the physician's dose within the recommended safe range?

   d. How many milliliters will be prepared for one prescribed dose if the product is available as a 250 mg/5 mL suspension?

32. A pediatric patient weighs 28.6 kg and is 50 in. in height. The manufacturer of acetaminophen has a recommended dose of 10 to 15 mg/kg per day. The physician has ordered 325 mg/day.

   a. Calculate the minimum daily dose for this pediatric patient.

   b. Calculate the maximum daily dose for this pediatric patient.

   c. Is the physician's dose within the recommended safe range?

   d. How many milliliters will be prepared for one dose if the product is available as a 160 mg/5 mL suspension?

33. An 8-year-old child weighs 68 lb (30.9 kg) and is to take acyclovir, which has a normal adult dose of 600 mg.

   a. Using Young's Rule, what is the appropriate pediatric dose?

   b. Using Clark's Rule, what is the appropriate pediatric dose?

   Self-check your work in Appendix A.

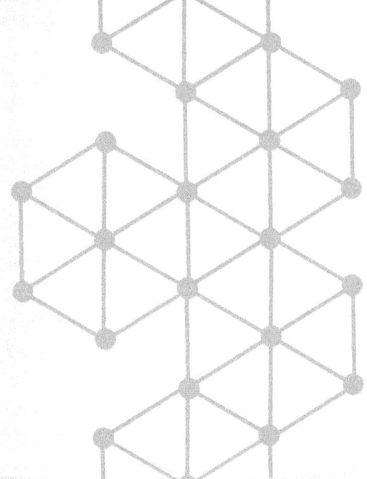

CHAPTER SUMMARY

- The basic units of measure in the metric system are meter (length), gram (weight), and liter (volume).

- The metric system uses prefixes that describe the value of the unit by multiples of 10, 100, or 1,000.

- The milligram and microgram are the two most common units of weight measure in the pharmacy.

- A gram weighs about the same as a large paper clip.

- The liter and milliliter are the two most common units of volumetric measure in the pharmacy.

- The meter and centimeter are the two most common units of measure used to describe lengths and heights in a healthcare setting.

- A meter is about the same length as a yard, or three feet.

- Converting units in the metric system often requires multiplying or dividing by 1,000, or moving the decimal point three places when changing the unit of measure.

- Use the ratio-proportion method to convert the unit if you need a foolproof way to perform the conversion—especially if you get confused as to which direction you should move the decimal point.

- The dimensional analysis method can be used to convert units of measure.

- When solving a story problem, remember to identify what the question is asking for. Then designate this unknown value with the letter x when writing your calculations.

- Always double-check that units in the numerators match on both sides of your ratio-proportion; the units in the denominators must match as well.

- When solving for x, cross out (cancel) your units to verify that you are left with the correct unit.

- You should always check your answer by multiplying the two means and the two extremes in your ratio. The two products should be equal.

- Pediatric patients often need a dose customized for them based on their weight.

- Body surface area is used to calculate some patients' doses, especially chemotherapy agents for pediatric patients.
- Clark's Rule and Young's Rule are older methods of calculating a pediatric dose based on what is normal for an adult dose.

Formulas for Success

Young's Rule	$\dfrac{\text{age (in years)}}{\text{age} + 12 \text{ years}} \times \text{adult dose} = \text{pediatric dose}$
Clark's Rule	$\dfrac{\text{weight (in lb)}}{150 \text{ lb}} \times \text{adult dose} = \text{pediatric dose}$

Important Equivalencies

TABLE 4.4 Metric Unit Equivalents

Kilo	Base	Milli	Micro
0.001 kg	1 g	1,000 mg	1,000,000 mcg
0.001 kL	1 L	1,000 mL	1,000,000 mcL
0.001 km	1 m	1,000 mm	1,000,000 mcm

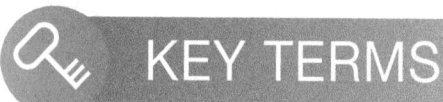 KEY TERMS

body surface area (BSA) a measurement related to a patient's weight and height, expressed in meters squared (m^2), and used to calculate patient-specific doses of medications

Clark's Rule a formula used to determine an appropriate pediatric dose by using the child's weight in pounds and the normal adult dose; weight in lb/150 lb $\times$ adult dose = pediatric dose

dimensional analysis method a conversion method in which the given number and unit are multiplied by the ratio of the desired unit to the given unit, which is equivalent to 1

gram the basic unit for measuring weight in the metric system

liter the basic unit for measuring volume in the metric system

meter the basic unit for measuring length in the metric system

metric system a measurement system based on subdivisions and multiples of 10; made up of three basic units: meter, gram, and liter

vehicle an inert medium, such as a syrup, in which a drug is administered

Young's Rule a formula used to determine an appropriate pediatric dose by using the child's age in years and the normal adult dose; age in years/(age in years + 12 years) × adult dose = pediatric dose

 CHAPTER REVIEW

Finding Solutions

To gain practice in handling challenging situations in the workplace, consider the following real-world scenarios, and then use the guiding questions to help you formulate your responses.

Scenario A: A mother approaches you and hands you a prescription for thioridazine for her son, who weighs 15 kg and is 41 in. tall. The manufacturer of thioridazine recommends a dose between 0.5 mg/kg and 3 mg/kg per day for children, to be given in divided doses. The boy's physician has prescribed 15 mg every 12 hours.

1. Calculate the minimum daily dose for this pediatric patient.

2. Calculate the maximum daily dose for this pediatric patient.

3. Is the physician's dose within the recommended safe range?

4. How many milliliters of 5 mg/mL strength thioridizine suspension will be given at each prescribed dose?

Scenario B: Your pharmacy just received a prescription from a pediatrician for acetaminophen 325 mg. The pediatric patient weighs 21.8 kg and is 52 in. in height. The manufacturer of acetaminophen has a recommended dose of 10 to 15 mg/kg per dose.

5. Calculate the minimum dose for this pediatric patient.

6. Calculate the maximum dose for this pediatric patient.

7. Is the physician's dose within the recommended safe range?

8. How many milliliters will be prepared for one prescribed dose if the product is available as a 160 mg/5 mL suspension?

 Scenario C: A 12-year-old child, who weighs 80 lb (36.36 kg), has been prescribed zidovudine. The normal adult dose is 600 mg.

9. Using Young's Rule, what is the appropriate pediatric dose? Round to the nearest milligram.

10. Using Clark's Rule, what is the appropriate pediatric dose? Round to the nearest milligram.

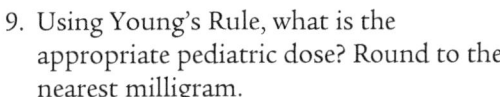 **Scenario D:** An e-prescription for Flumadine arrived at your pharmacy for a 9-year-old child who weighs 62 lb (28.2 kg). Flumadine has a normal adult dose of 100 mg twice daily for 7 days.

11. Using Young's Rule, what is the appropriate pediatric dose? Round to the nearest milligram.

12. Using Clark's Rule, what is the appropriate pediatric dose? Round to the nearest milligram.

Scenario E: You are working in a hospital pharmacy and you receive an order that is part of a pre-written protocol for doxorubicin (a chemotherapy agent) 96 mg. The protocol shows that doxorubicin is dosed at 60 mg/m².

13. Your hospital has a policy that the patient's body surface area (BSA) must be included with all chemotherapy orders. You notice this is not included and realize the patient's BSA must be obtained. If the dose for doxorubicin was ordered correctly, what do you expect the patient's BSA to be?

14. The patient's BSA is verified and it is determined that the ordered dose is appropriate. Your pharmacy stocks doxorubicin as 2 mg/mL in 10-mL, 25-mL, and 100-mL containers. How many milliliters of doxorubicin are needed for the dose? Which container should you select?

Scenario F: You are working in a hospital pharmacy where you receive an order for atropine 15 mcg/kg. Your pharmacy has atropine 400 mcg/mL in stock. The patient weights 196 pounds.

NDC 0000-0000-00
20 mL Multiple Dose Vial

ATROPINE
SULFATE INJECTION, USP

400 mcg/mL

(0.4 mg/mL)
FOR SC, IM, OR IV USE

15. How many micrograms of atropine are needed for the dose? Round to the nearest tenth.

16. How many milliliters of atropine solution are needed to supply the dose? Round to the nearest tenth.

Navigator

Access interactive chapter review exercises, practice activities, flash cards, and study games.

5

Using Household Measure in Pharmacy Calculations

Learning Objectives

1 Identify units of household measure and convert between them.

2 Apply the household measure and the metric systems to pharmacy calculations.

3 Convert body weight between kilograms and pounds.

4 Determine pediatric doses using dosing tables.

5 Calculate the amount of medication to be dispensed.

6 Convert temperature between Celsius and Fahrenheit.

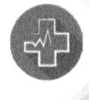 Preview chapter terms and definitions.

5.1 Household Measure

 Household measure is a measurement system used in homes, particularly in kitchens, in the United States. The units of household measure for volume are teaspoonful, tablespoonful, cup, pint, quart, and gallon. The units of household measure for weight are ounces and pounds. Table 5.1 lists the household measure equivalents and their abbreviations. Figure 5.1 on the following page illustrates household measure equivalents.

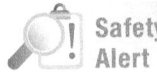 **Safety Alert**

To avoid misreading c for c̄ or 0, do not abbreviate *cup* using a lower-case c.

TABLE 5.1 Household Measure Equivalents

Volume		Weight	
3 teaspoonsful (tsp)	= 1 tablespoonful (tbsp)	1 pound (lb)	= 16 ounces (oz)
2 tablespoonsful (tbsp)	= 1 fluid ounce (fl oz)		
8 fluid ounces (fl oz)	= 1 cup		
2 cups	= 1 pint (pt)		
2 pints (pt)	= 1 quart (qt)		
4 quarts (qt)	= 1 gallon (gal)		

FIGURE 5.1 **Household Measure Equivalents**

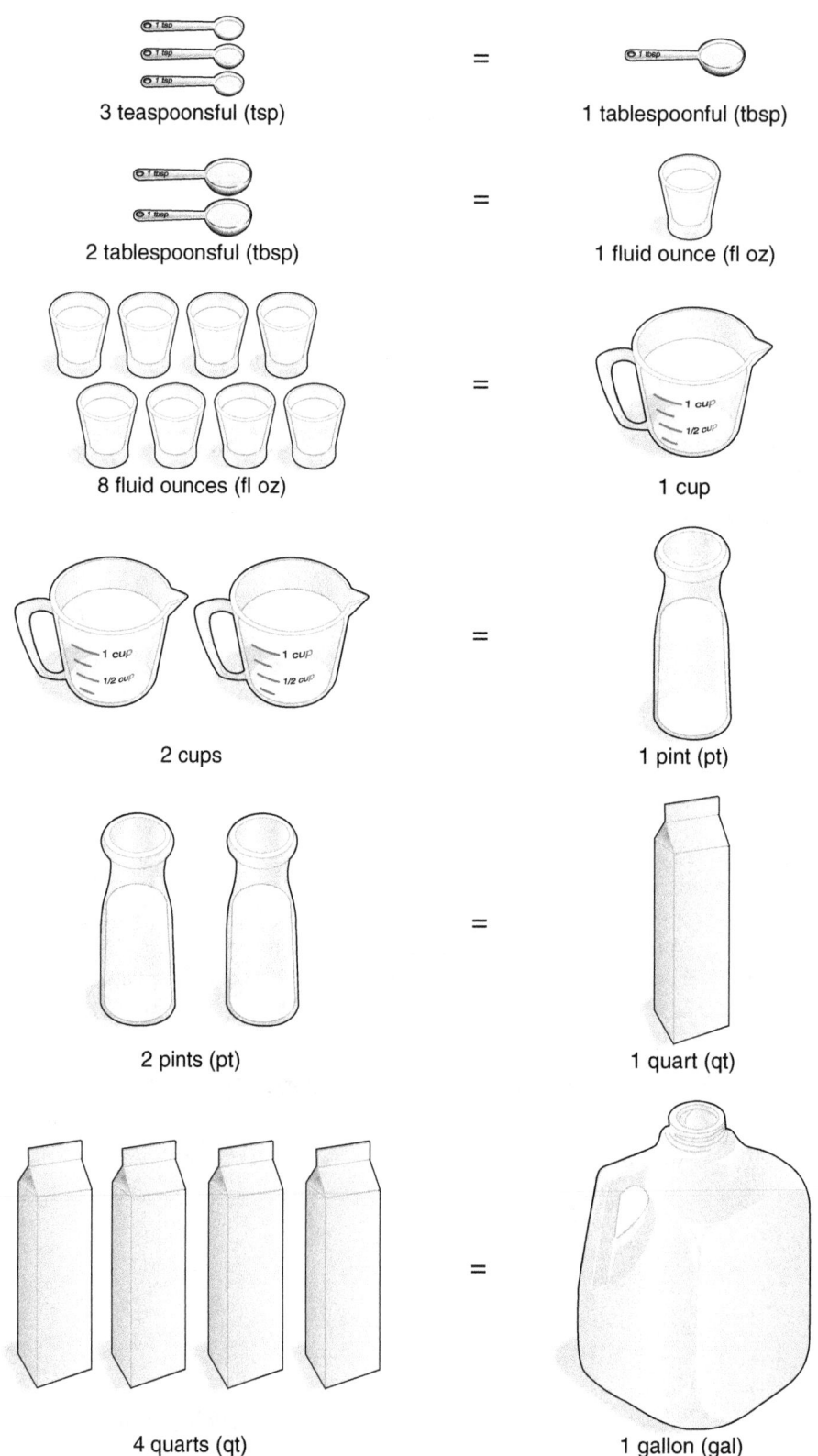

3 teaspoonsful (tsp) = 1 tablespoonful (tbsp)

2 tablespoonsful (tbsp) = 1 fluid ounce (fl oz)

8 fluid ounces (fl oz) = 1 cup

2 cups = 1 pint (pt)

2 pints (pt) = 1 quart (qt)

4 quarts (qt) = 1 gallon (gal)

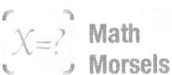
Measuring volume using household measure can be less accurate than using other systems because the measuring utensils can vary in size. Nevertheless, household volume measurement may be used in community pharmacy practice when dispensing drugs that will be administered in the patient's home because patients may not have other measuring devices at their disposal. Labels instructing patients on how to take a medication often use household measure units for this reason.

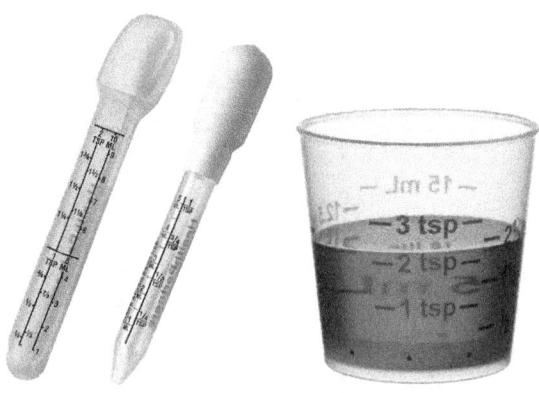

Dosing spoons, droppers, and cups are frequently marked with both metric and household measures.

However, there is a growing trend among prescribers and pharmacies to use the preferred metric system for medication dosage. To that end, pharmacies often give patients dosing spoons, droppers, and cups marked with both metric and household measurements at minimal or no cost.

Converting Household Volume Measures

Like all systems, units of household measures can be converted to larger or smaller units. The following examples demonstrate converting units of volume.

Example 5.1.1

How many teaspoonsful are in 2 tablespoonsful?

Begin the solution by noting the appropriate equivalents indicated in Table 5.1 and Figure 5.1.

$$3 \text{ tsp} = 1 \text{ tbsp}$$

Using these equivalents, you can find the solution in two ways.

Using the ratio-proportion method:

$$\frac{x \text{ tsp}}{2 \text{ tbsp}} = \frac{3 \text{ tsp}}{1 \text{ tbsp}}$$

$$x \text{ tsp} (1 \text{ tbsp}) = 3 \text{ tsp} (2 \text{ tbsp})$$

$$x = 6 \text{ tsp}$$

Using the dimensional analysis method:

$$2 \text{ tbsp} \times \frac{3 \text{ tsp}}{1 \text{ tbsp}} = 6 \text{ tsp}$$

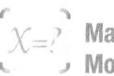
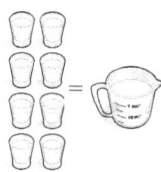
Example 5.1.2

How many tablespoonsful are in 2 cups of medication?

Begin the solution by noting the appropriate equivalents indicated in Table 5.1 and Figure 5.1.

$$2 \text{ tbsp} = 1 \text{ fl oz}$$

$$1 \text{ cup} = 8 \text{ fl oz}$$

Using these equivalents, you can find the solution in two ways.

Using the ratio-proportion method:

First determine the number of fluid ounces in 2 cups.

$$\frac{x \text{ fl oz}}{2 \text{ cups}} = \frac{8 \text{ fl oz}}{1 \text{ cup}}$$

$$x \text{ fl oz } (1 \text{ cup}) = 8 \text{ fl oz } (2 \text{ cups})$$

$$x \text{ fl oz} = 16 \text{ fl oz}$$

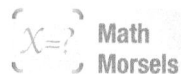
Second, determine the number of tablespoonsful in 16 fl oz.

$$\frac{x \text{ tbsp}}{16 \text{ fl oz}} = \frac{2 \text{ tbsp}}{1 \text{ fl oz}}$$

$$x \text{ tbsp } (1 \text{ fl oz}) = 2 \text{ tbsp } (16 \text{ fl oz})$$

$$x \text{ tbsp} = 32 \text{ tbsp}$$

Using the dimensional analysis method:

$$2 \text{ cups} \times \frac{8 \text{ fl oz}}{1 \text{ cup}} \times \frac{2 \text{ tbsp}}{1 \text{ fl oz}} = 32 \text{ tbsp}$$

Note that the cups units cancel, the fluid ounces units cancel, and the tablespoonsful unit remains.

Example 5.1.3

How many 1 tsp doses are in 3 cups of liquid medication?

Begin the solution by noting the appropriate equivalents indicated in Table 5.1.

$$3 \text{ tsp} = 1 \text{ tbsp}$$

$$2 \text{ tbsp} = 1 \text{ fl oz}$$

$$8 \text{ fl oz} = 1 \text{ cup}$$

Using these equivalents, you can find the solution in two ways.

Using the ratio-proportion method:

First, determine the number of fluid ounces in 3 cups.

$$\frac{x \text{ fl oz}}{3 \text{ cups}} = \frac{8 \text{ fl oz}}{1 \text{ cup}}$$

$$x \text{ fl oz } (1 \text{ cup}) = 8 \text{ fl oz } (3 \text{ cups})$$

$$x \text{ fl oz} = 24 \text{ fl oz}$$

Second, calculate the number of tablespoonsful in 24 fl oz.

$$\frac{x \text{ tbsp}}{24 \text{ fl oz}} = \frac{2 \text{ tbsp}}{1 \text{ fl oz}}$$

$$x \text{ tbsp } (1 \text{ fl oz}) = 2 \text{ tbsp } (24 \text{ fl oz})$$

$$x \text{ tbsp} = 48 \text{ tbsp}$$

Third, determine the number of teaspoonsful in 48 tablespoonsful.

$$\frac{x \text{ tsp}}{48 \text{ tbsp}} = \frac{3 \text{ tsp}}{1 \text{ tbsp}}$$

$$x \text{ tsp } (1 \text{ tbsp}) = 3 \text{ tsp } (48 \text{ tbsp})$$

$$x \text{ tsp} = 144 \text{ tsp}$$

Using the dimensional analysis method:

$$3 \text{ cups} \times \frac{8 \text{ fl oz}}{1 \text{ cup}} \times \frac{2 \text{ tbsp}}{1 \text{ fl oz}} \times \frac{3 \text{ tsp}}{1 \text{ tbsp}} = 144 \text{ tsp}$$

Note that the cups units cancel, the fluid ounces units cancel, the tablespoon units cancel, and the teaspoon unit remains.

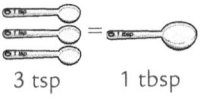

8 fl oz = 1 cup

2 tbsp = 1 fl oz

3 tsp = 1 tbsp

2 cups = 1 pt

Example 5.1.4

How many 1 fl oz doses are in 3 pt of liquid medication?

Begin the solution by noting the appropriate equivalents indicated in Table 5.1.

$$8 \text{ fl oz} = 1 \text{ cup}$$

$$2 \text{ cups} = 1 \text{ pt}$$

$$2 \text{ pt} = 1 \text{ qt}$$

Using these equivalents, the solution can be determined in two ways.

Using the ratio-proportion method:

First determine the number of cups in 3 pt.

$$\frac{x \text{ cups}}{3 \text{ pt}} = \frac{2 \text{ cups}}{1 \text{ pt}}$$

$$x \text{ cups } (1 \text{ pt}) = 2 \text{ cups } (3 \text{ pt})$$

$$x \text{ cups} = 6 \text{ cups}$$

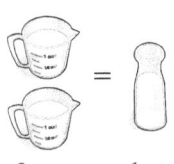

2 cups = 1 pt

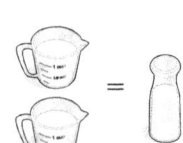

8 fl oz   1 cup

Second, calculate the number of fluid ounces in 6 cups.

$$\frac{x \text{ fl oz}}{6 \text{ cups}} = \frac{8 \text{ fl oz}}{1 \text{ cup}}$$

$$x \text{ fl oz} (1 \text{ cup}) = 8 \text{ fl oz} (6 \text{ cups})$$

$$x \text{ fl oz} = 48 \text{ fl oz}$$

Using the dimensional analysis method:

$$3 \text{ pt} \times \frac{2 \text{ cups}}{1 \text{ pt}} \times \frac{8 \text{ fl oz}}{1 \text{ cup}} = 48 \text{ fl oz}$$

Example 5.1.5

How many 1 fl oz doses are in 2 qt of liquid medication?

Begin the solution by noting the appropriate equivalents indicated in Table 5.1.

$$8 \text{ fl oz} = 1 \text{ cup}$$

$$2 \text{ cups} = 1 \text{ pt}$$

$$2 \text{ pt} = 1 \text{ qt}$$

Using these equivalents, the solution can be determined in two ways:

Using the ratio-proportion method:

First, determine the number of pints in 2 qt.

$$\frac{x \text{ pt}}{2 \text{ qt}} = \frac{2 \text{ pt}}{1 \text{ qt}}$$

$$x \text{ pt} (1 \text{ qt}) = 2 \text{ pt} (2 \text{ qt})$$

$$x \text{ pt} = 4 \text{ pt}$$

2 pt   1 qt

Second, calculate the number of cups in 4 pt.

$$\frac{x \text{ cup}}{4 \text{ pt}} = \frac{2 \text{ cups}}{1 \text{ pt}}$$

$$x \text{ cup} (1 \text{ pt}) = 2 \text{ cups} (4 \text{ pt})$$

$$x \text{ cup} = 8 \text{ cups}$$

2 cups   1 pt

Third, determine the number of fluid ounces in 8 cups.

$$\frac{x \text{ fl oz}}{8 \text{ cups}} = \frac{8 \text{ fl oz}}{1 \text{ cup}}$$

$$x \text{ fl oz} (1 \text{ cup}) = 8 \text{ fl oz} (8 \text{ cups})$$

$$x \text{ fl oz} = 64 \text{ fl oz}$$

8 fl oz   1 cup

Using the dimensional analysis method:

$$2 \text{ qt} \times \frac{2 \text{ pt}}{1 \text{ qt}} \times \frac{2 \text{ cups}}{1 \text{ pt}} \times \frac{8 \text{ fl oz}}{1 \text{ cup}} = 64 \text{ fl oz}$$

Converting between Household Measure and the Metric System

Because of the inaccuracy of the measuring tools used in household measure, it is often preferable to convert all quantities to the metric system. These conversions may seem like additional work, but using the metric system is more accurate than the household system, which is declining in use.

Prescriptions that are interpreted and entered into a computer as part of the patient's record need to be converted to the metric system. Typically, such computer programs are set up to accept quantity measurements using milliliters for liquid prescriptions and grams for solid prescriptions, such as for creams or ointments. When a prescription is written for a liquid, the volume to be dispensed and the quantity to be given at each dose is used to calculate the amount of medication needed for 24 hours, or 1 day. Calculating the volume to be dispensed and days' supply are important steps in the processing of each prescription. These calculations provide the pharmacist and pharmacy technician with the information needed to accurately fill the prescription, ensuring that the patient is getting the prescribed therapy.

Although some references list exact values for conversions between the household measure and the metric system, the equivalents shown in Table 5.2 below and Figure 5.2 on the following page are generally accepted for use for these conversions in daily pharmacy practice. You should commit all of these conversion values to memory.

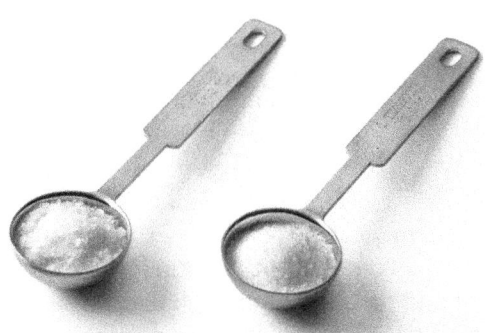

The volume held by a household teaspoonful may vary, but a true teaspoonful equals 5 mL.

 **Work Wise**

Certain household measures are commonly used in the pharmacy setting. You may find it useful to commit many conversions to memory. This task may seem daunting at first, but a good place to start is to remember that 1 tsp = 5 mL, 3 tsp = 1 tbsp = 15 mL, and 2.2 lb = 1 kg.

TABLE 5.2   Household Measure and Metric System Conversion Values

Volume		Weight	
1 tsp	= 5 mL	1 oz	= 30 g†
1 tbsp	= 15 mL	1 lb	= 450 g†
1 fl oz	= 30 mL*	2.2 lb	= 1 kg
1 cup	= 240 mL		
1 pt	= 480 mL*		
1 qt	= 960 mL		
1 gal	= 3,840 mL		

* There are actually 29.57 mL in 1 fl oz, but 30 mL is usually used. When packaging a pint, companies will typically include 473 mL, rather than the full 480 mL. Additionally, 1 gal is actually equivalent to 3,785 mL.

† There are actually 28.34952 g in a household ounce; however, pharmacy personnel often round up to 30 g. It iscommon practice to use 454 g as the equivalent for a pound (28.35 g × 16 oz/lb = 453.6 g/lb, rounded to 454 g/lb).

FIGURE 5.1 **Household Measure and Metric System Conversion Volume Values**

Most common household measure and metric system approximate equivalents for volume

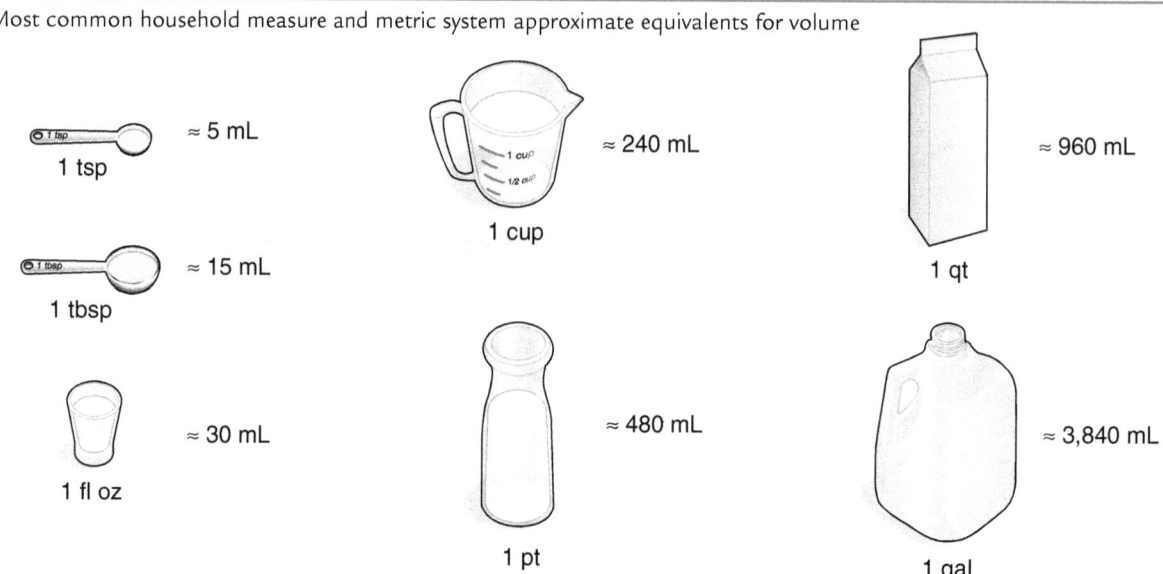

1 tsp ≈ 5 mL

1 tbsp ≈ 15 mL

1 fl oz ≈ 30 mL

1 cup ≈ 240 mL

1 pt ≈ 480 mL

1 qt ≈ 960 mL

1 gal ≈ 3,840 mL

As seen in Table 5.2 and Figure 5.2, it is common practice to round a household fluid ounce (29.57 mL) up to 30 mL. When measuring this amount, this estimation is often appropriate because the volume differs by such a small amount. When measuring multiple fluid ounces that have been rounded up to 30 mL, however, the discrepancy becomes far more apparent. For example, if asked to measure a pint (16 fl oz), you would measure roughly 480 mL. This measurement becomes problematic because 29.57 mL multiplied by 16 is equal to only 473.12 mL, not 480 mL. Most stock bottles are labeled 473 mL, yet pharmacies bill according to the estimation of 480 mL and measure out fluid ounces in 30 mL increments. For the purposes of this chapter, use the rounded 30 mL and 480 mL values.

The following examples show some typical conversion problems the pharmacy technician must be able to solve.

Example 5.1.6

You are to dispense 300 mL of morphine sulfate 100 mg per 5 mL solution. The prescription states the patient is to take ¹/₂ tsp four times daily. How many doses will the dispensed volume contain?

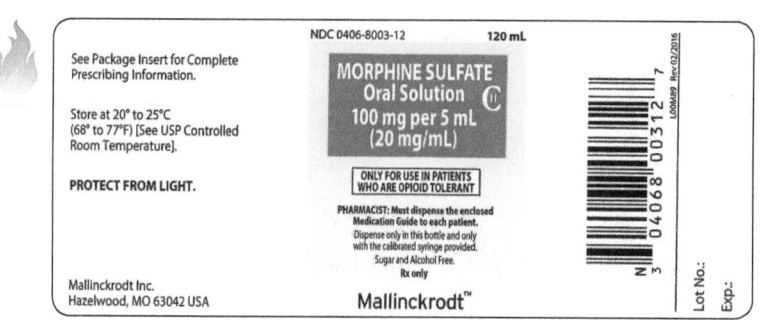

Using the ratio-proportion method:

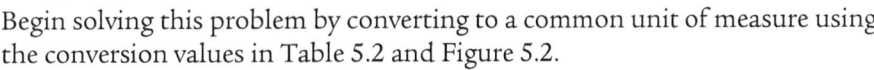

Begin solving this problem by converting to a common unit of measure using the conversion values in Table 5.2 and Figure 5.2.

$$1 \text{ dose} = 2 \text{ tsp} = 2 \times 5 \text{ mL} = 10 \text{ mL}$$

Determine the number of doses needed.

$$\frac{x \text{ doses}}{300 \text{ mL}} = \frac{1 \text{ dose}}{10 \text{ mL}}$$

$$x \text{ doses } (10 \text{ mL}) = 1 \text{ dose } (300 \text{ mL})$$

$$x \text{ doses} = 30 \text{ doses}$$

Using the dimensional analysis method:

$$\frac{300 \text{ mL}}{1} \times \frac{\text{dose}}{2 \text{ tsp}} \times \frac{1 \text{ tsp}}{5 \text{ mL}} = 30 \text{ doses}$$

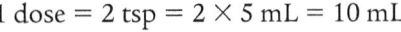
2 tsp = 10 mL

Example 5.1.7

Using the medication and dosing instructions in Example 5.1.6, how many days will the 300 mL last?

The patient is to take 1 dose twice daily (BID), and, as calculated in Example 5.1.6, there are 30 doses in the dispensed volume.

Using the ratio-proportion method:

$$\frac{x \text{ days}}{30 \text{ doses}} = \frac{1 \text{ day}}{2 \text{ doses}}$$

$$x \text{ days } (2 \text{ doses}) = 1 \text{ day } (30 \text{ doses})$$

$$x \text{ days} = 15 \text{ days}$$

Using the dimensional analysis method:

$$30 \text{ doses} \times \frac{1 \text{ day}}{2 \text{ doses}} = 15 \text{ days}$$

Example 5.1.8

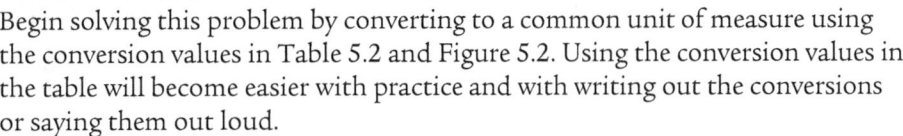

A patient is to purchase a 12 fl oz bottle of antacid. The patient is to take 15 mL before each meal and at bedtime. How many doses does the bottle contain?

Using the ratio-proportion method:

Begin solving this problem by converting to a common unit of measure using the conversion values in Table 5.2 and Figure 5.2. Using the conversion values in the table will become easier with practice and with writing out the conversions or saying them out loud.

$$1 \text{ fl oz} = 30 \text{ mL, so } 0.5 \text{ fl oz} = 15 \text{ mL, and } 12 \text{ fl oz} = 360 \text{ mL}$$

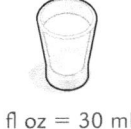
1 fl oz = 30 mL

Use this information to set up a ratio proportion.

$$\frac{x \text{ doses}}{360 \text{ mL}} = \frac{1 \text{ dose}}{15 \text{ mL}}$$

$$x \text{ doses} (15 \text{ mL}) = 1 \text{ dose} (360 \text{ mL})$$

$$x \text{ dose} = 24 \text{ doses}$$

Using the dimensional analysis method:

$$\frac{12 \text{ fl oz}}{1} \times \frac{30 \text{ mL}}{1 \text{ fl oz}} \times \frac{\text{dose}}{15 \text{ mL}} = 24 \text{ doses}$$

Example 5.1.9

Using the medication and dosing instructions in Example 5.1.8, if the patient eats three times a day, how many days will the 12 fl oz bottle last?

The patient is to take 1 dose with every meal and at bedtime, so a daily dose is

$$\left(\frac{1 \text{ dose}}{\text{meal}} \times \frac{3 \text{ meals}}{\text{day}} \right) + 1 \text{ dose at bedtime} = \frac{4 \text{ doses}}{\text{day}}$$

If 24 doses are dispensed, as calculated in Example 5.1.7,

$$24 \text{ doses} \times \frac{1 \text{ day}}{4 \text{ doses}} = 6 \text{ days}$$

Example 5.1.10

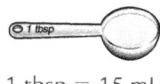

1 tbsp = 15 mL

How many 2 tbsp doses are in 480 mL?

Using the ratio-proportion method:

Using the conversion values in Table 5.2 and Figure 5.2, 1 tbsp = 15 mL. Because 1 dose equals 2 tbsp,

$$1 \text{ dose} = 2 \text{ tbsp} = 2 \times 15 \text{ mL} = 30 \text{ mL}$$

Use these converted measurements to set up a ratio proportion.

$$\frac{x \text{ doses}}{480 \text{ mL}} = \frac{1 \text{ dose}}{30 \text{ mL}}$$

$$x \text{ doses} (30 \text{ mL}) = 1 \text{ dose} (480 \text{ mL})$$

$$x \text{ dose} = 16 \text{ doses}$$

Using the dimensional analysis method:

$$\frac{480 \text{ mL}}{1} \times \frac{1 \text{ tbsp}}{15 \text{ mL}} \times \frac{1 \text{ dose}}{2 \text{ tbsp}} = 16 \text{ doses}$$

Example 5.1.11

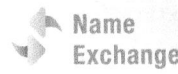
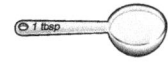
Theophylline elixir contains 80 mg/15 mL. One dose is 2 tbsp. How many milligrams are in 1 dose of the theophylline elixir?

Using the ratio-proportion method:

Using the conversion values in Table 5.2 and Figure 5.2,

$$1 \text{ dose} = 2 \text{ tbsp} = 2 \times 15 \text{ mL} = 30 \text{ mL}$$

Use these conversions to create a ratio proportion.

$$\frac{x \text{ mg}}{30 \text{ mL}} = \frac{80 \text{ mg}}{15 \text{ mL}}$$

$$x \text{ mg (15 mL)} = 80 \text{ mg (30 mL)}$$

$$x \text{ mg} = 160 \text{ mg}$$

Using the dimensional analysis method:

$$\frac{2 \text{ tbsp}}{1} \times \frac{15 \text{ mL}}{1 \text{ tbsp}} \times \frac{80 \text{ mg}}{15 \text{ mL}} = 160 \text{ mg}$$

NDC 0000-0000-00

THEOPHYLLINE ELIXIR

Contains 80 mg/15 mL

480 mL

Dispense in tight, light-resistant container.

R_x only

Like volumes, weights can be converted between household measure and metric measure. The most common conversions are between the household measurements of pounds and ounces and the metric measurements of kilograms and grams. These conversions were presented in Table 5.2.

Example 5.1.12

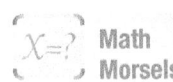
A physician has written a prescription for a 1.5 oz tube of ointment. How many grams is this?

Since 1 oz equals 30 g, this problem can be solved in two ways.

Using the ratio-proportion method:

$$\frac{x \text{ g}}{1.5 \text{ oz}} = \frac{30 \text{ g}}{1 \text{ oz}}$$

$$x \text{ g (1 oz)} = 30 \text{ g (1.5 oz)}$$

$$x \text{ g} = 45 \text{ g}$$

Using the dimensional analysis method:

$$1.5 \text{ oz} \times \frac{30 \text{ g}}{1 \text{ oz}} = 45 \text{ g}$$

Example 5.1.13

You have a 1 lb jar of ointment available. You are instructed to use this stock to fill smaller jars with 20 g of ointment each. How many jars can you fill?

Because 1 lb equals 454 g, this problem can be solved in two ways.

Using the ratio-proportion method:

$$\frac{x \text{ jars}}{454 \text{ g}} = \frac{1 \text{ jar}}{20 \text{ g}}$$

$$x \text{ jars } (20 \text{ g}) = 1 \text{ jar } (454 \text{ g})$$

$$x \text{ jar} = 22.7 \text{ jars, or } 22 \text{ full jars}$$

Using the dimensional analysis method:

$$454 \text{ g} \times \frac{1 \text{ jar}}{20 \text{ g}} = 22.7 \text{ jars, or } 22 \text{ full jars}$$

In both solutions, there is 0.7 jar of ointment remaining. You can determine how many grams of ointment are left over with the following calculation:

$$\frac{20 \text{ g}}{\text{jar}} \times 0.7 \text{ jar leftover ointment} = 14 \text{ g leftover ointment}$$

Converting Body Weight

As discussed in the previous chapter, medications are sometimes dosed based on the weight of the patient. Increasingly, drug manufacturers are providing a recommended dose based on a specific dose in milligrams per kilogram of the patient's weight. Because most medications are dosed on the basis of kilograms, if a patient's weight is documented in pounds, the weight will have to be converted to kilograms before calculating the appropriate dose.

☑ TAKE NOTE

Many medications are dosed by weight (usually mg per kg). However, you may find that patients or medical records record weight in pounds or kilograms. If a weight is not labeled with units, it is important to verify with the patient or caregiver. It may be tempting to make assumptions about weight, but you should resist. Mistaking pounds for kilograms can result in a patient receiving more than double the intended dose. With some medications, a dose increase of that magnitude could result in harm or even death.

Example 5.1.14

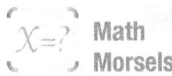

Math Morsels

Pharmacy technicians should memorize the following conversion:
2.2 lb = 1 kg

A patient weighs 134 lb. What is this patient's weight in kilograms?

Since 1 kg equals 2.2 lb, this problem can be solved in two ways.

Using the ratio-proportion method:

$$\frac{x \text{ kg}}{134 \text{ lb}} = \frac{1 \text{ kg}}{2.2 \text{ lb}}$$

$$x \text{ kg } (2.2 \text{ lb}) = 1 \text{ kg } (134 \text{ lb})$$

$$x \text{ kg} = 60.909 \text{ kg, rounded to } 60.9 \text{ kg}$$

Using the dimensional analysis method:

$$134 \text{ lb} \times \frac{1 \text{ kg}}{2.2 \text{ lb}} = 60.909 \text{ kg, rounded to } 60.9 \text{ kg}$$

Example 5.1.15

A patient weighs 76 lb. What is this patient's weight in kilograms?

To convert the patient's weight from pounds to kilograms, recall that 1 kg equals 2.2 lb. You can then solve this problem in two ways.

Using the ratio-proportion method:

$$\frac{x \text{ kg}}{76 \text{ lb}} = \frac{1 \text{ kg}}{2.2 \text{ lb}}$$

$$x \text{ kg } (2.2 \text{ lb}) = 1 \text{ kg } (76 \text{ lb})$$

$$x \text{ kg} = 34.545 \text{ kg, rounded to } 34.5 \text{ kg}$$

Using the dimensional analysis method:

$$76 \text{ lb} \times \frac{1 \text{ kg}}{2.2 \text{ lb}} = 34.545 \text{ kg, rounded to } 34.5 \text{ kg}$$

One kilogram is approximately equal to 2.2 lb, which is slightly more than two boxes of pasta.

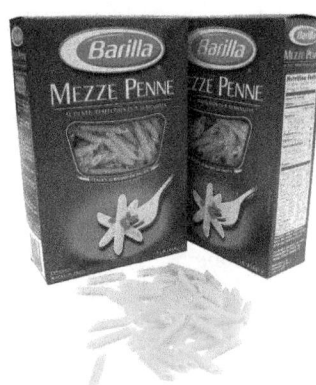

Although it is important to understand the conversion using both the ratio-proportion and the dimensional analysis methods, a shorthand method for converting a patient's weight from pounds to kilograms is to divide the patient's weight by 2.2 lb/1 kg. Similarly, you can convert a patient's weight from kilograms to pounds by multiplying it by 2.2 lb/1 kg.

Example 5.1.16

A patient weighs 58 kg. What is this patient's weight in pounds?

$$58 \text{ kg} \times \frac{2.2 \text{ lb}}{1 \text{ kg}} = 127.6 \text{ lb}$$

Check this answer by converting the answer from pounds back to kilograms.

$$127.6 \text{ lb} \times \frac{1 \text{ kg}}{2.2 \text{ lb}} = 58 \text{ kg}$$

Example 5.1.17

A patient in the neonatal ICU weighs 1,250 g. How many pounds is this?
First, convert grams to kilograms.

$$1,250 \text{ g} = 1.25 \text{ kg}$$

Second, convert kilograms to pounds.

$$1.25 \text{ kg} \times \frac{2.2 \text{ lb}}{1 \text{ kg}} = 2.75 \text{ lb}$$

Check the answer by converting the answer from pounds back to kilograms.

$$2.75 \text{ lb} \times \frac{1 \text{ kg}}{2.2 \text{ lb}} = 1.25 \text{ kg}$$

Example 5.1.18

A patient's weight is recorded as 150 and does not include units. The pharmacy technician incorrectly assumes the weight is in pounds. If the weight was reported in kg, how many pounds does the patient weigh?

$$150 \text{ kg} \times \frac{2.2 \text{ lb}}{1 \text{ kg}} = 330 \text{ lb}$$

The patient's actual weight is 180 lb more than the pharmacy technician assumed.

5.1 Problem Set

Convert the given volumes within the household measure system. Round your answer to the nearest tenth unless otherwise indicated.

1. 8 cups = _____ pt

2. 3 pt = _____ fl oz

3. 1 pt = _____ tbsp

4. 3 qt = _____ fl oz

5. 28 tsp = _____ fl oz

6. 1 pt = _____ qt

7. 6 cups = _____ tsp

Convert the given volumes between the household measure and metric systems. Round your answer to the nearest tenth unless otherwise indicated.

8. 80 mL = _____ tbsp

9. 6 fl oz = _____ mL

10. 90 mL = _____ fl oz

11. 800 mL = _____ pt

12. 53 mL = _____ tsp

13. 35 mL = _____ tsp

14. 10 L = _____ gal

15. 4 tbsp = _____ mL

16. 15 mL = _____ tsp

17. 720 mL = _____ pt

18. 30 tsp = _____ mL

19. 120 mL = _____ fl oz

20. ½ gal = _____ mL

21. 2 L = _____ pt

Convert the following commonly used volumes to milliliters. Round your answer to the nearest tenth unless otherwise indicated.

22. 3 tbsp = _____ mL

23. 1 fl oz = _____ mL

24. 2 fl oz = _____ mL

25. 3 fl oz = _____ mL

26. 4 fl oz = _____ mL

27. 5 fl oz = _____ mL

28. 6 fl oz = _____ mL

29. 7 fl oz = _____ mL

30. 8 fl oz = _____ mL

31. 12 fl oz = _____ mL

32. 16 fl oz = _____ mL

Convert the following weights between the household measure and metric systems. Round your answer to the nearest tenth unless otherwise indicated.

33. 2 oz = _____ g

34. 1.5 oz = _____ g

35. 8 oz = _____ g

36. 906 g = _____ lb

37. 30 g = _____ lb

38. 0.8 oz = _____ g

Convert the following patient weights from pounds to kilograms. Round your answer to the nearest tenth unless otherwise indicated.

39. 3.5 lb

40. 14 lb

41. 42 lb

42. 97 lb

43. 112 lb

44. 165 lb

45. 178 lb

46. 247 lb

Applications

In solving these problems, convert all quantities to the metric system. Round your answer to the nearest tenth unless otherwise indicated.

47. How many 1 tsp doses are in 2 pt, 6 fl oz?

48. How many 2 tsp doses are in 3 cups?

49. How many 1 tbsp doses are in 12 bottles containing 16 fl oz each?

50. How many 5 mL doses are in a 5 fl oz bottle?

51. How many 3 tsp doses are in 1 pt?

52. A dose of 1.5 fl oz is to be given three times daily. How many milliliters will be given in one day?

53. How many 1½ tsp doses are in an 8 fl oz bottle of cough syrup?

Use the following label to answer questions 54 and 55. Round your answer to the nearest tenth unless otherwise indicated.

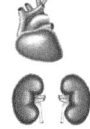
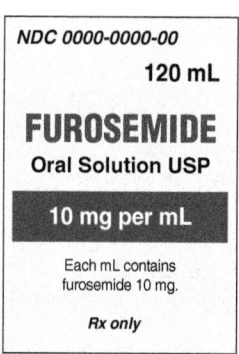

NDC 0000-0000-00

120 mL

FUROSEMIDE
Oral Solution USP

10 mg per mL

Each mL contains
furosemide 10 mg.

Rx only

54. A prescription states that a patient is to take ½ tsp of furosemide oral solution daily. Using the furosemide label shown above, how many milligrams are in a dose?

55. Using the furosemide label shown above, how many days will a 4 fl oz bottle last a patient taking 20 mg daily?

Use the following label to answer questions 56 and 57. Round your answer to the nearest tenth unless otherwise indicated.

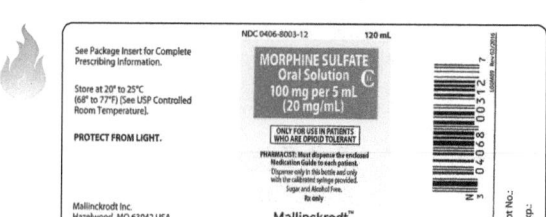

56. A prescription states that a patient is to take 2.5 mL morphine sulfate oral solution four times daily as needed for pain. Using the provided label, calculate the equivalent dose measured in teaspoonsful.

57. How many days will 320 mL of morphine sulfate oral solution last if a patient is using 3 tsp daily?

58. A physician prescribes the following dose of medication for an adult patient: 2 tsp/68 kg/day. How many doses would you get in a 300 mL bottle for a patient who weighs 180 lb?

59. A physician prescribes the following dose of medication for a pediatric patient: 1 tsp/20 kg/day. How many doses will a 4 fl oz bottle provide for a 52 lb patient?

60. A nurse practitioner writes the following prescription for a laxative medication: 2 tbsp/50 kg. How many doses will a 12 fl oz bottle last for a patient who weighs 172 lb?

Self-check your work in Appendix A.

5.2 Oral Doses

It is important that pharmacy technicians master the ability to perform calculations involving oral dosing of medications. Oral medications are prescribed over other dosage forms whenever possible and appropriate because oral medications are typically safe and cost-effective. Most prescriptions taken orally come in tablet or capsule form, but liquid forms are also common. Liquid medications are used most commonly by children and adults with a disease that impairs swallowing. For all dosing calculations, accuracy of conversions from the metric to the household system, dosing amounts, and dispensing amounts need to be checked for safety as well as billing purposes.

Determining Pediatric Doses Using Dosing Tables

Not all medications that are safe and effective for adult use are appropriate for the pediatric population. As discussed in Chapter 4, formulas using the child's weight or age were used to reduce the normal adult dose to a smaller amount appropriate for the pediatric patient. Today, prescribers are reluctant to use a medication for a child unless the pharmaceutical manufacturer indicates the proper dose. A manufacturer will provide specific age- and/or weight-related prescribing guidelines for pediatric-appropriate doses of a medication as soon as its safety and effectiveness for the pediatric population have been established. These guidelines are provided in dosing tables as a dose range that is a function of the patient's weight and/or age. When a recommended dose is not provided, the reason is often that the Food and Drug Administration has not approved the particular drug for use in children. The dosing tables are satisfactory for many purposes, but when a more accurate calculation is needed, you must use either the weight-based dosing method or the body surface area (BSA) dosing method (discussed in Chapter 4).

A typical **dosing table** includes an age range and/or a weight range with corresponding doses. Dosing tables are used for both oral liquids and solid dosage forms, but oral liquids are easier for young patients to take and thus are more common.

Dosing tables often appear on over-the-counter (OTC) packaging for products used for children older than age two. For medications used for children under age two, the instruction "Consult your physician" appears. The table for children under age two is available to healthcare providers in pharmacies and physicians' offices. Physicians often instruct parents to purchase OTC medications for small children, so appropriate dosing instructions must be provided for these patients. Dosing may need to be translated from metric units to household measure units. Use the dosing information in Tables 5.3 and 5.4 to complete the following examples.

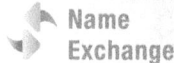

Name Exchange

The generic drug acetaminophen is commonly known by the brand name Tylenol.

TABLE 5.3 Pediatric Acetaminophen Dosing

Age	Dose
0–3 mo	40 mg
4–11 mo	80 mg
1–2 yr	120 mg
2–3 yr	160 mg
4–5 yr	240 mg
6–8 yr	320 mg
9–10 yr	400 mg
11 yr to adult	480 mg
adult maximum	4,000 mg daily

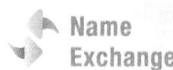

Name Exchange

The generic drug ibuprofen is commonly known by the brand name Ibuprofen or Motrin.

TABLE 5.4 Pediatric Ibuprofen Dosing

Age	Weight	Dose
6–11 mo	12–17 lb	50 mg
12–23 mo	18–23 lb	75 mg
2–3 yr	24–35 lb	100 mg
4–5 yr	36–47 lb	150 mg
6–8 yr	48–59 lb	200 mg
9–10 yr	60–71 lb	250 mg
11 yr	72–95 lb	300 mg

Example 5.2.1

A 12-month-old child weighing 22 lb is to receive one dose of acetaminophen. According to the dosing information in Table 5.3, what is an appropriate dose?

Because the acetaminophen dosing is by age, not weight, use dosing for the age category 1–2 yr. The appropriate dose would be 120 mg.

Example 5.2.2

A parent wants to give her 15-month-old child, who weighs 21 lb, an appropriate dose of OTC ibuprofen. The package provides the dosing information in Table 5.4. What is the appropriate dose?

The dose can be determined by either age or weight, and for this child, the dosing would be the same. The appropriate dose would be 75 mg.

Example 5.2.3

A parent is instructed to give his 4-year-old child acetaminophen alternating with ibuprofen. What is an appropriate dose for each drug?

The acetaminophen dose would be 240 mg, and the ibuprofen dose would be 150 mg.

Dispensing Liquid Medications

Many oral liquid medications are actually solids, suspended in a liquid. These suspensions are often indicated by the number of milligrams of solid drug particle per milliliter of solution. For example, amoxicillin is available as a 125 mg/5 mL oral liquid. In other words, 5 mL of the liquid contains 125 mg of amoxicillin.

Oral liquid medications are most often dosed by teaspoonful, tablespoonful, fluid ounces, or—in the metric system—milliliters. Being able to convert accurately between household measure and the metric measure system is, therefore, a necessary skill for the pharmacy technician when working with liquid medications. When calculating volumes of oral medication, it is best to convert everything into the same units. The preferred method is to use the metric system. Patient instructions will usually indicate teaspoonsful if the amount is an even half or full teaspoonful. However, the instructions should indicate milliliters if the dose is not easily measured using the household system. An oral syringe, as shown in Figure 5.3, is helpful to patients dosing oral liquids using the metric or household system.

Usually, an oral liquid medication's written prescription includes a specific volume to be given at each dose, as well as the total volume to be dispensed. It is important to have a working knowledge of the volumes of oral liquid medications that are commonly prescribed. Most frequently, the dosage amount is between 2 mL and 60 mL, or roughly 1/2 tsp to 2 fl oz.

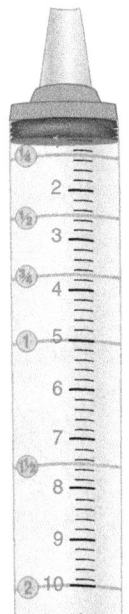

FIGURE 5.3
Oral Syringe

This oral syringe is marked with both household and metric units of measure.

Example 5.2.4

The pharmacy receives a prescription for 100 mg of amoxicillin to be taken three times daily for 10 days. The pharmacy has a 150 mL bottle of 125 mg/5 mL amoxicillin. How many milliliters of the suspension will be dispensed, and what will the patient's dosing instructions on the label state?

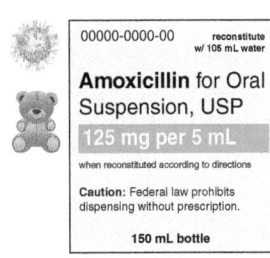

Determine what quantity of suspension contains 100 mg amoxicillin. This can be solved in two ways.

Using the ratio-proportion method:

$$\frac{x \text{ mL}}{100 \text{ mg}} = \frac{5 \text{ mL}}{125 \text{ mg}}$$

$$x \text{ mL} = 4 \text{ mL}$$

Using the amount determined for a single dose, calculate the total amount of suspension to be dispensed for 10 days.

$$\frac{4 \text{ mL}}{\text{dose}} \times \frac{3 \text{ doses}}{\text{day}} \times 10 \text{ days} = 120 \text{ mL}$$

Using the dimensional analysis method:

$$\frac{100 \text{ mg}}{\text{dose}} \times \frac{3 \text{ doses}}{\text{day}} \times \frac{10 \text{ days}}{1} \times \frac{5 \text{ mL}}{125 \text{ mg}} = 120 \text{ mL}$$

The patient's instructions will state, "Take 4 mL three times daily for 10 days." The patient will need a dosing syringe to dispense the required amount of medication.

Example 5.2.5

If a 12 fl oz bottle of mouthwash contains 0.75 g of the active ingredient, how many milligrams will be in a 1 tbsp dose?

This problem can be solved in two ways.

Using the ratio-proportion method:

Begin to solve the problem by converting all of the household measure units to metric units.

$$12 \text{ fl oz} = 360 \text{ mL}$$

$$1 \text{ tbsp} = 15 \text{ mL}$$

Also, convert 0.75 g to 750 mg. Using these converted values, set up a proportion.

$$\frac{x \text{ mg}}{15 \text{ mL}} = \frac{750 \text{ mg}}{360 \text{ mL}}$$

$$x \text{ mg} = 31.25 \text{ mg}$$

Using the dimensional analysis method:

$$\frac{1 \text{ tbsp}}{1} \times \frac{0.75 \text{ g}}{12 \text{ fl oz}} \times \frac{1 \text{ fl oz}}{2 \text{ tbsp}} \times \frac{1000 \text{ mg}}{\text{g}} = 31.25 \text{ mg, rounded to } 31.2 \text{ mg}$$

Example 5.2.6

The pharmacy receives a prescription for amoxicillin suspension 1 g bid. The pharmacy has a supply of amoxicillin 250 mg/5 mL. How many milliliters are in one dose? What will the patient's dosing instructions on the bottle label indicate?

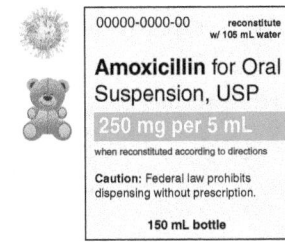

Using the ratio-proportion method:

First, determine how many milligrams are needed for one dose.

$$1 \text{ g} = 1{,}000 \text{ mg}$$

Then calculate what quantity of suspension contains 1,000 mg.

$$\frac{x \text{ mL}}{1{,}000 \text{ mg}} = \frac{5 \text{ mL}}{250 \text{ mg}}$$

$$x \text{ mL} = 20 \text{ mL}$$

Using the dimensional analysis method:

$$\frac{1 \cancel{\text{ g}}}{\text{dose}} \times \frac{1{,}000 \cancel{\text{ mg}}}{1 \cancel{\text{ g}}} \times \frac{5 \text{ mL}}{250 \cancel{\text{ mg}}} = 20 \text{ mL}$$

Convert the amount in milliliters to teaspoonsful: 5 mL = 1 tsp, so 20 mL = 4 tsp. The patient's instructions will state, "Take 20 mL (or 4 teaspoonsful) two times daily."

Example 5.2.7

A patient is to take 7 mL of amoxicillin 250 mg/5 mL. How many milligrams are present in one dose?

Using the ratio-proportion method:

$$\frac{x \text{ mg}}{7 \text{ mL}} = \frac{250 \text{ mg}}{5 \text{ mL}}$$

$$x \text{ mg} = 350 \text{ mg}$$

Using the dimensional analysis method:

$$7 \cancel{\text{ mL}} \times \frac{250 \text{ mg}}{5 \cancel{\text{ mL}}} = 350 \text{ mg}$$

Example 5.2.8

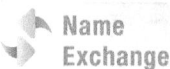
A patient is taking 4 tsp of diphenhydramine elixir at bedtime. He wishes to take oral capsules instead of the elixir. The 12.5 mg/5 mL elixir comes in a 4 fl oz bottle and is 14% alcohol. The 25 mg capsules come in a 100 count bottle. How many capsules will he need to take to equal the dose in the 4 tsp of elixir?

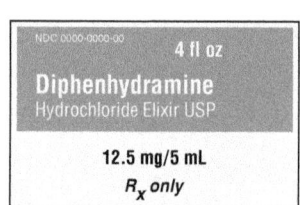

Using the ratio-proportion method:

$$\frac{x \text{ mg}}{20 \text{ mL}} = \frac{12.5 \text{ mg}}{5 \text{ mL}}$$

$$x \text{ mg} = 50 \text{ mg}$$

Now, compare the milligrams to the alternative capsule product.

$$\frac{x \text{ capsules}}{50 \text{ mg}} = \frac{1 \text{ capsule}}{25 \text{ mg}}$$

$$x \text{ capsule} = 2 \text{ capsules}$$

Using the dimensional analysis method:

$$\frac{4 \text{ tsp}}{1} \times \frac{5 \text{ mL}}{1 \text{ tsp}} \times \frac{12.5 \text{ mg}}{5 \text{ mL}} \times \frac{1 \text{ capsule}}{25 \text{ mg}} = 2 \text{ capsules}$$

Because the patient's dose is 50 mg, and the capsules come in 25 mg, he will need to take two capsules to provide the proper amount of the drug.

Example 5.2.9

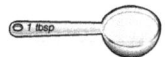
How many milligrams of medication are in 1 tbsp of clarithromycin that contains 125 mg/tsp?

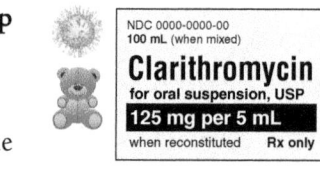

Using the ratio-proportion method:

Convert both volumes to the metric system using the following values from Table 5.2.

$$1 \text{ tbsp} = 15 \text{ mL}$$

$$1 \text{ tsp} = 5 \text{ mL}$$

$$\frac{x \text{ mg}}{15 \text{ mL}} = \frac{125 \text{ mg}}{5 \text{ mL}}$$

$$x \text{ mg} = 375 \text{ mg}$$

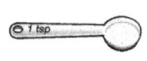

1 tbsp ≈ 15 mL

1 tsp ≈ 5 mL

Using the dimensional analysis method:

$$\frac{1 \text{ tbsp}}{1} \times \frac{15 \text{ mL}}{1 \text{ tbsp}} \times \frac{125 \text{ mg}}{5 \text{ mL}} = 375 \text{ mg}$$

Calculating the Volume to Dispense

The length of time that a volume of dispensed medication will last the patient must be determined when the prescription is entered into the patient's computerized record. Pharmacies typically bill liquid medications by the milliliter and solid medications by the unit, such as a tablet. Insurance companies require claims for reimbursement for prescription drugs to include the volume of the medication dispensed as well as the number of days that the dispensed volume should last. The volume dispensed is usually indicated by the prescriber; however, if it is not indicated, the volume to be dispensed is calculated by multiplying the volume of the medication needed for a single day by the number of days of treatment. Not only is the dispensed volume needed for insurance purposes, but the pharmacy also needs to ensure that the patient is receiving enough medication to last for the duration of treatment, whether the medication is in liquid or solid form.

Example 5.2.10

A patient is taking 2 tsp of medication every 8 hours. He has a 6 fl oz bottle of medication. How much medication will the patient take in one day, and how many days will the medication last?

Using dimensional analysis:

Multiple Step Method

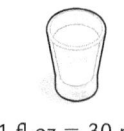

1 tsp = 5 mL

1 fl oz = 30 mL

Begin by converting all of the stated volumes to the metric system using the conversion values in Table 5.2.

$$1 \text{ tsp} = 5 \text{ mL}; \text{ therefore, } 2 \text{ tsp/dose} = 10 \text{ mL/dose}$$

$$1 \text{ fl oz} = 30 \text{ mL}; \text{ therefore, } 6 \text{ fl oz/bottle} = 180 \text{ mL/bottle}$$

Next, determine how much medication is needed for one day of treatment. The dose is every 8 hours, and there are 24 hours in a day, so

$$\frac{24 \text{ hours}}{\text{day}} \times \frac{1 \text{ dose}}{8 \text{ hours}} = \frac{3 \text{ doses}}{\text{day}}$$

$$\frac{3 \text{ doses}}{\text{day}} \times \frac{10 \text{ mL}}{\text{dose}} = \frac{30 \text{ mL}}{\text{day}}$$

Finally, calculate the number of days the medication will last.

$$\frac{180 \text{ mL}}{\text{bottle}} \times \frac{1 \text{ day}}{30 \text{ mL}} = \frac{6 \text{ days}}{\text{bottle}}$$

One Step Method

$$\frac{6 \text{ fl oz}}{\text{bottle}} \times \frac{30 \text{ mL}}{1 \text{ fl oz}} \times \frac{1 \text{ tsp}}{5 \text{ mL}} \times \frac{8 \text{ hr}}{2 \text{ tsp}} \times \frac{1 \text{ day}}{24 \text{ hours}} = \frac{6 \text{ days}}{\text{bottle}}$$

Example 5.2.11

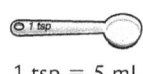

1 tsp = 5 mL

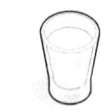

1 fl oz = 30 mL

A patient is to take 1 tsp of a medication twice daily, and she has a 4 fl oz bottle of medication. How many milliliters of medication will the patient take in one day, and how many days will the medication last?

Begin by converting all of the stated volumes to the metric system using the conversion values in Table 5.2.

$$1 \text{ tsp} = 5 \text{ mL; therefore, } 1 \text{ tsp/dose} = 5 \text{ mL/dose}$$

$$1 \text{ fl oz} = 30 \text{ mL; therefore, } 4 \text{ fl oz/bottle} = 120 \text{ mL/bottle}$$

Next, determine how much medication is needed for one day.

The dose is taken twice daily, so there are 2 doses/day.

$$\frac{2 \text{ doses}}{\text{day}} \times \frac{5 \text{ mL}}{\text{dose}} = \frac{10 \text{ mL}}{\text{day}}$$

Finally, calculate the number of days the medication will last.

$$\frac{120 \text{ mL}}{\text{bottle}} \times \frac{1 \text{ day}}{10 \text{ mL}} = \frac{12 \text{ days}}{\text{bottle}}$$

Example 5.2.12

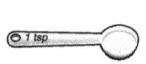

1 tsp = 5 mL

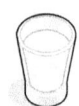

1 fl oz = 30 mL

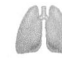

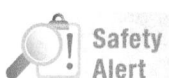

Safety Alert

The professional judgment of the pharmacist must be used in assigning a days' supply to a prescription with a prn or "as needed" instruction.

A patient has a prescription that states the following: "Take Magic Cough Syrup 1–2 tsp every 4–6 hours prn cough. Disp: 8 fl oz."
How many days will the cough syrup last?

Using dimensional analysis:

Multiple Step Method

Begin by converting all of the stated volumes to the metric system using the conversion values in Table 5.2.

$$1 \text{ tsp} = 5 \text{ mL; therefore, } 1\text{–}2 \text{ tsp/dose} = 5\text{–}10 \text{ mL/dose}$$

$$1 \text{ fl oz} = 30 \text{ mL; therefore, for this prescription calculation,}$$
$$8 \text{ fl oz/bottle} = 240 \text{ mL/bottle}$$

Next, determine how much medication is needed for one day. As prescribed, the patient will take the medication up to 6 times a day (every 4 hours). Using 6 doses a day for the calculation will give the minimum number of days the medication will last.

$$\frac{6 \text{ doses}}{\text{day}} \times \frac{10 \text{ mL}}{\text{dose}} = \frac{60 \text{ mL}}{\text{day}}$$

Finally, determine the number of days the medication will last.

$$\frac{240 \text{ mL}}{\text{bottle}} \times \frac{1 \text{ day}}{60 \text{ mL}} = \frac{4 \text{ days}}{\text{bottle}}$$

The minimum number of days the medication will last is 4. Note that the medication may last longer if the patient uses the prescription less than 6 times a day or uses 1 teaspoonful a dose instead of 2 teaspoonsful).

One Step Method

$$\frac{8 \text{ fl oz}}{1} \times \frac{30 \text{ mL}}{1 \text{ fl oz}} \times \frac{1 \text{ tsp}}{5 \text{ mL}} \times \frac{4 \text{ hr}}{2 \text{ tsp}} \times \frac{1 \text{ day}}{24 \text{ hr}} = 4 \text{ days}$$

Some prescriptions do not come with explicit instructions about how much medication is to be dispensed. The prescription may state, "Take 2 tsp every morning for 10 days." The quantity indicated on the prescription may also state, "QS," which means to dispense a "quantity sufficient" to meet the needs of the patient with the instructions given. When the duration of treatment is indicated, the volume of medication needed for a single day and the total volume to be dispensed can be calculated as demonstrated in the following examples.

Example 5.2.13

A patient comes to the pharmacy with a prescription that does not indicate a total dispensing quantity. It states, "Amoxicillin 125 mg/5 mL, 1 tsp tid for 10 days." What is the total volume of medication to be dispensed?

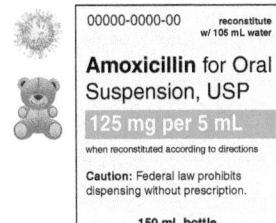

Using dimensional analysis:

Multiple Step Method

Begin by converting all of the dosage volumes to the metric system using the conversion values in Table 5.2.

$$1 \text{ tsp} = 5 \text{ mL; therefore, } 1 \text{ tsp/dose} = 5 \text{ mL/dose}$$

Next, calculate how much medication is needed for one day. Because "tid" means three times daily,

$$\frac{5 \text{ mL}}{\text{dose}} \times \frac{3 \text{ doses}}{\text{day}} = \frac{15 \text{ mL}}{\text{day}}$$

Finally, determine the volume of medication to dispense.

$$\frac{15 \text{ mL}}{\text{day}} \times 10 \text{ days} = 150 \text{ mL}$$

One Step Method

$$\frac{1 \text{ tsp}}{\text{dose}} \times \frac{3 \text{ dose}}{\text{day}} \times \frac{10 \text{ days}}{1} \times \frac{5 \text{ mL}}{1 \text{ tsp}} = 150 \text{ mL}$$

Example 5.2.14

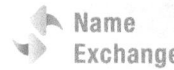
**Name
Exchange**

Fluoxetine, a
generic drug, is
widely known as
the brand name
Prozac and is
used to treat
depression.

**A patient is to take 2 tsp of fluoxetine each
morning for 30 days. How many milliliters
will be needed? How many bottles with the label
shown will be required to fill this prescription?**

Using dimensional analysis:

Multiple Step Method

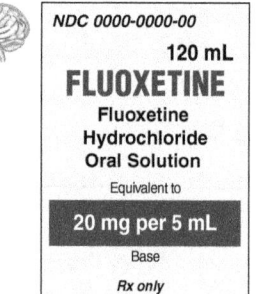

Begin by converting all of the dosage volumes to
the metric system using the conversion values in
Table 5.2 and Figure 5.2.

Because 1 tsp = 5 mL, 2 tsp/dose = 10 mL/dose.

Next, determine how many milliliters are needed for 30 days.

$$\frac{10 \text{ mL}}{\text{day}} \times 30 \text{ days} = 300 \text{ mL}$$

Finally, calculate the number of bottles of medication needed. The label indicates that each bottle contains 120 mL, so,

$$2 \text{ bottles} \times \frac{120 \text{ mL}}{\text{bottle}} = 240 \text{ mL}$$

$$3 \text{ bottles} \times \frac{120 \text{ mL}}{\text{bottle}} = 360 \text{ mL}$$

Therefore, two full bottles and part of a third bottle will be needed to fill this
prescription. (There will be 60 mL left over.)

One Step Method

This problem has two questions and therefore the one step method must be
used twice (each time to answer each question).

To find the milliliters needed,

$$\frac{2 \text{ tsp}}{\text{dose}} \times \frac{1 \text{ dose}}{\text{day}} \times \frac{30 \text{ day}}{1} \times \frac{5 \text{ mL}}{\text{tsp}} = 300 \text{ mL}$$

To find the number of bottles needed to fill the prescription,

$$\frac{300 \text{ mL}}{1} \times \frac{1 \text{ bottle}}{120 \text{ mL}} = 2.5 \text{ bottles}$$

You use the same procedure to calculate the number of tablets needed to fill a
prescription or the number of days a given prescription will last.

Example 5.2.15

 A patient has brought in a prescription for a diabetes medication. The prescription states, "Take 2 tablets before breakfast, 1 before lunch and supper, and 1 at bedtime." Determine the quantity needed for 30 days.

Begin by determining the number of tablets required for one day.

2 before breakfast + 1 before lunch + 1 before supper + 1 at bedtime = 5

The patient will take 5 tablets/day, so a 30-day supply will be

$$\frac{5\ tablets}{day} \times 30\ days = 150\ tablets$$

Example 5.2.16

A patient is to take a prescription for prednisone that uses a tapered dosing schedule. Determine the number of 5 mg tablets needed.

℞   **Prednisone 5 mg Oral Tablets**   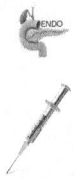
Take 40 mg for 2 days
Take 35 mg for 1 day
Take 30 mg for 2 days
Then decrease by 5 mg each day
for 5 days.

In this problem, the number of tablets taken each day changes, so the most straightforward way to determine the number of tablets needed is to make a list showing the number of tablets the patient will take each day of treatment.

$$Day\ 1:\ 40\ mg \times \frac{1\ tablet}{5\ mg} = 8\ tablets$$

$$Day\ 2:\ 40\ mg \times \frac{1\ tablet}{5\ mg} = 8\ tablets$$

$$Day\ 3:\ 35\ mg \times \frac{1\ tablet}{5\ mg} = 7\ tablets$$

$$Day\ 4:\ 30\ mg \times \frac{1\ tablet}{5\ mg} = 6\ tablets$$

$$Day\ 5:\ 30\ mg \times \frac{1\ tablet}{5\ mg} = 6\ tablets$$

$$Day\ 6:\ 25\ mg \times \frac{1\ tablet}{5\ mg} = 5\ tablets$$

$$Day\ 7:\ 20\ mg \times \frac{1\ tablet}{5\ mg} = 4\ tablets$$

$$Day\ 8:\ 15\ mg \times \frac{1\ tablet}{5\ mg} = 3\ tablets$$

$$\text{Day 9: } 10 \text{ mg} \times \frac{1 \text{ tablet}}{5 \text{ mg}} = 2 \text{ tablets}$$

$$\text{Day 10: } 5 \text{ mg} \times \frac{1 \text{ tablet}}{5 \text{ mg}} = 1 \text{ tablet}$$

The sum of the daily totals is 50 tablets for a 10-day regimen.

5.2 Problem Set

Complete the following calculations regarding aspirin dosing.

Aspirin is typically contraindicated in children. If a child is unable to take acetaminophen or ibuprofen, however, aspirin may be used. Additionally, aspirin is indicated for some conditions in children such as antiplatelet therapy and antirheumatic therapy. Items 1–4 identify the age of a child. For each child, determine the milligram dose of aspirin every 4 hours using the dosing table provided.

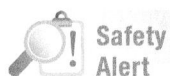

Safety Alert

Some manufacturers provide special dosing recommendations to account for patients that are overweight and in some cases, underweight.

Aspirin			
Age (years)	Weight		Dose (mg every 4 hr)
	lb	kg	
2–3	24–35	10.6–15.9	162
4–5	36–47	16–21.4	243
6–8	48–59	21.5–26.8	324
9–10	60–71	26.9–32.3	405
11	72–95	32.4–43.2	486
12–14	≥96	≥43.3	648

1. 4 years

2. 7 years

3. 10 years

4. 14 years

Complete the following calculations regarding levothyroxine dosing.

Levothyroxine is indicated for children with hypothyroidism. Many states require infants to be tested for hypothyroidism shortly after birth so that therapy can begin immediately if needed. In adult patients, the dose is adjusted up or down based on blood titers and clinical signs and symptoms. Newborn patients are more difficult to assess, so a standard dosing table based on kilograms has been developed. For items 5–8, determine the daily dose of levothyroxine for each child using the dosing table provided.

Levothyroxine	
Age	Daily dose per kg (mcg)
0–3 mo	10–15
3–6 mo	8–10
6–12 mo	6–8
1–5 yr	5–6
6–12 yr	4–5
>12 yr	2–3

5. newborn (6 lb)

6. newborn (7 lb, 12 oz)

7. 11-month-old (23 lb)

8. 15-month-old (18 lb)

Applications

Calculate the following using either the dimensional analysis method or the ratio-proportion method.

9. A patient takes 1 tsp daily of a medication with the concentration 80 mg/15 mL. How many milligrams are in one dose?

10. A patient needs to have 60 mg of medication, and the drug has the concentration 120 mg/5 mL. How many teaspoonsful will the patient take?

11. If there are 24 mg in a teaspoonful of liquid medication, how many grams are in 8 fl oz?

12. How many milligrams are in 4 fl oz of liquid medication with the concentration of 65 mg/tbsp?

13. How many milligrams are in a 2 tsp dose of liquid medication if there are 2.5 g in 2 fl oz?

14. How many milligrams are in a 1 tbsp dose of liquid medication if there are 260 mg in 600 mL?

15. A prescription is received for Drug YXZ to be taken 2 tsp bid. The required strength of the medication is 25 mg/tsp. How many grams are needed to prepare 20 fl oz?

16. A prescription is received for Drug YXZ to be taken 1 tbsp qam. The required strength of the drug is 30 mg/5 mL. How many milligrams are in a 1 tbsp dose?

17. A prescription is received for Drug YXZ to be taken 1 tbsp bid. The required strength of the medication is 40 mg/mL. How many grams are needed to prepare 1 pint of medication?

18. A patient is taking ¾ tsp of an antibiotic suspension three times a day.

    a. How long will a 150 mL bottle of antibiotic suspension last this patient?

    b. How many milliliters will be left after 10 days?

19. An antibiotic suspension is available in 80 mL, 150 mL, and 200 mL bottles.

a. What size bottle of antibiotic suspension will a patient need in order to take 1 tsp twice daily for 14 days?

b. How much antibiotic suspension will remain after 14 days?

20. How many days will a 12 fl oz bottle last if a patient takes 1 tbsp tid?

21. A patient is on an alternate-day therapy consisting of 2 tsp of a medication one day and 1 tbsp the next. How long will a 300 mL bottle last?

22. If there are 25 mg in a tablespoonful of liquid medication, how many grams are in 20 fl oz?

23. A patient uses an antacid 1 fl oz tid and hs. How many 12 fl oz bottles will this patient need to last 14 days?

24. How many prednisone 5 mg tablets are needed to fill the following prescription?

℞ **Prednisone 5 mg**
Take 4 tab × 2 days
Take 3 tab × 2 days
Take 1 tab × 1 day

25. How many milliliters of nystatin must be dispensed for the following prescription?

℞ **Nystatin Suspension**
Use 1 mL in each cheek pouch q3 h, dispense qs 10 days

26. There are 25 mg in a teaspoonful of medication. You are dispensing 12 fl oz.

a. How many milligrams will be in the bottle?

b. If the patient is to get a total of 9 g for a full therapy program, how many refills will be needed?

27. For the prescription below, how many fluid ounces of nystatin must be dispensed?

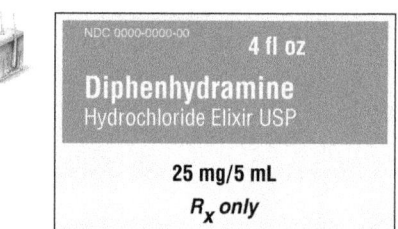

℞ **Nystatin Oral Suspension**
Take ii teaspoonsful 3 times daily for 15 days.

28. A prescription states, "Take 2 tbsp of an oral elixir three times daily for 20 days." How many milliliters should be dispensed?

Use the label below to answer questions 29 and 30.

NDC 0000-0000-00
4 fl oz
Diphenhydramine
Hydrochloride Elixir USP

25 mg/5 mL
R_x only

29. A mother has two children with poison ivy. One child takes 1 tsp tid, and the other child takes 2 tsp tid. How many bottles of diphenhydramine elixir will be needed to supply both children for 4 days?

30. How many milligrams are contained in each child's dose?

Use the label below to answer questions 31–34.

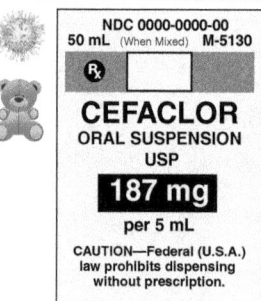

NDC 0000-0000-00
50 mL (When Mixed) M-5130
℞
CEFACLOR
ORAL SUSPENSION
USP
187 mg
per 5 mL
CAUTION—Federal (U.S.A.) law prohibits dispensing without prescription.

31. How many milligrams are in ¾ tsp?

32. How many milligrams are in 1½ tsp?

33. How many milliliters are needed to provide 125 mg?

34. How many milliliters are needed to provide 500 mg?

35. The following prescription for buttocks cream has been brought into the compounding pharmacy for compounding on January 3, 2018.

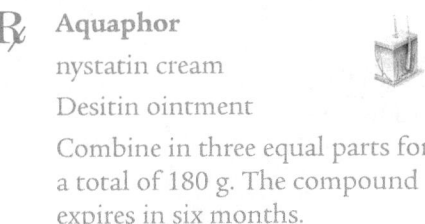

℞ **Aquaphor**

nystatin cream

Desitin ointment

Combine in three equal parts for a total of 180 g. The compound expires in six months.

a. How much of each ingredient will you use?

b. What size of ointment jar (ounces) will you use to store the compound?

c. What expiration date will you put on the compound?

36. The following order for absolute (dehydrated) alcohol has been brought into the compounding pharmacy. How many syringes will be sent to the floor?

℞ 1. Obtain a 12 fl oz bottle of absolute alcohol from the narcotics cabinet.

2. Filter through a 0.2 micron filter.

3. Send to the floor in 60 mL syringes.

Self-check your work in Appendix A.

5.3 Temperature Measurement

Temperature is a factor in dealing with chemical compounds. Two temperature scales are used to measure temperatures: the Celsius system and the Fahrenheit system. Both were developed almost 300 years ago.

Understanding Temperature Measurement Systems

Daniel Fahrenheit, a German physicist, invented an alcohol thermometer in 1709, a mercury thermometer in 1714, and a temperature scale in 1724. This temperature scale was based on ice water and salt as a low point (0 °F) and the human body temperature as the high point (100 °F). Fahrenheit used his own body temperature as the standard, but in the years that followed, scientists learned that body temperature varied. Therefore, the **Fahrenheit** scale was keyed to water for both the low point and the high point. The freezing point of water at sea level was set at 32 °F, and the boiling point of water at sea level was set at 212 °F.

In the early 1740s, Anders Celsius, a Swedish astronomer, developed what became the **Celsius**, or *centigrade*, thermometer. In Celsius measurement, water freezes at 0 °C and boils at 100 °C.

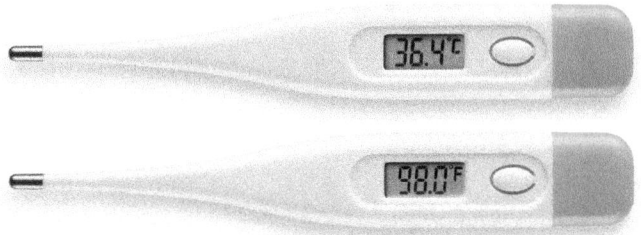

Pharmacy technicians may be asked to help patients convert between temperature readings in degrees Celsius and Fahrenheit. As with all conversions, this calculation must be done accurately.

Converting Celsius and Fahrenheit Temperatures

Both measurement systems are commonly used today. Pharmacy personnel must know the two systems and be able to convert between them. The formulas for converting from one temperature measuring system to another are based on the fact that each Celsius degree equals 1.8 or $\frac{9}{5}$ of each Fahrenheit degree. Below are the conversion formulas. Note that temperatures should be rounded to the nearest tenth.

Degrees Celsius to degrees Fahrenheit:

$$°F = \left(\frac{9 \times °C}{5}\right) + 32°$$

or

$$°F = (1.8 \times °C) + 32°$$

Degrees Fahrenheit to degrees Celsius:

$$°C = (°F - 32°) \times \frac{5}{9}$$

or

$$°C = \frac{°F - 32°}{1.8}$$

Example 5.3.1

Convert 40 °C to its equivalent in the Fahrenheit scale.

Solution 1:

$$°F = \left(\frac{9 \times °C}{5}\right) + 32°$$

$$= \left(\frac{9 \times 40°}{5}\right) + 32°$$

$$= \frac{360°}{5} + 32°$$

$$= 72° + 32°$$

$$= 104 °F$$

Solution 2:

$$°F = (1.8 \times °C) + 32°$$

$$= (1.8 \times 40°) + 32°$$

$$= 72° + 32°$$

$$= 104 °F$$

Example 5.3.2

Convert 82 °F to its equivalent in the Celsius scale.

Solution 1:

$$°C = (°F - 32°) \times \frac{5}{9}$$

$$= (82° - 32°) \times \frac{5}{9}$$

$$= 50° \times \frac{5}{9}$$

$$= 27.777 \text{ °C, rounded to } 27.8 \text{ °C}$$

Solution 2:

$$°C = \frac{(°F - 32°)}{1.8}$$

$$= \frac{(82° - 32°)}{1.8}$$

$$= \frac{50°}{1.8}$$

$$= 27.777 \text{ °C, rounded to } 27.8 \text{ °C}$$

Monitoring Temperature in Pharmacy Practice

Medications are required to be stored under specific temperature conditions. Some medication must be stored in refrigerated conditions. Refrigerated conditions are defined as being between 2 °C and 5 °C (35.6 °F and 41 °F). Other medications must be stored in freezing conditions. Freezers for medication storage should be maintained at temperatures between −25 °C and −10 °C (−13 °F and 14 °F). Storing drugs outside of recommended temperature conditions compromises quality and safety. Pharmacy refrigerators and freezers for medication storage should be monitored and the temperatures should be logged daily.

Many pharmacies use specific charts for recording temperatures of refrigerators and freezers used for drug storage. See Figure 5.4 and Figure 5.5 on the following page for examples of these charts.

FIGURE 5.4 Drug Storage Refrigerator Temperature Chart (Celsius)

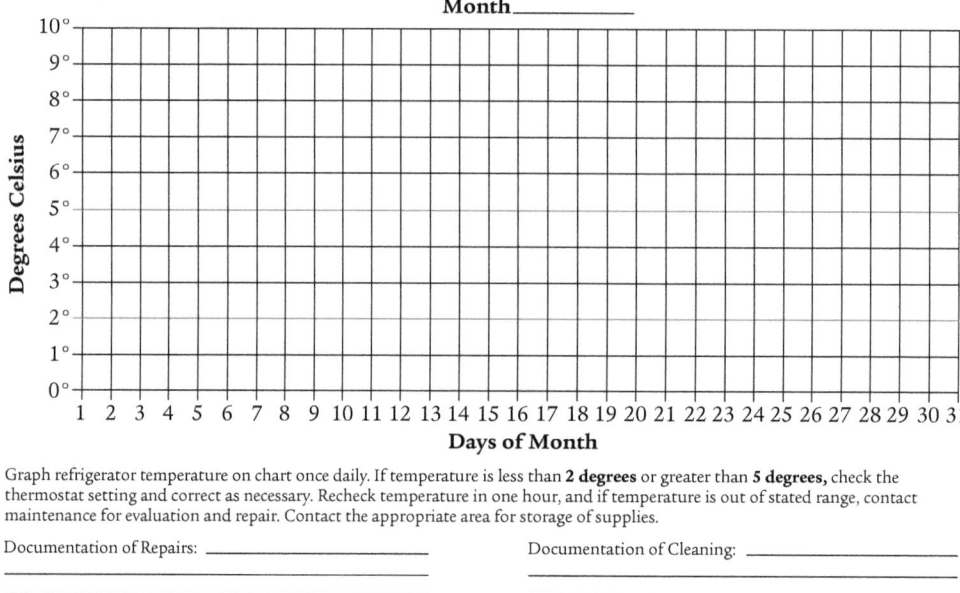

Graph refrigerator temperature on chart once daily. If temperature is less than **2 degrees** or greater than **5 degrees,** check the thermostat setting and correct as necessary. Recheck temperature in one hour, and if temperature is out of stated range, contact maintenance for evaluation and repair. Contact the appropriate area for storage of supplies.

Documentation of Repairs: _____   Documentation of Cleaning: _____

FIGURE 5.5 Drug Storage Refrigerator Temperature Chart (Fahrenheit)

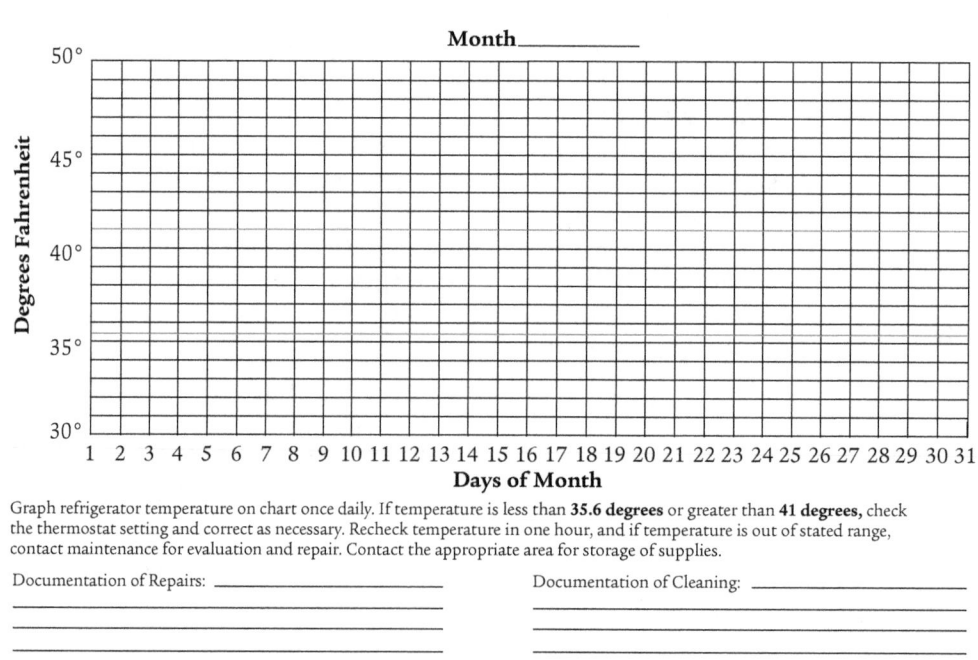

Graph refrigerator temperature on chart once daily. If temperature is less than **35.6 degrees** or greater than **41 degrees,** check the thermostat setting and correct as necessary. Recheck temperature in one hour, and if temperature is out of stated range, contact maintenance for evaluation and repair. Contact the appropriate area for storage of supplies.

Documentation of Repairs: _____   Documentation of Cleaning: _____

Convert the following Fahrenheit temperatures to Celsius. Round the temperatures to the nearest tenth.

1. 0 °F

2. 23 °F

3. 36 °F

4. 40 °F

5. 64 °F

6. 72 °F

7. 98.6 °F

8. 100.5 °F

9. 102.8 °F

10. 105 °F

Convert the following Celsius temperatures to Fahrenheit. Round the temperatures to the nearest tenth.

11. −15 °C

12. 18 °C

13. 27 °C

14. 31 °C

15. 38 °C

16. 40 °C

17. 49 °C

18. 63 °C

19. 99.8 °C

20. 101.4 °C

Applications

21. When making a mixture, you are instructed to heat the mixture to 130 °C. You have only a Fahrenheit thermometer. What is the equivalent temperature on the Fahrenheit scale?

22. The following prescription is sent to the hospital pharmacy:

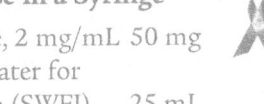

R̸   **Alteplase in a Syringe**

alteplase, 2 mg/mL 50 mg
sterile water for
injection (SWFI)   25 mL

1. Reconstitute the alteplase with SWFI.

2. Draw up 5 mL in 10 mL syringes.

3. Label syringes with contents, concentration, and date of preparation.

4. Place syringes in freezer.

The syringes are stable for six months, or 180 days, −20° C.

a. What is the Fahrenheit temperature at which you should store this product?

b. What expiration date should you put on this compound if today is February 1, 2018?

23. A compounding pharmacy is required to dry heat sterilize some of their supplies in a 300 °F oven for 12 hours. At what Celsius temperature does the oven need to be set?

24. Convert the following refrigerator temperatures and log them on the Celsius chart. Round the temperatures to the nearest tenth, and note any temperatures out of the safe range.

Date	Degrees F	Degrees C
5/5	36.1°	a. _____
5/6	37.7°	b._____
5/7	39.0°	c. _____
5/8	35.7°	d._____
5/9	36.9°	e. _____
5/10	34.9°	f. _____
5/11	36.4°	g._____
5/12	36.8°	h._____
5/13	35.5°	i. _____
5/14	38.8°	j. _____

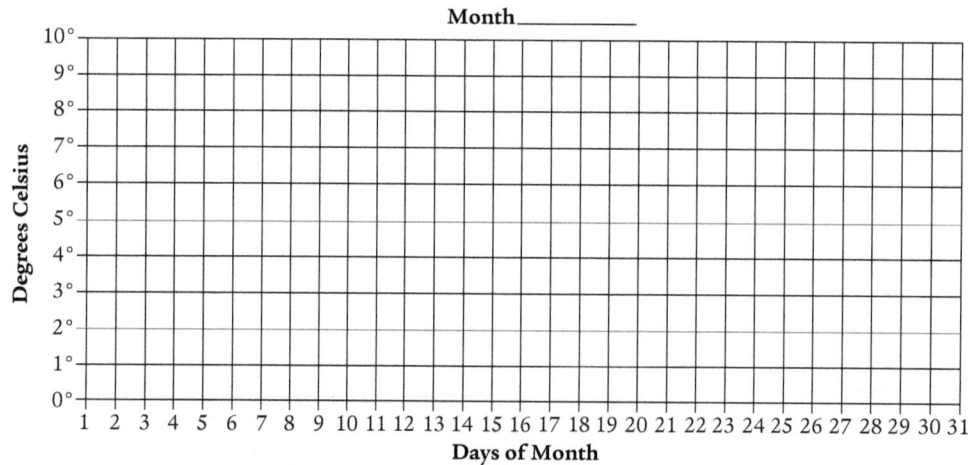

25. Convert the following refrigerator temperatures and log them on the Fahrenheit chart. Round the temperatures to the nearest tenth, and note any temperatures out of the safe range.

Date	Degrees C	Degrees F
7/12	1.8°	a. _____
7/13	3.1°	b. _____
7/14	2.8°	c. _____
7/15	3.0°	d. _____
7/16	4.5°	e. _____
7/17	3.2°	f. _____
7/18	3.9°	g. _____
7/19	2.5°	h. _____
7/20	4.1°	i. _____
7/21	4.7°	j. _____

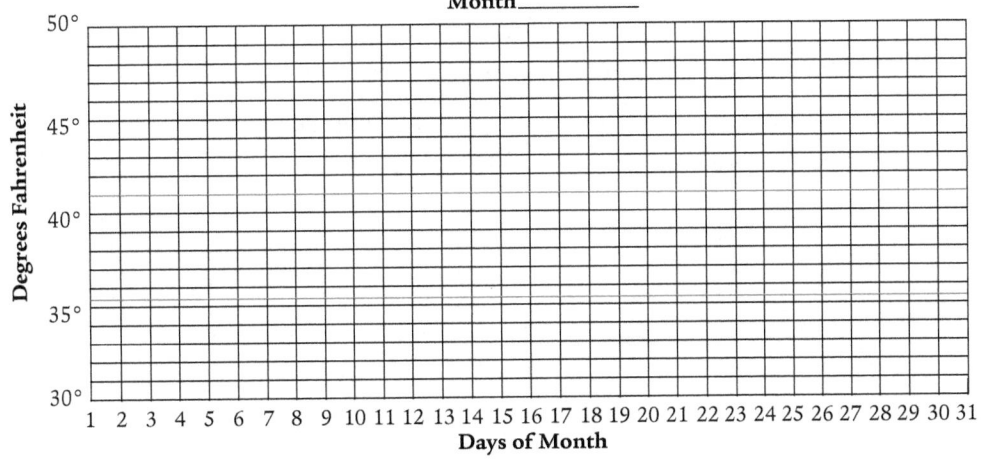

Month_____

Self-check your work in Appendix A.

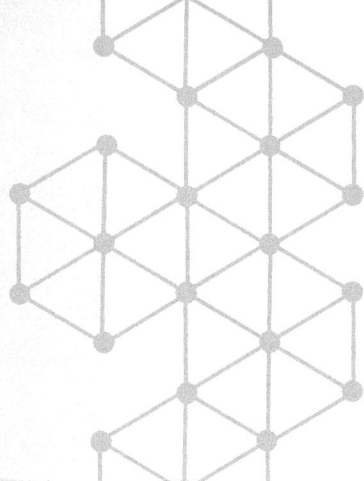

CHAPTER SUMMARY

- Patients are most familiar with household measurements such as teaspoonsful and cups.

- Household measuring devices are often less accurate than the measuring devices used in the pharmacy.

- Household measurements may be easily converted to metric using either the ratio-proportion method or the dimensional analysis method.

- Some drugs are dosed based on a patient's weight in kilograms.

- Weights measured in pounds may be converted to kilograms by dividing the pounds by 2.2.

- The preferred measurement for liquid oral doses is milliliters.

- Most oral doses are between 2 mL and 60 mL (or roughly ½ tsp to 2 fluid ounces).

- Teaspoonful and fluid ounce conversions should be memorized: 1 tsp = 5 mL, and 1 fl oz = 30 mL.

- Celsius uses a measurement system in which 0° is freezing and 100° is boiling.

- Fahrenheit uses a measurement system in which 32° is freezing and 212° is boiling.

- Temperatures in pharmacy refrigerators and freezers must be checked daily to ensure medications are being stored within the appropriate temperature ranges.

Formulas for Success

3 teaspoonsful (tsp) = 1 tablespoon (tbsp)	2 cups = 1 pint (pt)
2 tablespoonsful (tbsp) = 1 fluid ounce (fl oz)	2 pints (pt) = 1 quart (qt)
8 fluid ounces (fl oz) = 1 cup	4 quarts (qt) = 1 gallon (gal)

Celsius a thermometric scale in which 100° is the boiling point of water and 0° is the freezing point of water

dosing table a table providing dose recommendations based on the age and/or the weight of the patient; often used for determining the safe dose for a pediatric patient

Fahrenheit a thermometric scale in which 212° is the boiling point of water and 32° is the freezing point of water

household measure a system of measure used in homes, particularly in kitchens, in the United States; units of measure for volume are teaspoonful, tablespoonful, cup, pint, quart, and gallon; units for weight are ounce and pound

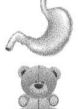

CHAPTER REVIEW

Finding Solutions

To gain practice in handling challenging situations in the workplace, consider the following real-world scenarios, and then use the guiding questions to help you formulate your responses.

Note: *To indicate your answer for Scenario A, Question 4, ask your instructor for the handout depicting an oral syringe; for Scenario B, Question 8, ask your instructor for the handout depicting a medicine cup.*

Scenario A: Lucy Ramirez, a 14-month-old patient in the pediatric unit, weighs 22 pounds. She has just been diagnosed with gastroesophageal reflux disease (GERD). Her physician has prescribed Pepcid Oral Suspension, which is dosed at 1 mg/kg per day, divided into two doses. Pepcid Oral Suspension is available in a 40 mg/5 mL strength.

1. How many kilograms does Lucy weigh?

2. How many milligrams should Lucy be taking each day?

3. How many milligrams will be given at each dose?

4. How many milliliters will be given at each dose? On the handout that you obtained from your instructor, indicate on the measuring device the amount of medication that should be administered to the child.

5. Is this dose more or less than a teaspoonful?

6. How will this volume of medication be measured accurately?

Scenario B: Antonio Rigoni has a severe skin infection that his physician wants to treat with cephalexin, an oral antibiotic. The physician wants him patient to receive a liquid suspension of cephalexin at a dosage of 4 g per day, in four divided doses. Cephalexin is available in a 250 mg/5 mL suspension.

7. How many milligrams will be given at each dose?

8. How many milliliters will be given at each dose? On the handout that you obtained from your instructor, indicate on the measuring device the amount of medication that should be administered to the patient.

9. How many teaspoonsful are in each dose?

10. How many milliliters will the patient need to complete a 10-day course of therapy?

Scenario C: A patient brings a prescription for fluoxetine 40 mg daily to the pharmacy. The patient requests the medication be filled as a liquid product. You check the pharmacy stock and see that you have fluoxetine 20 mg/5 mL.

11. How many milliliters are needed to make a 40 mg dose?

12. The patient realizes that her insurance will not pay for the liquid formula because she is an adult. You check the pharmacy stock and see you have fluoxetine 20 mg capsules in stock. How many capsules are needed to dispense a 30 days' supply?

Scenario D: You receive a prescription for a pediatric patient for cephalexin 100 mg/kg divided every 8 hours. The patient that will receive the cephalexin is 22 kg and requests a liquid dosage form. You have two concentrations of cephalexin available in the pharmacy: 250 mg/5 mL and 125 mg/5 mL.

13. How many milligrams will the patient receive with each dose?

14. What volume of each cephalexin concentration would be needed to deliver the ordered dose?

15. The manufacturer instructs cephalexin suspension be stored at 2 to 8 degrees Celsius once reconstituted. Convert this temperature range to Fahrenheit.

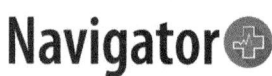

Navigator

Access interactive chapter review exercises, practice activities, flash cards, and study games.

6

Preparing Injectable Medications

Jennifer L. Babin, PharmD, BCPS

Learning Objectives

1 Calculate the volume to be measured when given a specific dose.

2 Calculate the amount of medication in a given volume.

3 Identify medications that use units as a dose designation.

4 Calculate the volume of a substance that has an electrolyte as its primary ingredient.

5 Determine the quantity of units in a given concentration and dose.

6 Calculate the volume of insulin to be administered.

 Preview chapter terms and definitions.

6.1 Parenteral Injections and Infusions

Rx Put Down Roots

Subcutaneous (Latin roots: *sub* ("under") and *cutis* ("skin") means "under the skin."
Intramuscular (Latin roots *intra* (inward) and *musculus* ("little mouse" because the shape and movement of the biceps resemble a mouse) means "within the muscle."

An **injection** is a method of administering medications in which a needle or cannula (a small tube) attached to a syringe penetrates the skin or a membrane to deposit medication into the tissue, muscle, or vessel below. An **infusion** is a type of injection in which a large volume of fluid is administered over a long period through a needle, usually into a vein. Medications given as injections or infusions are considered **parenteral**, which literally means "occurring outside the intestines." In other words, the medications do not pass through the gastrointestinal (GI) system.

There are three main types of injections: subcutaneous injections, intramuscular injections, and intravenous infusions. All three types of injections are given by healthcare professionals on a regular basis. A **subcutaneous (SC) injection** is given into the vascular, fatty layer of tissue under the layers of skin. Most medications given by this route are quickly absorbed. Patients can self-administer medications such as insulin by SC injection. An **intramuscular (IM) injection** is given into the muscle tissue. Water-soluble medications are absorbed rapidly when given intramuscularly, whereas oil-based medications are absorbed slowly. With proper training, patients can self-administer medications by IM injection, but this route requires more skill and coordination than the subcutaneous route. An **intravenous (IV) infusion** is given into a vein. Large-volume IV infusions, such as 500–1,000 mL, may be administered over a period of hours. IV infusions of

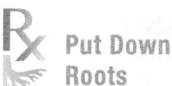

Put Down Roots

The term *intra-venous* has Latin roots. The root word *intra* means "inward," and the root word *venous* means "vein." Thus, *intravenous* describes something that occurs within the vein.

50–100 mL are often given over a period of 30–60 minutes. Smaller volumes, such as 5–30 mL, may be given via a syringe as an IV push medication over a few minutes. Most IV infusions are administered to inpatients, although they can also be given in a clinic or at home with proper training.

Medications given by injection are often ordered in milligrams, and the pharmacy or nursing staff must select and prepare an appropriate concentration of medication from available stock. The amount of medication is determined using the same methods for calculating liquid oral solutions (see Chapter 5).

When calculating the dose, personnel should choose a barrel size that will hold a total volume of 1 mL, 3 mL, 5 mL, 10 mL, 20 mL, or 50 mL. Smaller syringes are marked to indicate volume using fifths, tenths, or other fractions of a millimeter. Larger syringes are marked in one to two millimeter increments.

TAKE NOTE

Ideally, you should choose the syringe that provides the most accurate volume measurement. Typically, the smaller the syringe, the more accurate its measure. The total volume to be prepared should generally fill at least half of the syringe barrel. For example, when measuring 2.8 mL of medication, the selection of a 3 mL or 5 mL syringe would be appropriate because the 2.8 mL would fill half or more of either syringe. If you chose the 10 mL syringe for dispensing 2.8 mL, the volume of fluid might not be measured as accurately as it would be in the smaller syringes.

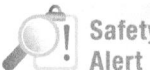

Safety Alert

Because all syringes are not marked using the same increments, become familiar with the demarcations before using a syringe to measure volume.

Calculating the Volume of an Injectable Solution

The volume of medication to be administered is calculated by both the pharmacy staff and the nursing staff who administer the medication. Some facilities prepare syringes ahead of time for the nursing staff, but others provide the vial and syringe for the nursing staff to draw up just before administration.

The following examples demonstrate how to calculate the volume of medication using the ratio-proportion and dimensional analysis methods. A small volume (less than 20 mL) is rounded to the nearest tenth or hundredth, depending on the size of the syringe barrel and its degree of accuracy. Larger volumes are rounded to the nearest tenth or whole milliliter.

Example 6.1.1

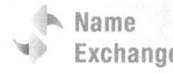

Name Exchange

The generic medication midazolam is commonly known as the brand name Versed.

How many milliliters of the medication shown in the label below must be prepared to provide 12.5 mg to a patient?

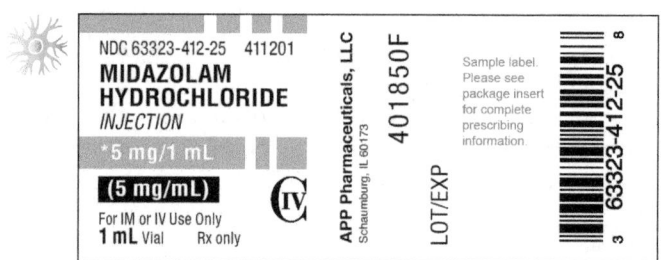

Using the ratio-proportion method:

$$\frac{12.5 \text{ mg}}{x \text{ mL}} = \frac{5 \text{ mg}}{1 \text{ mL}}$$

$$x \text{ mL} (5 \text{ mg}) = 1 \text{ mL} (12.5 \text{ mg})$$

$$\frac{x \text{ mL} (\cancel{5 \text{ mg}})}{\cancel{5 \text{ mg}}} = \frac{1 \text{ mL} (12.5 \cancel{\text{ mg}})}{5 \cancel{\text{ mg}}}$$

$$x = 2.5 \text{ mL}$$

Using the dimensional analysis method:

$$12.5 \cancel{\text{ mg}} \times \frac{1 \text{ mL}}{5 \cancel{\text{ mg}}} = 2.5 \text{ mL}$$

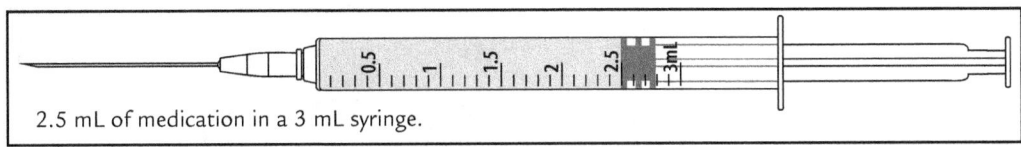

2.5 mL of medication in a 3 mL syringe.

Example 6.1.2

Name Exchange

The generic medication ondansetron is commonly known by the brand name Zofran.

How many milliliters of the medication shown in the label below must be prepared to provide 8 mg of ondansetron to a patient?

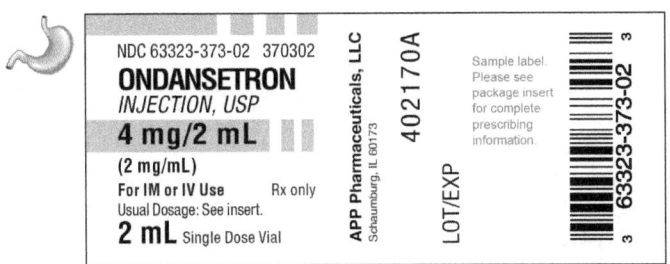

Using the ratio-proportion method:

$$\frac{8 \text{ mg}}{x \text{ mL}} = \frac{4 \text{ mg}}{2 \text{ mL}}$$

$$x \text{ mL} (4 \text{ mg}) = 2 \text{ mL} (8 \text{ mg})$$

$$\frac{x \text{ mL} (\cancel{4 \text{ mg}})}{\cancel{4 \text{ mg}}} = \frac{2 \text{ mL} (8 \cancel{\text{ mg}})}{4 \cancel{\text{ mg}}}$$

$$x = 4 \text{ mL}$$

Using the dimensional analysis method:

$$8 \cancel{\text{ mg}} \times \frac{2 \text{ mL}}{4 \cancel{\text{ mg}}} = 4 \text{ mL}$$

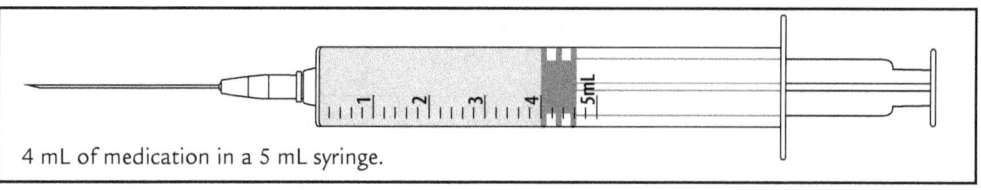

4 mL of medication in a 5 mL syringe.

Example 6.1.3

How many milliliters of medication shown in the label below must be prepared to provide 10 mg of adenosine?

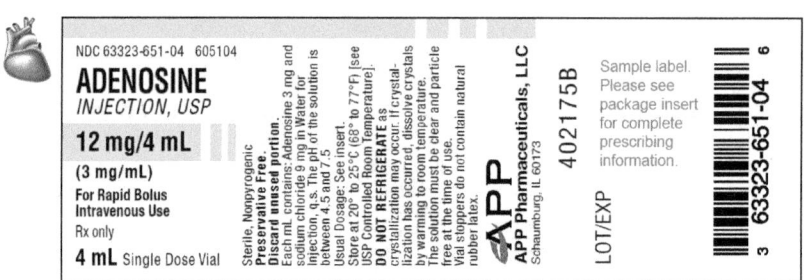

NDC 63323-651-04 605104

ADENOSINE
INJECTION, USP

12 mg/4 mL

(3 mg/mL)

For Rapid Bolus
Intravenous Use

Rx only

4 mL Single Dose Vial

Sterile, Nonpyrogenic.
Preservative Free.
Discard unused portion.
Each mL contains Adenosine 3 mg and
sodium chloride 9 mg in Water for
Injection, q.s. The pH of the solution is
between 4.5 and 7.5
Usual Dosage: See insert.
Store at 20° to 25°C (68° to 77°F) [see
USP Controlled Room Temperature].
DO NOT REFRIGERATE as
crystallization may occur: If crystal-
lization has occurred, dissolve crystals
by warming to room temperature.
The solution must be clear and particle
free at the time of use.
Vial stoppers do not contain natural
rubber latex.

APP
APP Pharmaceuticals, LLC
Schaumburg, IL 60173

402175B

LOT/EXP

Sample label.
Please see
package insert
for complete
prescribing
information.

3 63323-651-04 6

Using the ratio-proportion method:

$$\frac{10 \text{ mg}}{x \text{ mL}} = \frac{12 \text{ mg}}{4 \text{ mL}}$$

$$x \text{ mL} (12 \text{ mg}) = 4 \text{ mL} (10 \text{ mg})$$

$$\frac{x \text{ mL} (\cancel{12 \text{ mg}})}{\cancel{12 \text{ mg}}} = \frac{4 \text{ mL} (10 \cancel{\text{ mg}})}{12 \cancel{\text{ mg}}}$$

$$x = 3.3 \text{ mL}$$

Using the dimensional analysis method:

$$10 \cancel{\text{ mg}} \times \frac{4 \text{ mL}}{12 \cancel{\text{ mg}}} = 3.3 \text{ mL}$$

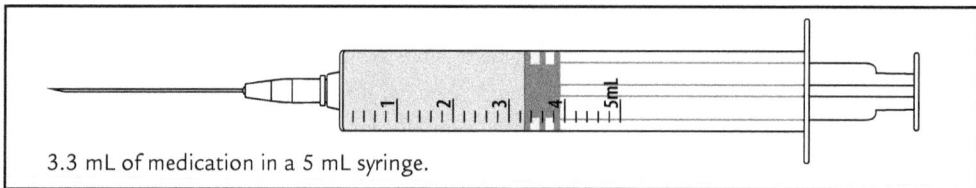

3.3 mL of medication in a 5 mL syringe.

Calculating the Quantity of Medication in an Injectable Solution

You can also use the ratio-proportion and dimensional analysis methods to determine the amount of medication in an injectable solution. The following examples demonstrate these calculations.

Example 6.1.4

How many milligrams of progesterone are in 2 mL of the solution shown in the label below?

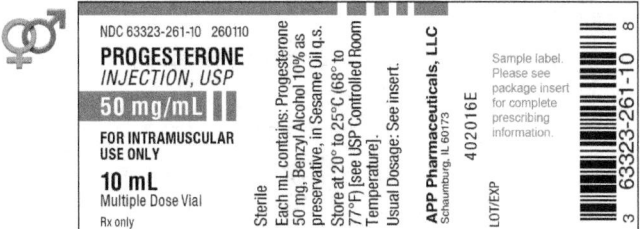

Using the ratio-proportion method:

$$\frac{2\ \text{mL}}{x\ \text{mg}} = \frac{1\ \text{mL}}{50\ \text{mg}}$$

$$x\ \text{mg}\ (1\ \text{mL}) = 50\ \text{mg}\ (2\ \text{mL})$$

$$\frac{x\ \text{mg}\ (\cancel{1\ \text{mL}})}{\cancel{1\ \text{mL}}} = \frac{50\ \text{mg}\ (2\ \cancel{\text{mL}})}{\cancel{1\ \text{mL}}}$$

$$x = 100\ \text{mg}$$

Using the dimensional analysis method:

$$2\ \cancel{\text{mL}} \times \frac{50\ \text{mg}}{1\ \cancel{\text{mL}}} = 100\ \text{mg}$$

Example 6.1.5

How many milligrams of carboplatin are in 30 mL of the solution shown in the label below?

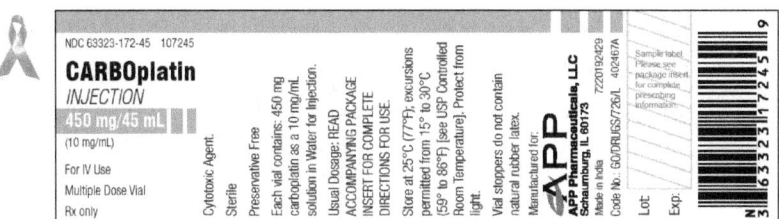

Using the ratio-proportion method:

$$\frac{30\ \text{mL}}{x\ \text{mg}} = \frac{45\ \text{mL}}{450\ \text{mg}}$$

$$x\ \text{mg}\ (45\ \text{mL}) = 450\ \text{mg}\ (30\ \text{mL})$$

$$\frac{x\ \text{mg}\ (\cancel{45\ \text{mL}})}{\cancel{45\ \text{mL}}} = \frac{450\ \text{mg}\ (30\ \cancel{\text{mL}})}{\cancel{45\ \text{mL}}}$$

$$x = 300\ \text{mg}$$

Using the dimensional analysis method:

$$30 \, \cancel{mL} \times \frac{450 \, mg}{45 \, \cancel{mL}} = 300 \, mg$$

Example 6.1.6

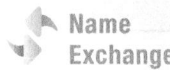

How many milligrams of furosemide are in 6 mL of the solution shown in the label below?

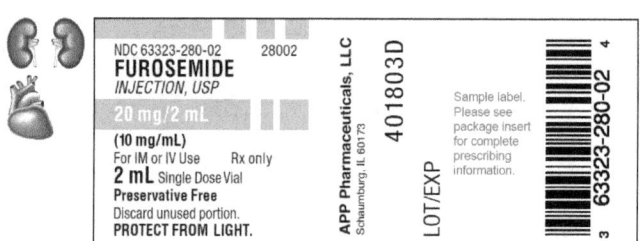

Using the ratio-proportion method:

$$\frac{6 \, mL}{x \, mg} = \frac{2 \, mL}{20 \, mg}$$

$$x \, mg \, (2 \, mL) = 20 \, mg \, (6 \, mL)$$

$$\frac{x \, mg \, (\cancel{2 \, mL})}{\cancel{2 \, mL}} = \frac{20 \, mg \, (6 \, \cancel{mL})}{2 \, \cancel{mL}}$$

$$x = 60 \, mg$$

Using the dimensional analysis method:

$$6 \, \cancel{mL} \times \frac{20 \, mg}{2 \, \cancel{mL}} = 60 \, mg$$

Calculating Ratio Strength

The **ratio strength** $a{:}b$ (read as "a to b") means there are a parts of a pure medication in b parts of a liquid solution. The units indicated in a ratio strength are always a grams:b milliliters. This formula is the same unit rule that is used to indicate the percent strength of medications (see Chapter 2). For example, a 1% solution could be written as 1:100, and the units would be 1 g:100 mL.

Example 6.1.7

How many grams of pure medication are in 500 mL of a 1:200 solution?

Using the ratio-proportion method:

$$\frac{500 \, mL}{x \, g} = \frac{200 \, mL}{1 \, g}$$

$$x \text{ g } (200 \text{ mL}) = 1 \text{ g } (500 \text{ mL})$$

$$\frac{x \text{ g } (200 \text{ mL})}{200 \text{ mL}} = \frac{1 \text{ g } (500 \text{ mL})}{200 \text{ mL}}$$

$$x = 2.5 \text{ g}$$

Using the dimensional analysis method:

$$500 \text{ mL} \times \frac{1 \text{ g}}{200 \text{ mL}} = 2.5 \text{ g}$$

Example 6.1.8

How many grams of pure medication are in 500 mL of a 1:3,000 solution?

Using the ratio-proportion method:

$$\frac{500 \text{ mL}}{x \text{ g}} = \frac{3,000 \text{ mL}}{1 \text{ g}}$$

$$x \text{ g } (3,000 \text{ mL}) = 1 \text{ g } (500 \text{ mL})$$

$$\frac{x \text{ g } (3,000 \text{ mL})}{3,000 \text{ mL}} = \frac{1 \text{ g } (500 \text{ mL})}{3,000 \text{ mL}}$$

$$x = 0.17 \text{ g}$$

Using the dimensional analysis method

$$500 \text{ mL} \times \frac{1 \text{ g}}{3,000 \text{ mL}} = 0.17 \text{ g}$$

Example 6.1.9

 How many milligrams of pure medication are in 1.5 mL of a 1:1,000 solution of epinephrine?

Using the ratio-proportion method:

First solve the problem in grams.

$$\frac{1.5 \text{ mL}}{x \text{ g}} = \frac{1,000 \text{ mL}}{1 \text{ g}}$$

$$x \text{ g } (1,000 \text{ mL}) = 1 \text{ g } (1.5 \text{ mL})$$

$$\frac{x \text{ g } (1,000 \text{ mL})}{1,000 \text{ mL}} = \frac{1 \text{ g } (1.5 \text{ mL})}{1,000 \text{ mL}}$$

$$x = 0.0015 \text{ g}$$

Next, convert to milligrams.

$$\frac{0.0015 \text{ g}}{x \text{ mg}} = \frac{1 \text{ g}}{1,000 \text{ mg}}$$

$$x \text{ mg } (1 \text{ g}) = 1,000 \text{ mg } (0.0015 \text{ g})$$

$$\frac{x \text{ mg } (\cancel{1 \text{ g}})}{\cancel{1 \text{ g}}} = \frac{1,000 \text{ mg } (0.0015 \cancel{\text{ g}})}{1 \cancel{\text{ g}}}$$

$$x = 1.5 \text{ mg}$$

Or simply move the decimal point three places to the right:

$$0.0015 \text{ g} = 1.5 \text{ mg}$$

Using the dimensional analysis method:

$$1.5 \cancel{\text{ mL}} \times \frac{1 \cancel{\text{ g}}}{1,000 \cancel{\text{ mL}}} \times \frac{1,000 \text{ mg}}{1 \cancel{\text{ g}}} = 1.5 \text{ mg}$$

Example 6.1.10

How many milligrams of pure medication are in 3 mL of a 1:2,500 solution?

Using the ratio-proportion method:

First solve the problem in grams.

$$\frac{3 \text{ mL}}{x \text{ g}} = \frac{2,500 \text{ mL}}{1 \text{ g}}$$

$$x \text{ g } (2,500 \text{ mL}) = 1 \text{ g } (3 \text{ mL})$$

$$\frac{x \text{ g } (\cancel{2,500 \text{ mL}})}{\cancel{2,500 \text{ mL}}} = \frac{1 \text{ g } (3 \cancel{\text{ mL}})}{2,500 \cancel{\text{ mL}}}$$

$$x = 0.0012 \text{ g}$$

Now convert to milligrams.

$$\frac{0.0012 \text{ g}}{x \text{ mg}} = \frac{1 \text{ g}}{1,000 \text{ mg}}$$

$$x \text{ mg } (1 \text{ g}) = 1,000 \text{ mg } (0.0012 \text{ g})$$

$$\frac{x \text{ mg } (\cancel{1 \text{ g}})}{\cancel{1 \text{ g}}} = \frac{1,000 \text{ mg } (0.0012 \cancel{\text{ g}})}{1 \cancel{\text{ g}}}$$

$$x = 1.2 \text{ mg}$$

Or simply move the decimal three places to the right:

$$0.0012 \text{ g} = 1.2 \text{ mg}$$

Using the dimensional analysis method:

$$3\ \text{mL} \times \frac{1\ \text{g}}{2,500\ \text{mL}} \times \frac{1,000\ \text{mg}}{1\ \text{g}} = 1.2\ \text{mg}$$

Example 6.1.11

How many milliliters are needed to provide 0.75 g of a medication if the solution available is 1:2,000?

Using the ratio-proportion method:

$$\frac{0.75\ \text{g}}{x\ \text{mL}} = \frac{1\ \text{g}}{2,000\ \text{mL}}$$

$$x\ \text{mL}\ (1\ \text{g}) = 2,000\ \text{mL}\ (0.75\ \text{g})$$

$$\frac{x\ \text{mL}\ (1\ \text{g})}{1\ \text{g}} = \frac{2,000\ \text{mL}\ (0.75\ \text{g})}{1\ \text{g}}$$

$$x = 1,500\ \text{mL}$$

Using the dimensional analysis method:

$$0.75\ \text{g} \times \frac{2,000\ \text{mL}}{1\ \text{g}} = 1,500\ \text{mL}$$

Example 6.1.12

How many milliliters are needed to provide 20 mg of a medication if the solution available is 1:500?

Begin by converting 20 mg to 0.02 g.

Using the ratio-proportion method:

$$\frac{0.02\ \text{g}}{x\ \text{mL}} = \frac{1\ \text{g}}{500\ \text{mL}}$$

$$x\ \text{mL}\ (1\ \text{g}) = 500\ \text{mL}\ (0.02\ \text{g})$$

$$\frac{x\ \text{mL}\ (1\ \text{g})}{1\ \text{g}} = \frac{500\ \text{mL}\ (0.02\ \text{g})}{1\ \text{g}}$$

$$x = 10\ \text{mL}$$

Using the dimensional analysis method:

$$0.02\ \text{g} \times \frac{500\ \text{mL}}{1\ \text{g}} = 10\ \text{mL}$$

6.1 Problem Set

Determine the volume to be prepared for each ordered injectable solution using the labels provided. (Round to the nearest hundredth.)

Note: *Questions 1–10 have accompanying handouts that you must obtain from your instructor.*

1. How many milliliters of solution are needed to provide 50 mg of Xylocaine? On the handout that you obtained from your instructor, indicate the correct volume on the measuring device.

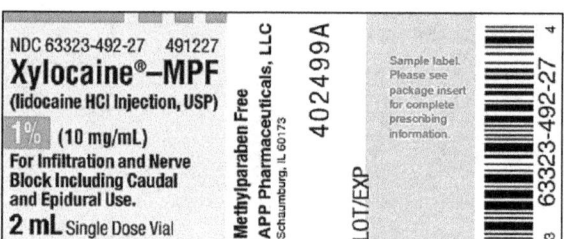

2. How many milliliters of solution are needed to provide 60 mg of furosemide? On the handout that you obtained from your instructor, indicate the correct volume on the measuring device.

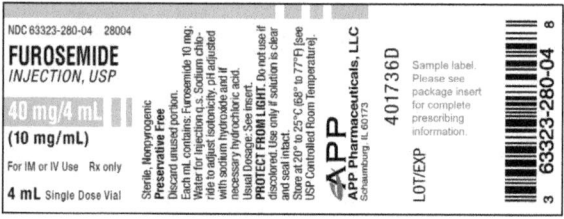

3. How many milliliters of solution are needed to provide 80 mg of furosemide? On the handout that you obtained from your instructor, indicate the correct volume on the measuring device.

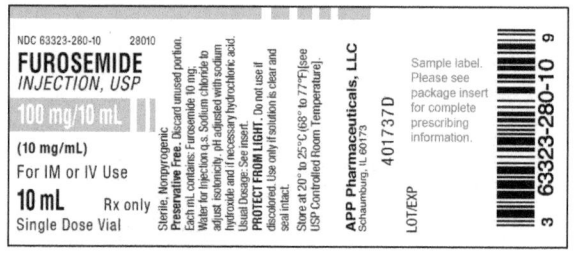

4. How many milliliters of solution are needed to provide 0.75 mg of indomethacin in this 1 mg/1 mL vial? On the handout that you obtained from your instructor, indicate the correct volume on the measuring device.

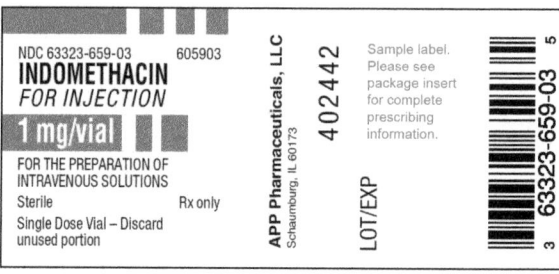

5. How many milliliters of solution are needed to provide 100 mg of diphenhydramine? On the handout that you obtained from your instructor, indicate the correct volume on the measuring device.

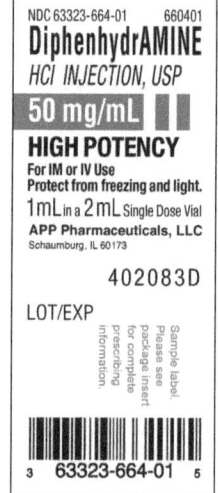

6. How many milliliters of solution are needed to provide 30 mg of famotidine? On the handout that you obtained from your instructor, indicate the correct volume on the measuring device.

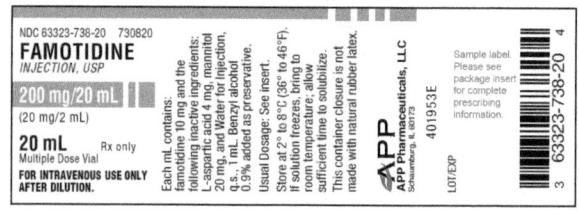

7. How many milliliters of solution are needed to provide 40 mg of famotidine? On the handout that you obtained from your instructor, indicate the correct volume on the measuring device.

8. How many milliliters of solution are needed to provide 250 mg of azithromycin? On the handout that you obtained from your instructor, indicate the correct volume on the measuring device.

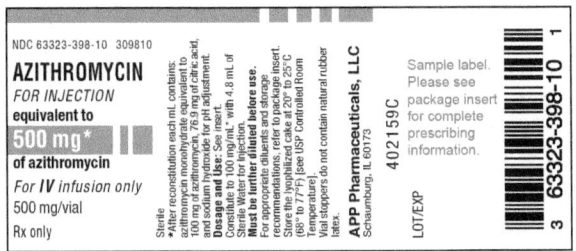

9. How many milliliters of solution are needed to provide 400 mg of azithromycin? On the handout that you obtained from your instructor, indicate the correct volume on the measuring device.

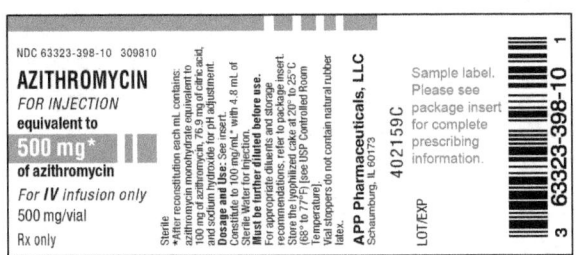

10. How many milliliters of solution are needed to provide 50 mg of cisplatin? On the handout that you obtained from your instructor, indicate the correct volume on the measuring device.

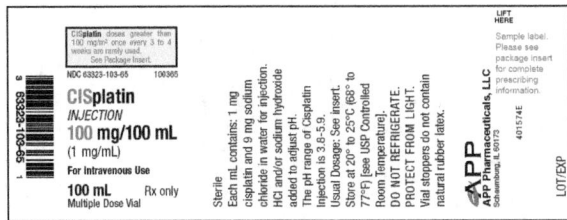

Calculate the quantity of medication in the injectable solution using the provided vial labels.

11. How many milligrams of ketorolac are contained in 0.5 mL?

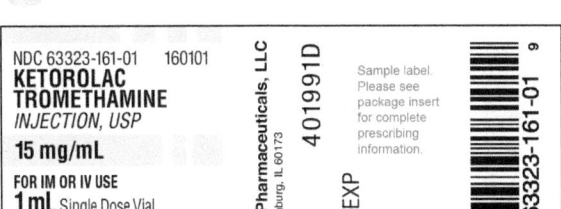

12. How many milligrams of ketorolac are contained in 1.75 mL?

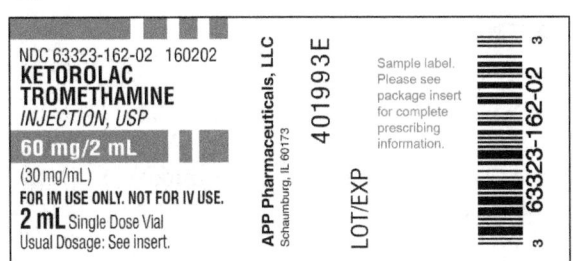

13. How many milligrams of lidocaine HCl are contained in 3.75 mL?

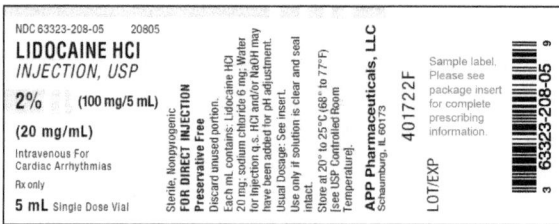

14. How many milligrams of midazolam HCl are contained in 1.3 mL?

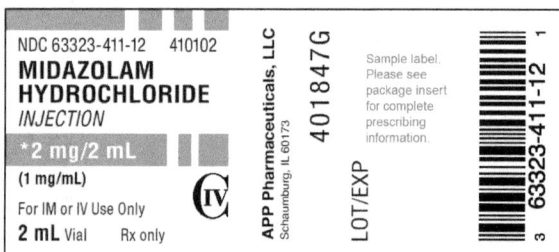

15. How many milligrams of midazolam HCl are contained in 5 mL?

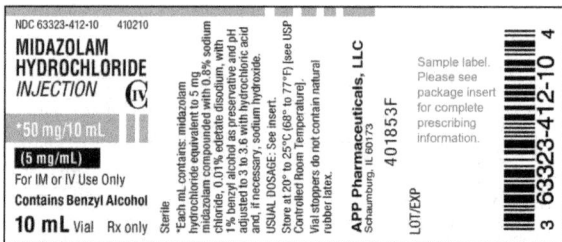

16. How many milligrams of midazolam HCl are contained in 5 mL?

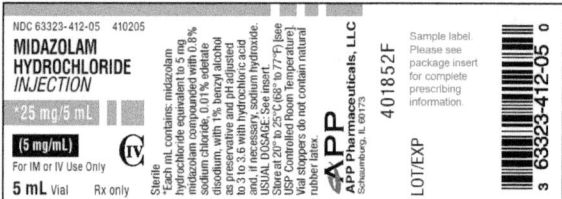

17. How many milligrams of midazolam HCl are contained in 5 mL?

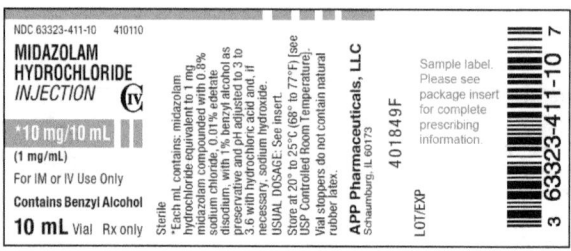

18. How many milligrams of dexamethasone are contained in 8 mL?

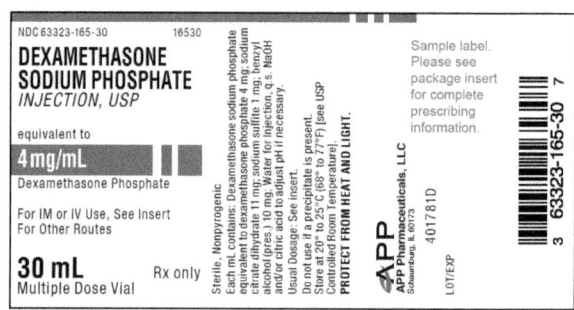

19. How many milligrams of ondansetron are contained in 1.5 mL?

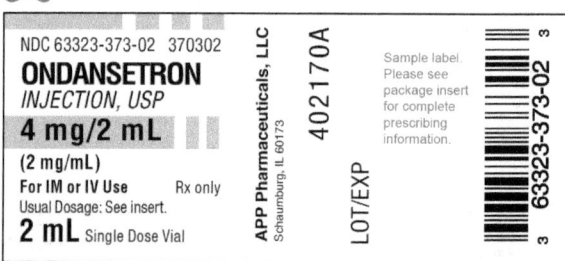

20. How many milligrams of progesterone are contained in 2.5 mL?

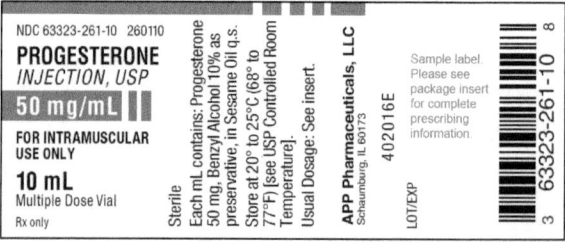

Calculate the amount of pure medication in a ratio solution.

21. How many milligrams are in 2 mL of a 1:1,000 solution?

22. How many micrograms are in 1 mL of a 1:5,000 solution?

23. How many micrograms are in 1.5 mL of a 1:10,000 solution?

24. How many micrograms are in 1.4 mL of a 1:2,000 solution?

25. How many micrograms are in 2.5 mL of a 1:10,000 solution?

Calculate the volume of solution needed for each requested dose to be infused intravenously.

26. How many milliliters of 1:1,000 solution are needed to provide a 500 mg dose?

27. How many milliliters of 1:10,000 solution are needed to provide a 50 mg dose?

28. How many milliliters of 1:300 solution are needed to provide a 600 mg dose?

29. How many milliliters of 1:500 solution are needed to provide a 250 mg dose?

30. How many milliliters of 1:750 solution are needed to provide a 0.01 g dose?

Self-check your work in Appendix A.

6.2 Other Units of Measure

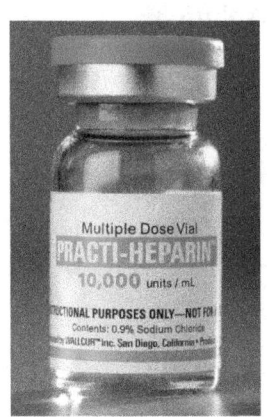

Heparin is a medication that is dosed in units.

Although most medications are dosed using the units of the metric system, such as milligrams or grams, doses of some medications are calculated using other units of measure. Some of these substances are as simple as vitamins, such as ergocalciferol, but others are complicated proteins, such as epoetin alfa, or hormones, such as insulin. Other examples include penicillin G, an antibiotic with units based on the number of bacteria affected, and heparin, an anticoagulant with units based on the amount of anticoagulant property present. Although these substances do have weights, they are dosed based on their activity, and their weights are often disregarded.

Calculating Milliequivalents and Millimoles

Many fluids in the pharmacy contain dissolved mineral salts known as **electrolytes**. They are so named because they conduct a charge through a solution.

Electrolytes are required for normal body functions and are typically obtained through nutrition. When administered as medications, they are used to restore a natural electrolyte balance and may affect many body systems.

Electrolytes are not measured using standard metric system units. The units used to measure electrolytes are particularly important when working with IV solutions. Knowledge of a few basic chemistry concepts is helpful in understanding these types of measure.

An **element** is a substance that cannot be chemically broken down into a simpler substance. The **atomic weight** of an element is the weight of a single atom of that element compared with the weight of a single atom of hydrogen. The **molecular weight** is the sum of the atomic weights of all atoms in one molecule of a compound. A **mole (mol)** is a unit of measurement based on the number of particles in a given substance. The mass of one mole of a substance is its molecular weight in grams. The number of grams in one mole differs between substances. A **millimole (mmol)** is one-thousandth of a mole, or the molecular weight expressed in milligrams. Medications such as phosphate are commonly measured in millimoles.

An **equivalent** is a unit that takes into account both moles and **valence**, the charge or ability to bond with other charged molecules. Valence is most familiar as the positive or negative symbols next to chemical abbreviations or symbols such as Na^+, Cl^-, or Ca^{++}. The valence of substances used in pharmacy preparations is most commonly plus or minus 1, 2, or 3. An equivalent gives you information about how one substance interacts with another.

An equivalent represents both the amount of active substance and the likelihood that the substance, once in the body, will cause a change in the way two compounds are bonded. An equivalent can be calculated by multiplying the number of moles of charged particles in a substance by the valence of those particles. A **milliequivalent (mEq)** is one-thousandth of an equivalent. Potassium is a common medication that is measured in milliequivalents.

Fortunately, medications commonly used today are standardized. The calculations needed in the pharmacy will involve determining the volume of a substance that has an electrolyte as its primary ingredient rather than calculating the number of millimoles or milliequivalents in a substance.

Example 6.2.1

 You are asked to add 44 mEq of sodium chloride (NaCl) to an IV bag. Sodium chloride is available as a 4 mEq/mL solution. How many milliliters will you add to the bag?

Using the ratio-proportion method:

$$\frac{44 \text{ mEq}}{x \text{ ml}} = \frac{4 \text{ mEq}}{1 \text{ ml}}$$

$$x \text{ mL } (4 \text{ mEq}) = 1 \text{ mL } (44 \text{ mEq})$$

$$\frac{x \text{ mL } (4 \text{ mEq})}{4 \text{ mEq}} = \frac{1 \text{ mL } (44 \text{ mEq})}{4 \text{ mEq}}$$

$$x = 11 \text{ mL}$$

Using the dimensional analysis method:

$$44 \text{ mEq} \times \frac{1 \text{ mL}}{4 \text{ mEq}} = 11 \text{ mL}$$

Example 6.2.2

A patient needs to take a solution of potassium chloride to replace potassium lost due to diuresis. The available solution is shown in the label below. The physician has indicated that the patient needs 15 mEq. How many milliliters should you prepare for the patient?

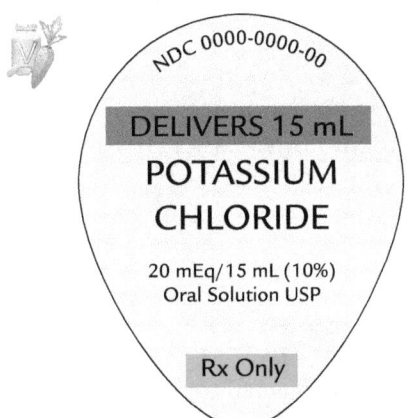

Using the ratio-proportion method:

$$\frac{15 \text{ mEq}}{x \text{ mL}} = \frac{20 \text{ mEq}}{15 \text{ mL}}$$

$$x \text{ mL} (20 \text{ mEq}) = 15 \text{ mL} (15 \text{ mEq})$$

$$\frac{x \text{ mL} (20 \text{ mEq})}{20 \text{ mEq}} = \frac{15 \text{ mL} (15 \text{ mEq})}{20 \text{ mEq}}$$

$$x = 11.25 \text{ mL, rounded to 11 mL}$$

Using the dimensional analysis method:

$$15 \text{ mEq} \times \frac{15 \text{ mL}}{20 \text{ mEq}} = 11.25 \text{ mL, rounded to 11 mL}$$

Example 6.2.3

You are instructed to add 20 mEq of potassium chloride to a patient's IV solution bag. Using the multiple-dose vial label provided, how many milliliters should be prepared?

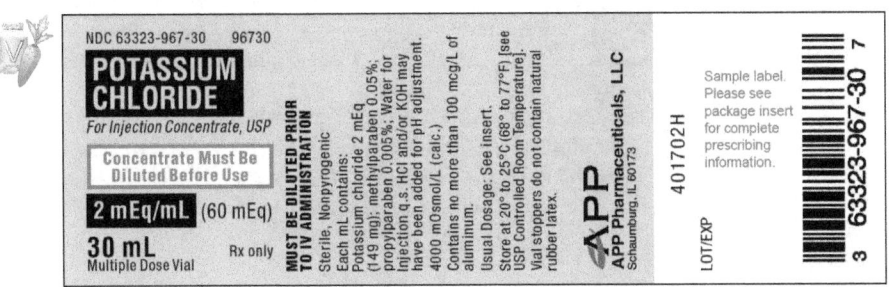

Using the ratio-proportion method:

$$\frac{20 \text{ mEq}}{x \text{ mL}} = \frac{2 \text{ mEq}}{1 \text{ mL}}$$

$$x \text{ mL} (2 \text{ mEq}) = 1 \text{ mL} (20 \text{ mEq})$$

$$\frac{x \text{ mL} (2 \text{ mEq})}{2 \text{ mEq}} = \frac{1 \text{ mL} (20 \text{ mEq})}{2 \text{ mEq}}$$

$$x = 10 \text{ mL}$$

Using the dimensional analysis method:

$$20 \text{ mEq} \times \frac{1 \text{ mL}}{2 \text{ mEq}} = 10 \text{ mL}$$

Example 6.2.4

You are instructed to add 16 mEq of potassium chloride to a patient's IV bag. Using the single-dose vial labels, select the correct vial and then calculate how many milliliters you will prepare.

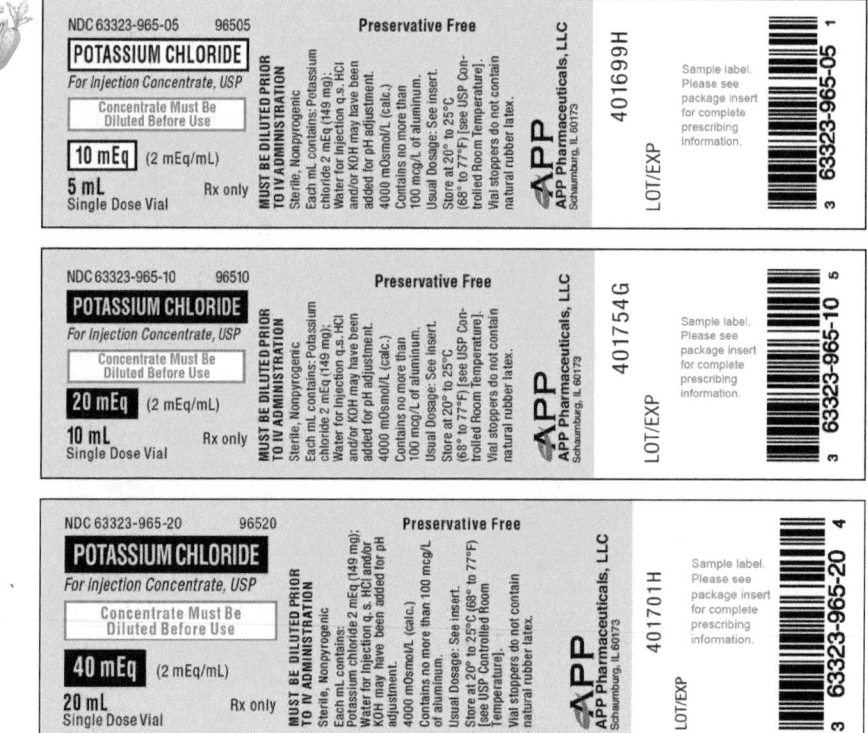

Part I. Analyze the total milliequivalents in each vial to choose the correct vial. In the labels shown, the manufacturer has highlighted the milliequivalents in each vial. Because your order calls for 16 mEq, you will select the potassium chloride vial labeled "20 mEq." The total volume is 10 mL.

Part II. Determine the number of milliliters needed to fill the order.

Using the ratio-proportion method:

$$\frac{16 \text{ mEq}}{x \text{ mL}} = \frac{20 \text{ mEq}}{10 \text{ mL}}$$

$$x \text{ mL} (20 \text{ mEq}) = 10 \text{ mL} (16 \text{ mEq})$$

$$\frac{x \text{ mL} (20 \text{ mEq})}{20 \text{ mEq}} = \frac{10 \text{ mL} (16 \text{ mEq})}{20 \text{ mEq}}$$

$$x = 8 \text{ mL}$$

Using the dimensional analysis method:

$$16 \text{ mEq} \times \frac{10 \text{ mL}}{20 \text{ mEq}} = 8 \text{ mL}$$

Example 6.2.5

 You have been instructed to add 15 mL of sodium chloride to a patient's IV bag for dilution. The medication label states that the concentration of sodium chloride is 4 mEq/mL. Calculate how many milliequivalents of sodium chloride will be in 15 mL of solution.

Using the ratio-proportion method:

$$\frac{15 \text{ mL}}{x \text{ mEq}} = \frac{1 \text{ mL}}{4 \text{ mEq}}$$

$$x \text{ mEq} (1 \text{ mL}) = 4 \text{ mEq} (15 \text{ mL})$$

$$\frac{x \text{ mEq} (1 \text{ mL})}{1 \text{ mL}} = \frac{4 \text{ mEq} (15 \text{ mL})}{1 \text{ mL}}$$

$$x = 60 \text{ mEq}$$

Using the dimensional analysis method:

$$15 \text{ mL} \times \frac{4 \text{ mEq}}{1 \text{ mL}} = 60 \text{ mEq}$$

Example 6.2.6

 You must add 9 mmol of an inorganic phosphate to an IV solution. You have 15 mmol/5 mL available. How many milliliters should you add?

Using the ratio-proportion method:

$$\frac{9 \text{ mmol}}{x \text{ mL}} = \frac{15 \text{ mmol}}{5 \text{ mL}}$$

$$x \text{ mL} (15 \text{ mmol}) = 5 \text{ mL} (9 \text{ mmol})$$

$$\frac{x \text{ mL} (\cancel{15 \text{ mmol}})}{\cancel{15 \text{ mmol}}} = \frac{5 \text{ mL} (9 \cancel{\text{ mmol}})}{15 \cancel{\text{ mmol}}}$$

$$x = 3 \text{ mL}$$

Using the dimensional analysis method:

$$9 \cancel{\text{ mmol}} \times \frac{5 \text{ mL}}{15 \cancel{\text{ mmol}}} = 3 \text{ mL}$$

Calculating Units

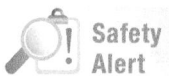

Safety Alert

Pharmacy technicians should not abbreviate international units as IU or U but should write out "units."

A number of medications are measured in units. A **unit** is a standardized measurement that describes medication activity irrespective of weight. Medications that are derived mainly from biological products, such as insulin, heparin, corticotropin (ACTH), Factor VIII, penicillin, and some vitamins, are expressed in international units or United States Pharmacopeia (USP) units. Both are expressed as "units."

Each of these medication's unique makeup defines its unit of activity. For example, insulin is dosed in units, and the units are based on the amount of glucose that a specific amount of insulin can make available to the cells in a living human being. The degree of activity in this case refers to the insulin's activity. When insulin is prescribed and administered, the dose is based on how much assistance the patient's body will need. Different types and brands of insulin have different weights, but all insulins are measured using a common unit of activity. Thus, the metric weight can be disregarded, and the unit becomes a universal dose for insulin. Insulin syringes are prepared and marked according to these standard units. Manufacturers maintain the same concentration of insulin from brand to brand so that the standard insulin syringe will measure out a uniform unit of insulin with a known activity level in the body.

Insulin doses are always calculated in units. Although it can be helpful to know the approximate volume in milliliters, the preparation will most likely involve the use of syringes that are specially marked with units instead of milliliters. Insulin syringes are available in standard unit sizes, as illustrated in Figure 6.1.

Safety Alert

Only insulin syringes should be used to administer the standard concentration of insulin.

FIGURE 6.1
Standard Insulin Syringe Sizes

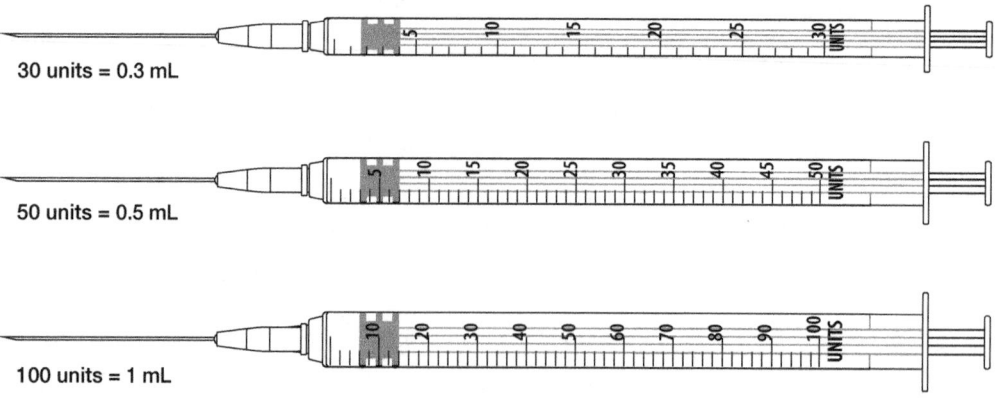

30 units = 0.3 mL

50 units = 0.5 mL

100 units = 1 mL

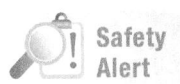

Example 6.2.7

A patient is to receive a bolus (concentrated) dose of heparin. If the dose is 7,500 units and you have a vial with the label shown below, how many milliliters will you prepare?

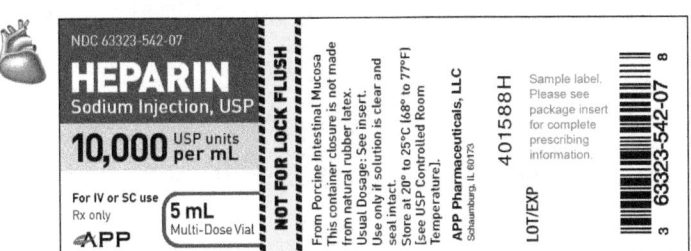

Using the ratio-proportion method:

$$\frac{7{,}500 \text{ units}}{x \text{ mL}} = \frac{10{,}000 \text{ units}}{1 \text{ mL}}$$

$$x \text{ mL} (10{,}000 \text{ units}) = 1 \text{ mL} (7{,}500 \text{ units})$$

$$\frac{x \text{ mL} (\cancel{10{,}000 \text{ units}})}{\cancel{10{,}000 \text{ units}}} = \frac{1 \text{ mL} (7{,}500 \cancel{\text{ units}})}{10{,}000 \cancel{\text{ units}}}$$

$$x = 0.75 \text{ mL}$$

Using the dimensional analysis method:

$$7{,}500 \cancel{\text{ units}} \times \frac{1 \text{ mL}}{10{,}000 \cancel{\text{ units}}} = 0.75 \text{ mL}$$

Example 6.2.8

An infant is to receive an injection of 75 units/kg of heparin. The infant weighs 6.4 kg. If you have a vial with the label shown below, how many milliliters will you prepare?

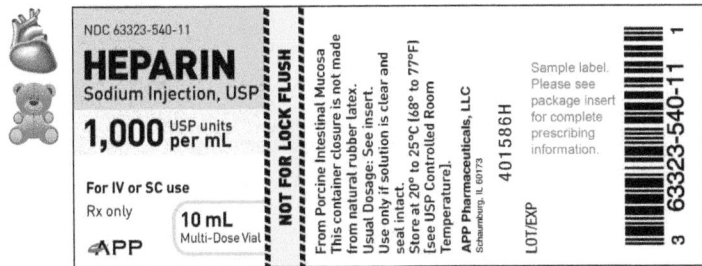

Begin by determining the number of units in the dose based on the patient's weight of 6.4 kg.

$$6.4 \cancel{\text{ kg}} \times \frac{75 \text{ units}}{\cancel{\text{ kg}}} = 480 \text{ units}$$

Then, calculate the amount of milliliters needed to prepare the dose.

Using the ratio-proportion method:

$$\frac{480 \text{ units}}{x \text{ mL}} = \frac{1{,}000 \text{ units}}{1 \text{ mL}}$$

$$x \text{ mL } (1{,}000 \text{ units}) = 1 \text{ mL } (480 \text{ units})$$

$$\frac{x \text{ mL } (1{,}000 \text{ units})}{1{,}000 \text{ units}} = \frac{1 \text{ mL } (480 \text{ units})}{1{,}000 \text{ units}}$$

$$x = 0.48 \text{ mL}$$

Using the dimensional analysis method:

$$480 \text{ units} \times \frac{1 \text{ mL}}{1{,}000 \text{ units}} = 0.48 \text{ mL}$$

Example 6.2.9

A patient is to receive 1,000 units/kg of bacitracin IM indicated on the label below. The patient weighs 15 kg. How many milliliters of bacitracin are needed?

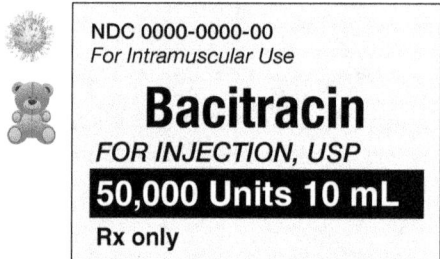

NDC 0000-0000-00
For Intramuscular Use

Bacitracin
FOR INJECTION, USP
50,000 Units 10 mL
Rx only

Begin by determining the number of units in the dose based on the patient's weight of 15 kg.

$$15 \text{ kg} \times \frac{1{,}000 \text{ units}}{1 \text{ kg}} = 15{,}000 \text{ units}$$

Then, calculate the amount of milliliters needed using either the ratio-proportion method or the dimensional analysis method.

Using the ratio-proportion method:

$$\frac{15{,}000 \text{ units}}{x \text{ mL}} = \frac{50{,}000 \text{ units}}{10 \text{ mL}}$$

$$x \text{ mL } (50{,}000 \text{ units}) = 10 \text{ mL } (15{,}000 \text{ units})$$

$$\frac{x \text{ mL } (50{,}000 \text{ units})}{50{,}000 \text{ units}} = \frac{10 \text{ mL } (15{,}000 \text{ units})}{50{,}000 \text{ units}}$$

$$x = 3 \text{ mL}$$

Using the dimensional analysis method:

$$15{,}000 \text{ units} \times \frac{10 \text{ mL}}{50{,}000 \text{ units}} = 3 \text{ mL}$$

Insulin is usually dosed with the concentration of 100 units/mL, and all insulin is always dosed in units. However, many types of insulin products are available. Some insulin products require the patient to withdraw medication from a vial into a syringe. Other insulin products come in a prefilled syringe or "pen" with a disposable needle on the tip. Only insulin syringes should be used to administer or dispense the standard concentration of insulin (100 units/mL).

Reading insulin labels can be challenging because there may be only slight differentiations from one product to another (see Figure 6.2). **It is important to select the correct insulin because they are not interchangeable.** They differ by onset and duration of action and have the potential to harm a patient who uses the wrong brand or type. When preparing an insulin dose or prescription, triple-check the medication's label against the printed label and the ordered medication. Confirm that the NDC numbers match. If the pharmacy is equipped with a bar-code scanner, the device helps to confirm that the correct medication is being used.

FIGURE 6.2 **Insulin Labels**

Although it is true for all medication labels, it is especially important to read insulin labels carefully.

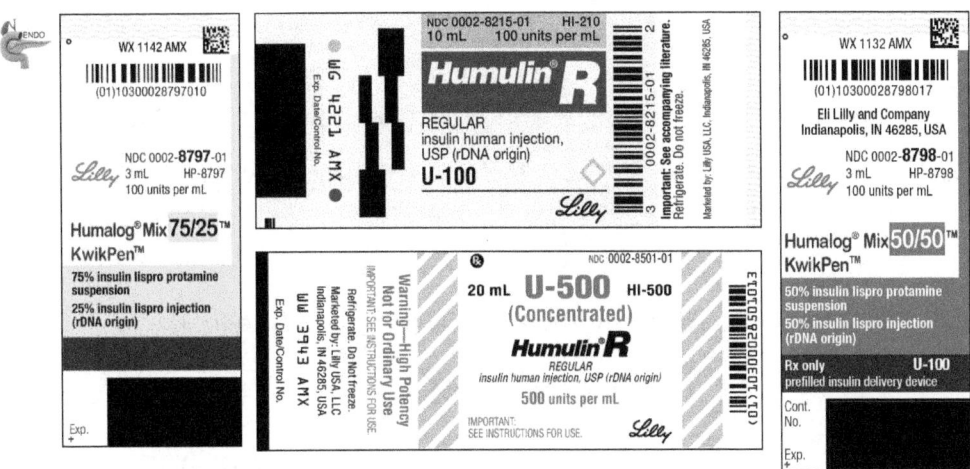

☑ TAKE NOTE

The most common insulin concentration is 100 units/mL (U-100). However, some types of insulin come in 200 units/mL (U-200), 300 units/mL (U-300), and 500 units/mL (U-500) formulations. When drawing up insulin into a syringe, be sure to choose the correct concentration. Patients can be harmed by receiving too much or too little insulin because the vial selected contained a concentration different from the concentration that was prescribed.

The following examples demonstrate how to calculate a volume of insulin in milliliters (vs. standard units). Calculating the volume of insulin in milliliters is helpful when determining how long an insulin vial or pen will last a patient.

Example 6.2.10

A patient is to receive 32 units of regular insulin each morning before breakfast. Insulin comes in a concentration of 100 units/mL. How many milliliters will the patient receive with each dose? How many days will the vial last?

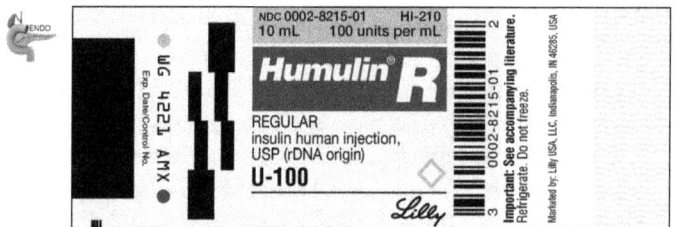

Part I. Calculate the volume the patient will receive with each dose by using either the ratio-proportion method or the dimensional analysis method.

Using the ratio-proportion method:

$$\frac{32 \text{ units}}{x \text{ mL}} = \frac{100 \text{ units}}{1 \text{ mL}}$$

$$x \text{ mL } (100 \text{ units}) = 1 \text{ mL } (32 \text{ units})$$

$$\frac{x \text{ mL } (100 \text{ units})}{100 \text{ units}} = \frac{1 \text{ mL } (32 \text{ units})}{100 \text{ units}}$$

$$x = 0.32 \text{ mL}$$

Using the dimensional analysis method:

$$32 \text{ units} \times \frac{1 \text{ mL}}{100 \text{ units}} = 0.32 \text{ mL}$$

Part II. Using the volume per dose just calculated, determine the number of days a single vial will last. In this example, the patient takes one dose a day.

Using the ratio-proportion method:

$$\frac{10 \text{ mL}}{x \text{ days}} = \frac{0.32 \text{ mL}}{1 \text{ day}}$$

$$x \text{ days } (0.32 \text{ mL}) = 1 \text{ day } (10 \text{ mL})$$

$$\frac{x \text{ days } (0.32 \text{ mL})}{0.32 \text{ mL}} = \frac{1 \text{ day } (10 \text{ mL})}{0.32 \text{ mL}}$$

$$x = 31.25 \text{ days, or rounded down to the}$$
$$\text{nearest whole day, 31 days}$$

Using the dimensional analysis method:

$$10 \, \text{mL} \times \frac{1 \text{ day}}{0.32 \, \text{mL}} = 31.25 \text{ days, or rounded down to}$$
$$\text{the nearest whole day, 31 days}$$

Example 6.2.11

A patient is to receive 49 units of Humulin 70/30 insulin twice daily. The insulin comes in a concentration of 100 units/mL. How many milliliters will the patient receive in each dose? How many vials will the patient need to last 30 days (1 month)?

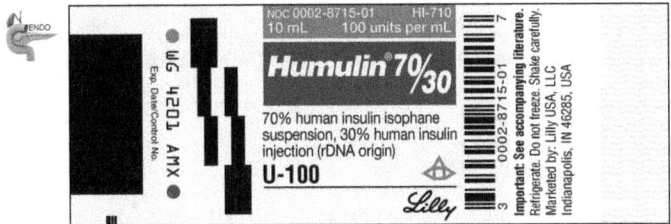

Part I. Calculate the volume the patient will receive with each dose by using either the ratio-proportion method or the dimensional analysis method.

Using the ratio-proportion method:

$$\frac{49 \text{ units}}{x \text{ mL}} = \frac{100 \text{ units}}{1 \text{ mL}}$$

$$x \text{ mL} (100 \text{ units}) = 1 \text{ mL} (49 \text{ units})$$

$$\frac{x \text{ mL} (100 \text{ units})}{100 \text{ units}} = \frac{1 \text{ mL} (49 \text{ units})}{100 \text{ units}}$$

$$x \text{ mL} = 0.49 \text{ mL}$$

Using the dimensional analysis method:

$$49 \text{ units} \times \frac{1 \text{ mL}}{100 \text{ units}} = 0.49 \text{ mL}$$

Part II. Using the volume per dose just calculated, determine the number of milliliters the patient will need for 30 days.

First, calculate the total milliliters used per day with twice daily dosing.

$$0.49 \text{ mL} \times 2 = 0.98 \text{ mL/day}$$

Then, calculate the number of milliliters needed.

Using the ratio-proportion method:

$$\frac{30 \text{ days}}{x \text{ mL}} = \frac{1 \text{ day}}{0.98 \text{ mL}}$$

$$x \text{ mL (1 day)} = 0.98 \text{ mL (30 days)}$$

$$\frac{x \text{ mL } (\cancel{1 \text{ day}})}{\cancel{1 \text{ day}}} = \frac{0.98 \text{ mL (30 } \cancel{\text{days}})}{\cancel{1 \text{ day}}}$$

$$x \text{ mL} = 29.4 \text{ mL}$$

Using the dimensional analysis method:

$$30 \ \cancel{\text{days}} \times \frac{0.98 \text{ mL}}{1 \ \cancel{\text{day}}} = 29.4 \text{ mL}$$

Because 1 vial = 10 mL, the patient will need 3 vials to last 30 days.

Example 6.2.12

How many units are in the Humalog Mix 75/25 KwikPen with the following label? If a patient uses 23 units daily, how many days will this KwikPen last?

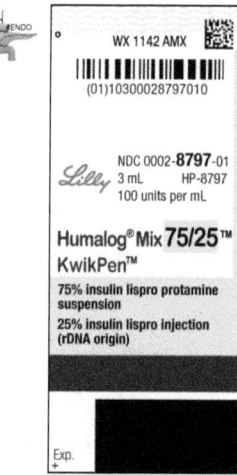

Part I. Calculate the total number of units in a single pen.

Using the ratio-proportion method:

$$\frac{3 \text{ mL}}{x \text{ units}} = \frac{1 \text{ mL}}{100 \text{ units}}$$

$$x \text{ units (1 mL)} = 100 \text{ units (3 mL)}$$

$$\frac{x \text{ units } (\cancel{1 \text{ mL}})}{\cancel{1 \text{ mL}}} = \frac{100 \text{ units (3 } \cancel{\text{mL}})}{\cancel{1 \text{ mL}}}$$

$$x = 300 \text{ units}$$

Using the dimensional analysis method:

$$3 \ \cancel{\text{mL}} \times \frac{100 \text{ units}}{1 \ \cancel{\text{mL}}} = 300 \text{ units}$$

Part II. Calculate the number of days a single pen will last using the patient's daily units. Again, you can use either the ratio-proportion method or the dimensional analysis method.

Using the ratio-proportion method:

$$\frac{300 \text{ units}}{x \text{ days}} = \frac{23 \text{ units}}{1 \text{ day}}$$

$$x \text{ days } (23 \text{ units}) = 1 \text{ day } (300 \text{ units})$$

$$\frac{x \text{ days } (23 \text{ units})}{23 \text{ units}} = \frac{1 \text{ day } (300 \text{ units})}{23 \text{ units}}$$

$$x = 13.04 \text{ days, or rounded down to the nearest whole day, 13 days}$$

Using the dimensional analysis method:

$$300 \text{ units} \times \frac{1 \text{ day}}{23 \text{ units}} = 13.04 \text{ days, or rounded down to the nearest whole day, 13 days}$$

Example 6.2.13

A patient is to receive 100 units of regular insulin twice daily. The insulin comes in a concentration of 500 units/mL. How many milliliters will the patient receive with each dose? Indicate the correct volume using a U-100 insulin syringe and a tuberculin (1 mL) syringe.

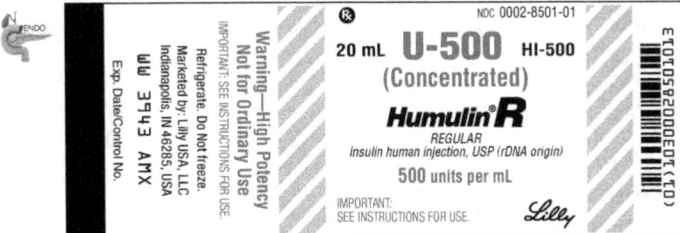

Using the ratio-proportion method:

$$\frac{100 \text{ units}}{x \text{ mL}} = \frac{500 \text{ units}}{1 \text{ mL}}$$

$$x \text{ mL } (500 \text{ units}) = 1 \text{ mL } (100 \text{ units})$$

$$\frac{x \text{ mL } (500 \text{ units})}{500 \text{ units}} = \frac{1 \text{ mL } (100 \text{ units})}{500 \text{ units}}$$

$$x \text{ mL} = 0.2 \text{ mL}$$

Using the dimensional analysis method:

$$100 \text{ units} \times \frac{1 \text{ mL}}{500 \text{ units}} = 0.2 \text{ mL}$$

Because U-500 insulin is five times more concentrated than U-100 insulin, every one unit of U-500 insulin is the same as five units of U-100 insulin. When using a U-100 syringe for U-500 insulin, divide the number of units of U-500 insulin by five to determine how much to fill the syringe. For this patient, 100 ÷ 5 is 20, so a U-100 insulin syringe would need to be filled to the 20 unit mark for the patient to receive the correct dose.

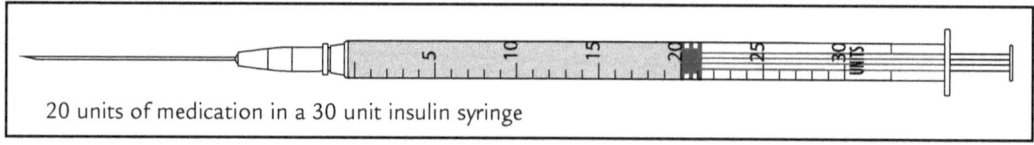

20 units of medication in a 30 unit insulin syringe

One-milliliter tuberculin syringes can also be used to administer U-500 insulin. Simply draw the insulin up to the calculated 0.2 mL mark to measure out the same dose.

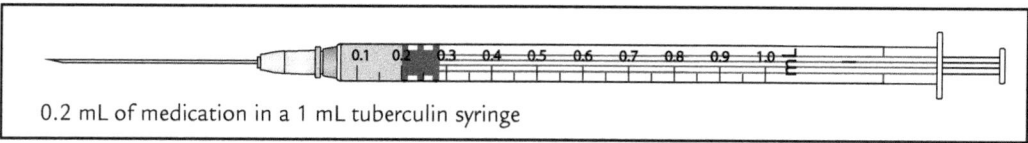

0.2 mL of medication in a 1 mL tuberculin syringe

6.2 Problem Set

Perform the necessary calculations to answer each of the following. (Round to the nearest hundredth.)

Note: *Questions 1, 2, 4, 6, 7, 8, 13, 14, and 16 have accompanying handouts that you must obtain from your instructor.*

1. An order requires 30 mEq of potassium phosphate. You have a 4.4 mEq/mL solution available. How many milliliters should you put in the IV bag? On the handout that you obtained from your instructor, indicate the correct volume on the measuring devices.

2. An order requires 45 mEq of potassium phosphate. You have a 4.4 mEq/mL solution available. How many milliliters should you put in the IV solution? On the handout that you obtained from your instructor, indicate the correct volume on the measuring devices.

3. A prescription states that a patient must take 32 mEq of potassium. The potassium replacement selected has 8 mEq per tablet. How many tablets would the patient need to take?

4. A patient is to use a sugar- and alcohol-free solution of potassium that contains 40 mEq/15 mL. The patient is to take 30 mEq daily in two equally divided doses. How many milliliters will each dose be? On the handout that you obtained from your instructor, indicate the correct volume on the measuring devices.

5. A prescription has been filled for 15 mL Rum-K with breakfast. Rum-K contains 20 mEq/10 mL. How many milliequivalents is the patient taking with each dose?

6. A patient needs to take 30 mEq of potassium orally. The solution on hand has 20 mEq/15 mL. How much should be prepared for the patient? On the handout that you obtained from your instructor, indicate the correct volume on the measuring device.

For questions 7–10, select the vial that is needed to fill each order with the required number of milliequivalents of potassium chloride, and then calculate the volume to be withdrawn from the selected vial for the order.

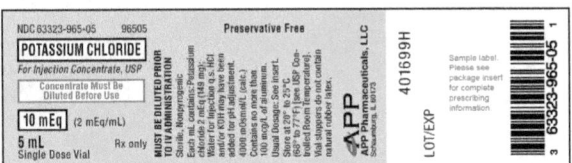

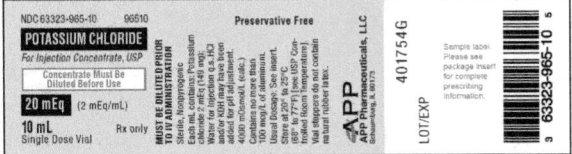

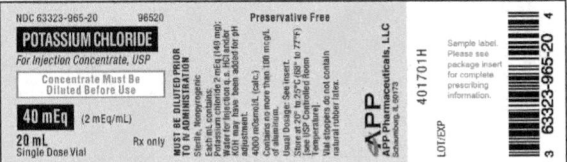

7. Add 14 mEq potassium chloride to the patient's IV solution. On the handout that you obtained from your instructor, indicate the correct volume on the measuring devices.

8. Add 19 mEq potassium chloride to the patient's IV solution. On the handout that you obtained from your instructor, indicate the correct volume on the measuring device.

9. Add 27 mEq potassium chloride to the patient's IV solution.

10. Add 50 mEq potassium chloride to the patient's IV solution.

For questions 11–12, use the label provided to calculate the volume or amount requested.

11. How many milliequivalents of potassium chloride are in 8 mL of the solution?

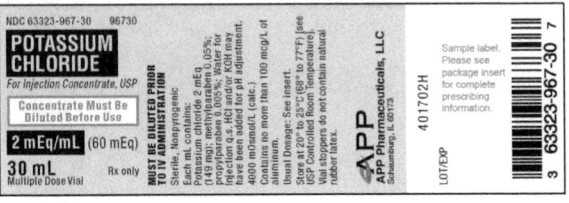

12. How many milliequivalents of potassium chloride are in 15 mL of the solution?

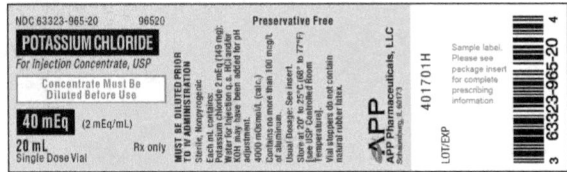

13. A pharmacy receives the following order. Sodium chloride is available as a 4 mEq/mL solution. How many milliliters should you add to the bag? On the handout that you obtained from your instructor, indicate the correct volume on the measuring device.

R_x Give 132 mEq of sodium chloride in 100 mL

Infuse at 62 mL/hour

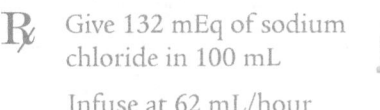

14. A pharmacy receives an order indicating that you should add 120 mEq sodium chloride to an IV bag of dextrose 5% in water (D_5W). Using a vial that is labeled 4 mEq/mL, how many milliliters should you add to the bag? On the handout that you obtained from your instructor, indicate the correct volume on the measuring device.

Use the following label to answer questions 15 and 16.

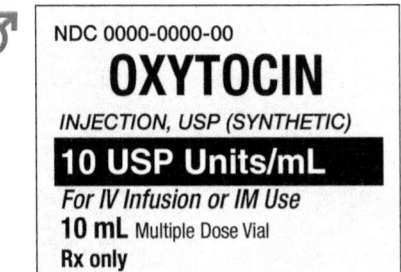

NDC 0000-0000-00
OXYTOCIN
INJECTION, USP (SYNTHETIC)
10 USP Units/mL
For IV Infusion or IM Use
10 mL Multiple Dose Vial
Rx only

15. A patient is to receive 4 units of oxytocin. Using the vial with the label shown above, how many milliliters will be needed?

16. A patient has received 2.8 mL of the oxytocin solution shown in the label above. How many units is this? On the handout that you obtained from your instructor, indicate the correct volume on the measuring device.

17. A patient is to receive 3,500 units heparin, and the following label shows the medication you are to dispense. How many milliliters is this?

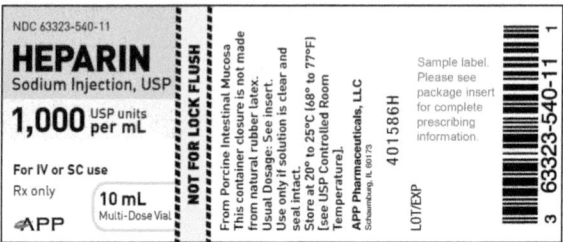

18. A patient needs an injection of heparin. An order for 0.43 mL has been prepared. How many units of heparin are in the dose if it contains 20,000 units/0.8 mL?

19. Prepare 7,000 units of heparin from the vial with the label shown below. How many milliliters is this?

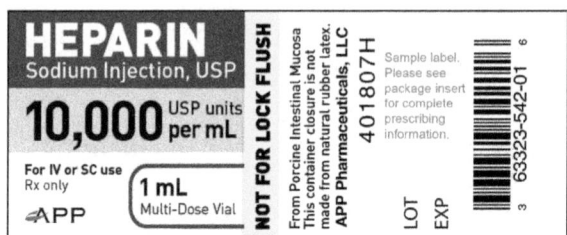

20. Prepare 24,000 units of heparin from the vial with the label shown below. How many milliliters is this?

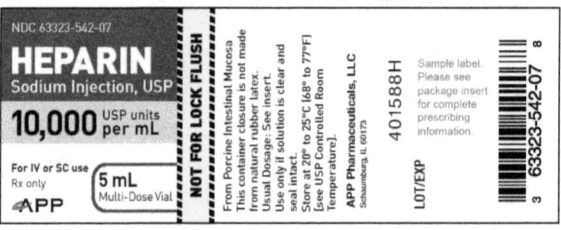

21. Prepare two syringes for a patient on the orthopedic floor. Each syringe should contain 30 mg of Lovenox. How many milliliters will be in each syringe?

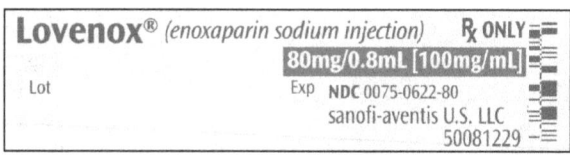

Calculate the following volumes or number of units.

22. Penicillin G can be reconstituted to many different concentrations. You are filling an order for 175,000 units and have available a concentration that has already been concentrated to 500,000 units/mL. How many milliliters is the dose?

23. Bicillin CR is given as an IM injection preparation. It comes as 600,000 units/mL, and the dose is 1.2 million units. What is the volume to be administered?

24. A physician has ordered 385,000 units of penicillin G for a patient. Your stock preparation has 50,000 units/mL. How many milliliters should the dose be?

25. A patient is to receive Humulin 70/30 insulin at a dose of 45 units at 8:00 every morning. Using the vial with the following label, how many milliliters should be drawn into the syringe?

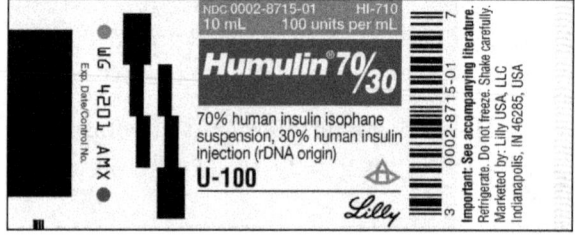

26. A patient uses 18 units of insulin each morning and 10 units at 7:00 p.m. How long will the volume shown in the following label last?

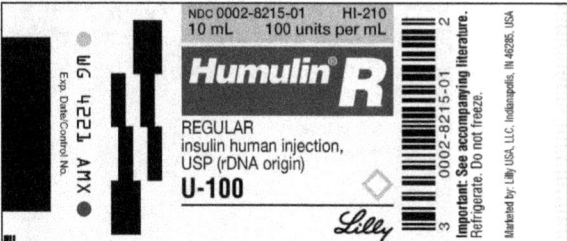

27. A patient uses 20 units of insulin every morning and 18 units of insulin every evening. Using the label below, answer the following questions.

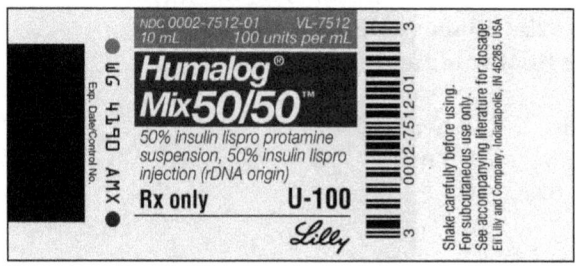

   a. How many total units does the patient use daily?

   b. How many vials does the patient need for 30 days?

28. A patient uses 10 units of Humulin R each morning and 15 units of Humulin 70/30 at lunch and dinner. Using the labels below, determine the number of vials of each type of Humulin the patient will need for 30 days.

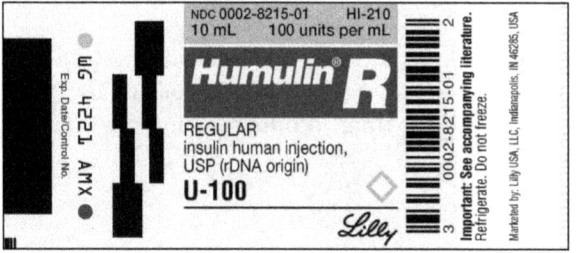

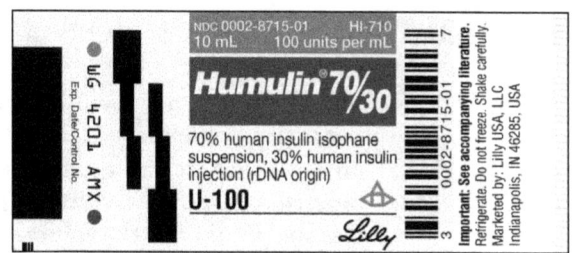

29. A patient uses 0.5 mL daily of Lantus shown in the following label. How many units is this?

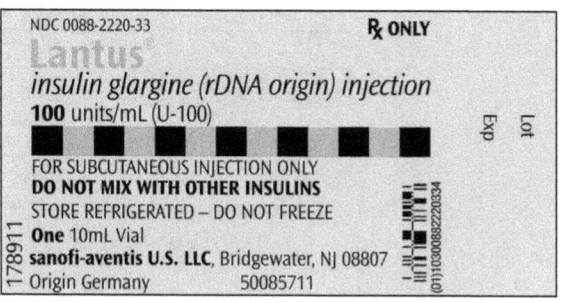

30. Using the label shown below, determine how long two vials of Apidra will last a patient who uses 20 units twice daily.

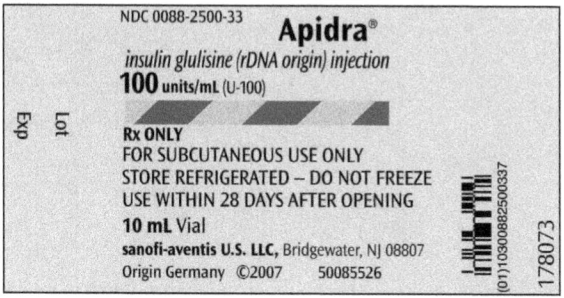

Self-check your work in Appendix A.

6.3 Solutions Using Powders

In the preparation of solutions, the active ingredient is discussed in terms of weight, but it also occupies a certain amount of space. For lyophilized (freeze-dried) pharmaceuticals that are packaged in a sterile vial and used for reconstitution, this space is referred to as **powder volume (pv)**. Powder volume equals the difference between the *final volume (fv)* and the volume of the diluting ingredient, or the *diluent volume (dv)*, as expressed in the following equation:

$$\text{powder volume (pv)} = \text{final volume (fv)} - \text{diluent volume (dv)}$$

or

$$pv = fv - dv$$

Example 6.3.1

 A powdered antibiotic must be reconstituted for use. The label states that the dry powder occupies 0.5 mL. Using the formula for solving for powder volume, determine the diluent volume (the amount of solvent added) for each of the final volumes listed below.

Final Volume	Powder Volume
2 mL	0.5 mL
5 mL	0.5 mL
10 mL	0.5 mL

Rearrange the formula to $dv = fv - pv$

$pv = fv - dv$
$pv + dv = fv$
$dv = fv - pv$

$dv = 2 \text{ mL} - 0.5 \text{ mL} = 1.5 \text{ mL}$
$dv = 5 \text{ mL} - 0.5 \text{ mL} = 4.5 \text{ mL}$
$dv = 10 \text{ mL} - 0.5 \text{ mL} = 9.5 \text{ mL}$

Example 6.3.2

You are to reconstitute 1 g of dry powder. The label states that you are to add 9.3 mL of diluent to make a final solution of 100 mg/mL. What is the powder volume?

To determine the powder volume, you must also know the final volume and diluent volume. The diluent volume has already been provided, so begin by calculating the final volume. You can find the final volume by using the final concentration of the solution.

Using the ratio-proportion method:

Convert 1 g to 1,000 mg.

$$\frac{1{,}000 \text{ mg}}{x \text{ mL}} = \frac{100 \text{ mg}}{1 \text{ mL}}$$

$$x \text{ mL } (100 \text{ mg}) = 1 \text{ mL } (1{,}000 \text{ mg})$$

$$\frac{x \text{ mL } (100 \text{ mg})}{100 \text{ mg}} = \frac{1 \text{ mL } (1{,}000 \text{ mg})}{100 \text{ mg}}$$

$$x = 10 \text{ mL}$$

Using the dimensional analysis method:

$$1 \text{ g} \times \frac{1{,}000 \text{ mg}}{1 \text{ g}} \times \frac{1 \text{ mL}}{100 \text{ mg}} = 10 \text{ mL}$$

Then, using the calculated final volume and the given diluent volume, determine the powder volume.

$$pv = fv - dv$$

$$pv = 10 \text{ mL} - 9.3 \text{ mL}$$

$$pv = 0.7 \text{ mL}$$

Example 6.3.3

 A label states that a 5 g quantity of an antibiotic in a bottle should be reconstituted with 8.7 mL saline for injection. The resulting concentration will be 500 mg/mL. What is the powder volume contained in the vial?

Begin by calculating the final volume using the final concentration of the solution.

Using the ratio-proportion method:

Convert 5 g to 5,000 mg

$$\frac{5{,}000 \text{ mg}}{x \text{ mL}} = \frac{500 \text{ mg}}{1 \text{ mL}}$$

$$x \text{ mL } (500 \text{ mg}) = 1 \text{ mL } (5{,}000 \text{ mg})$$

$$\frac{x \text{ mL } (500 \text{ mg})}{500 \text{ mg}} = \frac{1 \text{ mL } (5{,}000 \text{ mg})}{500 \text{ mg}}$$

$$x = 10 \text{ mL}$$

Using the dimensional analysis method:

$$5\,\cancel{g} \times \frac{1,000\,\cancel{mg}}{1\,\cancel{g}} \times \frac{1\,mL}{500\,\cancel{mg}} = 10\,mL$$

Then, using the calculated final volume and the given diluent volume, determine the powder volume.

$$pv = fv - dv$$

$$pv = 10\,mL - 8.7\,mL$$

$$pv = 1.3\,mL$$

Example 6.3.4

A 6 g vial must have 10 mL of diluent added to it. It has a powder volume of 2 mL. How many milligrams will be in each milliliter of the final solution?

First, determine the final volume of the solution.

$$pv = fv - dv$$

Therefore,

$$fv = pv + dv$$

$$fv = 2\,mL + 10\,mL$$

$$fv = 12\,mL$$

Next, determine the concentration of the solution.

Using the ratio-proportion method:

$$\frac{1\,mL}{x\,g} = \frac{12\,mL}{6\,g}$$

$$x\,g\,(12\,mL) = 6\,g\,(1\,mL)$$

$$\frac{x\,g\,(12\,\cancel{mL})}{12\,\cancel{mL}} = \frac{6\,g\,(1\,\cancel{mL})}{12\,\cancel{mL}}$$

$$x = 0.5\,g \text{ in each milliliter}$$

Convert 0.5 g to mg.

$$\frac{0.5\,g}{x\,mg} = \frac{1\,g}{1,000\,mg}$$

$$x\,mg\,(1\,g) = 1,000\,mg\,(0.5\,g)$$

$$\frac{x\,mg\,(1\,\cancel{g})}{1\,\cancel{g}} = \frac{1,000\,mg\,(0.5\,\cancel{g})}{1\,\cancel{g}}$$

$$x = 500\,mg \text{ in each milliliter}$$

Or simply move the decimal point three places to the right: $0.\underset{\smile}{500}$ g = 500 mg in each milliliter.

Using the dimensional analysis method:

$$\frac{6\,\cancel{g}}{12\ \text{mL}} \times \frac{1{,}000\ \text{mg}}{1\,\cancel{g}} = 500\ \text{mg/mL}$$

Example 6.3.5

The label of a 10 g vancomycin vial states that if you add 95 mL of sterile water to the vial's contents you will get a concentration of 1 g/10 mL. What concentration do you get if you add 45 mL?

First, determine the final volume of the solution.

$$\frac{10\ \text{g}}{x\ \text{mL}} = \frac{1\ \text{g}}{10\ \text{mL}}$$

$$x\ \text{mL}\ (1\ \text{g}) = 10\ \text{mL}\ (10\ \text{g})$$

$$\frac{x\ \text{mL}\ (\cancel{1\ \text{g}})}{\cancel{1\ \text{g}}} = \frac{10\ \text{mL}\ (10\,\cancel{\text{g}})}{1\,\cancel{\text{g}}}$$

$$x = 100\ \text{mL}$$

Next, determine the powder volume of the solution.

$$\text{pv} = \text{fv} - \text{dv}$$

$$\text{pv} = 100\ \text{mL} - 95\ \text{mL}$$

$$\text{pv} = 5\ \text{mL}$$

Then, determine the new final volume using 45 mL of diluent instead of 95 mL.

$$\text{pv} = \text{fv} - \text{dv}$$

Therefore,

$$\text{fv} = \text{pv} + \text{dv}$$

$$\text{fv} = 5\ \text{mL} + 45\ \text{mL}$$

$$\text{fv} = 50\ \text{mL}$$

Finally, determine the new concentration of the solution.

$$\frac{10\ \text{g}}{50\ \text{mL}} = 0.2\ \text{g/mL, or } 200\ \text{mg/mL}$$

1. You need to make an injectable solution with a final concentration of 375 mg/mL. After checking your supply, you see that you have a vial that contains 1.5 g with the instructions to add 3.3 mL. What is the powder volume?

2. You must add water to an oral suspension before it can be dispensed to the patient. The dose is to be 250 mg/tsp, and the dry powder is 5 g with a powder volume of 8.6 mL. How much water must you add?

3. An injectable preparation comes packaged as a 1 g vial, and you want a final concentration of 125 mg/2 mL. The vial states that you are to add 14.4 mL diluent. What is the powder volume?

4. The label of a 2 g vial states that you are to add 6.8 mL to get a concentration of 250 mg/mL. What is the powder volume?

5. In question 4, to make a final concentration of 125 mg/mL, how much diluent must you add?

6. The label of a 4 g vial states that you are to add 11.7 mL to get a concentration of 250 mg/mL. What is the powder volume?

7. The label of a 6 g vial says that if you add 12.5 mL of diluent to the vial's contents you will get a concentration of 1 g/2.5 mL. What concentration do you get if you add 2.5 mL?

8. You have added 3.3 mL of diluent to a 1 g vial and now have a final volume of 4 mL. What is the powder volume?

9. How many milliliters of the medication in question 8 do you need for a 100 mg dose?

10. If you add 8.8 mL of diluent to a 2 g vial and get a final concentration of 200 mg/mL, what is the powder volume?

11. A 10 g vial must have 45 mL of diluent added to it. It has a powder volume of 5 mL. How many milligrams will be in each milliliter of the final solution?

12. For an oral suspension, you add 170 mL of fluid and get a final volume of 200 mL. If it contains 8 g of medication, how many milligrams will be in 1 tsp?

13. A 20 g bulk vial label states that if you add 106 mL of diluent, the concentration will be 1 g/6 mL. How much diluent would you add to get a concentration of 1 g/3 mL?

14. You need a concentration of 375 mg/mL. Your vial contains 2 g with instructions to add 3.5 mL of diluent. What is the powder volume?

15. An oral medication requires reconstitution. The dose is 300 mg/tsp. The dry powder is 2.5 g with a volume of 9.6 mL. How much water do you add?

16. A 5 g vial requires that 8.6 mL diluent be added to get a concentration of 250 mg/mL. What is the powder volume?

17. A 10 g vial label says to add 20 mL of diluent to get 1 g per 2.5 mL. What concentration would you get if you added 35 mL?

18. You add 4.3 mL of diluent to a 1 g vial and have a final volume of 5 mL. What is the powder volume?

19. A 5 g vial requires 25 mL to be added. It has a powder volume of 5 mL. How many milligrams are in each milliliter of the final solution?

20. A 20 g vial must have 90 mL of diluent added. It has a powder volume of 10 mL. How many milligrams will be in each milliliter of the final solution?

21. A 3 g vial requires 20 mL of diluent to be added. It has a powder volume of 5 mL. How many milligrams are in each milliliter of the final solution?

22. A pediatric antibiotic requires 67 mL to be added to the bottle for reconstitution. The final volume will be 100 mL. What is the powder volume?

23. If the bottle in question 22 is reconstituted and there are 35 g of active ingredient in the bottle, what will the resulting strength be in milligrams per milliliters?

Solve the following compounding problems.

24. The pharmacy receives the following compound. What is the final concentration in milligrams per milliliters?

℞ **Vancomycin Ophthalmic Solution**

1. Remove and discard 9 mL of fluid from a commercial artificial tears bottle (15 mL).
2. Add 10 mL of sterile water for injection (SWFI) to a vancomycin 500 mg vial. There will be a dry volume of 0.2 mL.
3. Place 10.2 mL of reconstituted vancomycin into an amber tears bottle.

25. The pharmacy receives the following compound.

℞ **Cephalosporin Intravitreal Ophthalmic Antibiotic Preparation**

1. Reconstitute a 1 g vial with 4.4 mL of BSS Sterile Irrigating Solution.
2. Take 1 mL of this solution and add 9 mL of BSS Sterile Irrigating Solution.
3. Inject 0.1 mL intravitreally.

a. What concentration is the vial of cephalosporin when you reconstitute it in milligrams per milliliters?

b. What milligram dose is the patient receiving?

Self-check your work in Appendix A.

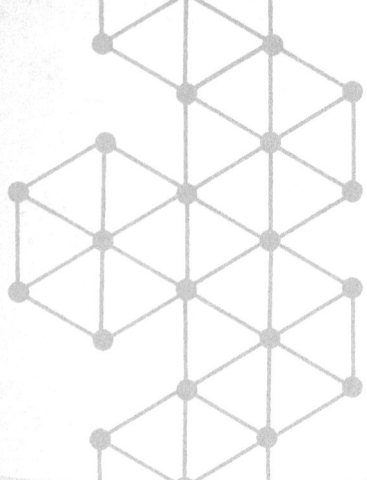

CHAPTER SUMMARY

- The three common types of injections are subcutaneous (SC), intramuscular (IM), and intravenous (IV).

- SC and IM injections are small-volume injections given over a short period.

- IV infusions typically range from 50 to 1,000 mL and are administered in a vein over a period of minutes to hours, depending on the volume.

- Syringe barrel size is selected by choosing the smallest volume barrel that will accurately measure the desired amount.

- Small volumes may be rounded to the nearest tenth or hundredth, depending on the accuracy of the measuring device available.

- Larger volumes may be rounded to the nearest tenth or whole milliliter, depending on the accuracy of the measuring device available.

- Ratio strength (example 1:1,000) is used to represent the concentration when the amount of medication in the vehicle is very small.

- When a solid medication has been dissolved in a liquid, the units of measure for a 1:100 ratio solution are 1 g:100 mL.

- Electrolytes are measured in milliequivalents or millimoles.

- Milliequivalents represent the amount of active, charged electrolytes, not the amount of medication by weight.

- Medications derived from biological sources are sometimes dosed in "units." Units may be used to measure medication doses instead of weight.

- When a medication is measured in units, weight is not used to measure the medication.

- Insulin and heparin are the two most common medications dosed in units.

- Insulin is most often concentrated as standard U-100, which means that there are 100 units in 1 mL.

- Even though there are many brands and types of insulin that use the standard U-100 concentration, they are not interchangeable.
- Powder volume is the amount of space taken up by the freeze-dried drug in a sterile vial. This type of medication is used for reconstitution.

Formulas for Success

powder volume (pv) = final volume (fv) − diluent volume (dv)

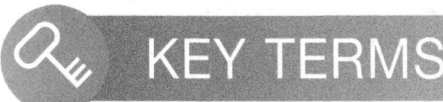

KEY TERMS

atomic weight the weight of a single atom of an element compared with the weight of a single atom of hydrogen

electrolytes substances such as mineral salts that carry an electrical charge when dissolved in a solution

element a substance that cannot be chemically broken down into a simpler substance.

equivalent a unit that takes into account both moles and valence

infusion the administration of a large volume of liquid medication given parenterally over a long period

injection a method of administering medications in which a needle or cannula attached to a syringe penetrates the skin or a membrane to deposit medication into the tissue, muscle, or vessel below

intramuscular (IM) injection an injection of fluid given into the aqueous muscle tissue

intravenous (IV) infusion an injection of fluid into the veins

milliequivalent (mEq) one thousandth of an equivalent; used to measure the concentration of electrolytes in a volume of solution; also an amount of medication that will provide the patient with a specific amount (equivalent amount) of an electrolyte

millimole (mmol) molecular weight expressed in milligrams

mole (mol) a unit of measurement based on the number of particles in a given substance

molecular weight the sum of the atomic weights of all atoms in one molecule of a compound

parenteral administered by injection or infusion and not by way of the GI system

powder volume (pv) the space occupied by dry pharmaceuticals, calculated as the difference between the final volume and the volume of the diluting ingredient, or the diluent volume; the amount of space occupied by lyophilized (freeze-dried) medication in a sterile vial, used for reconstitution

ratio strength a means of describing the concentration of a liquid medication based on a ratio such as *a* grams:*b* milliliters

subcutaneous (SC) injection an injection of fluid given into the vascular, fatty layer of tissue under the skin

unit a standardized measurement that describes medication activity irrespective of weight

valence the plus or minus signs next to chemical abbreviations or symbols such as Na^+, Cl^-, or Ca^{++} that represent the charge of the element

Finding Solutions

To gain practice in handling challenging situations in the workplace, consider the following real-world scenarios, and then use the guiding questions to help you formulate your responses.

Note: *To indicate your answer for Scenario A, Question 2, ask your instructor for the handout depicting 1 mL, 3 mL, and 5 mL syringes. For Scenario B, use the handout to select the correct insulin syringe.*

Scenario A: Lin Nguyen, a 23-year-old patient in the postsurgical unit, weighs 120 pounds. You have an order to prepare 100 mg of progesterone injection in a syringe for IM administration. You have a 50 mL multi-dose vial of progesterone 50 mg/mL as well as 1 mL, 3 mL, and 5 mL syringes on hand.

1. How many milliliters will be given at each dose?

2. On the handout that you obtained from your instructor, select the correct syringe size and indicate the amount of medication that should be administered to the patient.

3. How many milligrams are in the 50 mL multi-dose vial?

4. How many 100 mg doses can be obtained from this vial?

Scenario B: MaryEllen Wainwright is a patient who uses insulin to control her diabetes. She normally receives two vials of insulin each month, but the doctor has just reduced her dose of insulin from 55 units daily to 30 units daily. She also needs new insulin syringes that are smaller and easier to read.

5. How many 10 mL vials will be needed to administer the lowered dose for one month?

6. What size insulin syringe will the patient need? Select the insulin syringe to be used from the handout.

7. If the doctor has the patient reduce her dose by 2 units after 10 days, 2 units on day 20, and 2 units on day 30, how many units will she be using daily after 30 days? Fill in the correct amount that the patient will be using after 30 days.

Scenario C: Rahim Patel is a 56-year-old hospitalized male with labs indicating low potassium. The physician orders 40 mEq of IV potassium chloride and 40 mEq of oral potassium chloride.

8. You have a 10 mL vial of potassium chloride 20 mEq. How many milliliters will be needed for the patient's IV dose?

9. You have a 20 mEq/15 mL potassium chloride oral solution. How many milliliters will be needed for the patient's oral dose?

10. After receiving a total of 80 mEq of potassium chloride, the patient's potassium level is still low. An additional IV infusion is started with potassium chloride 10 mEq/5 mL added. How many milliequivalents of potassium chloride will the patient receive if the amount added was 15 mL?

Scenario D: Lauren Nickelson is a 38-year-old female weighing 83 kg who is being admitted to the hospital from the emergency department. Her admission orders include heparin 5000 units SC three times daily and vancomycin 15 mg/kg IV twice daily.

11. How many milliliters of heparin will the patient receive with each injection if the vial concentration is 10,000 units/mL?

12. How many milligrams of vancomycin will be given with each dose?

13. The label on the vancomycin 5 g vial states to reconstitute with 100 mL of sterile water for injection to create a concentration of 1 g/20 mL. How many milliliters of the reconstituted solution will be used for the patient's dose?

Navigator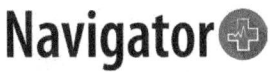

Access interactive chapter review exercises, practice activities, flash cards, and study games.

7

Preparing Parenteral Solutions

Jennifer L. Babin, PharmD, BCPS
Lisa McCartney, BAAS, CPhT, PhTR

Learning Objectives

1 Calculate the amount of medication in a solution based on a given percentage strength.

2 Calculate the percentage strength of medication in a given solution.

3 Describe the types of intravenous sets by drop factor.

4 Calculate intravenous drip rates and flow rates using various intravenous sets.

5 Estimate and calculate time for intravenous administration.

6 Calculate rates of intravenous infusion and intravenous piggyback infusion.

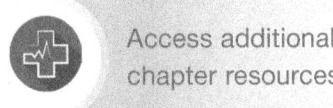 Access additional chapter resources.

7.1 Percentage and Ratio Strength Dilutions

A **solution** is a mixture of two or more substances. Solutions may comprise any of the three states of matter: gas, liquid, or solid. Some of the most common solutions exist in the following combinations of components:

- solid in a liquid (e.g., salt water)
- two liquids (e.g., a mixed drink)
- solid in a solid (e.g., fruit in gelatin)
- gas in a liquid (e.g., soda water)

In a solution, the substance dissolved in the liquid is called the **solute**, and the liquid is the **solvent**. If both substances are liquids, usually the component representing the greater amount is considered the solvent, and the component representing the smaller amount is the solute. In preparing pharmaceutical solutions, the goal is to mix concentrations that result in accurately measured doses.

In general, when comparing two solutions that contain the same components, the solution containing the smaller amount of solute is considered **dilute**. The solution containing the larger amount of solute is considered **concentrated**. As discussed in Chapter 6, the concentration of one substance dissolved in another substance may be expressed as either a percentage strength (e.g., 25%) or a ratio strength (e.g., $^{25}/_{100}$ or $^{1}/_{4}$). The percentage strength or ratio strength of a solution refers to the number of grams/100 mL. How the concentration of the solute in the solvent is expressed depends on which is a solid and/or which is a liquid.

Within the context of preparing sterile, parenteral solutions (solutions that are administered by injection or infusion), the percentage strength or ratio strength may be further classified as a solid in a liquid, sometimes referred to as weight in volume (w/v), or a liquid in a liquid, sometimes referred to as volume in volume (v/v). There are two common scenarios that require calculations based on percentage strength or ratio strength. These scenarios include the preparation of a solid-in-a-liquid solution and the preparation of a liquid-in-a-liquid solution.

Solid in a Liquid

$$\textbf{weight in volume (w/v)} = \text{number of grams of medication} = \frac{x \text{ g of medication}}{100 \text{ mL of final solution}}$$
$$\text{in 100 mL of final solution}$$

Liquid in a Liquid

$$\textbf{volume in volume (v/v)} = \text{number of milliliters of} = \frac{x \text{ mL medication}}{100 \text{ mL of final solution}}$$
$$\text{medication in 100 mL}$$
$$\text{of final solution}$$

Example 7.1.1

A 9% solution means there are 9 parts of the medication (or active ingredient) in 100 parts of the solution. Express this percentage strength as w/v and v/v.

w/v = 9 g of drug in 100 mL of final solution (or 9 g/100 mL)

v/v = 9 mL of drug in 100 mL of final solution (or 9 mL/100 mL)

Example 7.1.2

Express the components of a 4% solution of sodium chloride (NaCl) in the form of a w/v solution.

A 4% NaCl solution contains 4 g of NaCl in each 100 mL of fluid. Another way of saying this is that an IV solution with a concentration of 4% NaCl will provide 4 g of NaCl for every 100 mL of fluid that is administered to the patient.

$$\frac{4 \text{ g of NaCl}}{100 \text{ mL of fluid}}$$

For ease of understanding and computation, this type of ratio is usually expressed as:

$$\frac{4 \text{ g}}{100 \text{ mL}}$$

Example 7.1.3

Express the components of a 3% irrigation solution of acetic acid in the form of a v/v solution.

A 3% acetic acid irrigation solution contains 3 mL of pure acetic acid in each 100 mL of fluid. Another way of saying this is that an irrigation solution with a concentration of 3% acetic acid will provide 3 mL of pure acetic acid for every 100 mL of fluid that is administered to the patient.

$$\frac{3 \text{ mL of } 3\% \text{ acetic acid}}{100 \text{ mL of fluid}}$$

or

$$\frac{3 \text{ mL}}{100 \text{ mL}}$$

For Good Measure

Pharmacy technicians should be familiar with the frequently used abbreviation NS, which is short for normal saline, or NaCl 0.9%.

The following ratios are important to remember when setting up problems involving solutions.

Weight-in-volume (w/v) problems involve adding a solid medication (e.g., an active ingredient) to a liquid, such as water that has sodium chloride dissolved in it.

$$\text{percentage strength of w/v solution} = \frac{\text{g of active ingredient}}{100 \text{ mL of solution}} \times 100$$

Volume-in-volume (v/v) problems involve mixing a liquid in another liquid, such as pure acetic acid in water.

$$\text{percentage strength of v/v solution} = \frac{\text{mL of active ingredient}}{100 \text{ mL of solution}} \times 100$$

Intravenous (IV) solutions that are given in large quantities are labeled as a percentage strength, such as dextrose 5%, which is also written as D_5W or D5W. Normal saline (NS) is a solution of water and sodium chloride at 0.9% concentration. Water that is germ-free but has no dextrose or sodium chloride added to it is called *sterile water*. The following examples show how IV and injectable products are labeled. The most obvious difference between these labels and previous label examples is that there is no milligrams-per-milliliter designation.

Commercially available containers of IV solution are labeled with the following volumes: 25 mL, 50 mL, 100 mL, 250 mL, 500 mL, or 1000 mL. It is important to realize that the actual volume contained in each container is greater than the labeled amount. This is due to overfill. Manufacturers purposefully overfill IV solution containers to protect against potential volume loss, which may result from product evaporation. Therefore, there is variability in the actual volume contained in a commercially available IV solution container. For example, an IV solution of NS may be labeled as containing 100 mL. However, the actual volume in the container is likely greater than 100 mL.

In clinical practice, there are many circumstances in which the additional volume is considered negligible. However, there are other instances in which overfill volume must be accounted for. In this textbook, assume that given IV solution volumes are accurate and IV solution overfill is negligible.

There are several concentrations of sodium chloride available for intravenous use, including 0.45%, 0.9%, 3%, 14.6%, and 23.4%. It is also common for IV solutions to contain dextrose (a sugar) in addition to sodium chloride. Lactated Ringer's (LR) is another commonly used IV fluid that contains several electrolytes. Unlike sodium chloride, the label for LR is not written using a percentage strength. When preparing a solution, read labels carefully to ensure that the correct product and concentration are used. Patients can be harmed if their IV fluids are made incorrectly.

When the percentage concentration of a solution is known, that percentage can be used to determine the amount of active ingredient, as demonstrated in the following examples.

Example 7.1.4

How many grams of dextrose are in 1 L of D$_5$W?

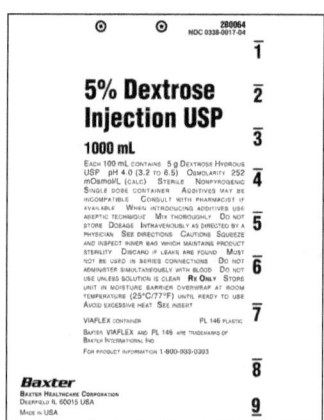

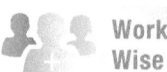

Work Wise

In practice, you will not typically be required to calculate the number of grams of dextrose or sodium chloride, but knowing how to solve these types of pharmacy calculations is important to your overall understanding of pharmacy math applications.

Remember that D$_5$W means 5% dextrose in water, or a concentration of 5 g/100 mL.

Using the ratio-proportion method:

Convert 1 L to 1,000 mL.

$$\frac{1{,}000 \text{ mL}}{x \text{ g}} = \frac{100 \text{ mL}}{5 \text{ g}}$$

$$x \text{ g} (100 \text{ mL}) = 5 \text{ g} (1{,}000 \text{ mL})$$

$$\frac{x \text{ g} (\cancel{100 \text{ mL}})}{\cancel{100 \text{ mL}}} = \frac{5 \text{ g} (1{,}000 \cancel{\text{ mL}})}{100 \cancel{\text{ mL}}}$$

$$x = 50 \text{ g}$$

Using the dimensional analysis method:

$$1 \cancel{\text{ L}} \times \frac{1{,}000 \cancel{\text{ mL}}}{1 \cancel{\text{ L}}} \times \frac{5 \text{ g}}{100 \cancel{\text{ mL}}} = 50 \text{ g}$$

Example 7.1.5

How many grams of sodium chloride (NaCl) are in 1 L of NS?

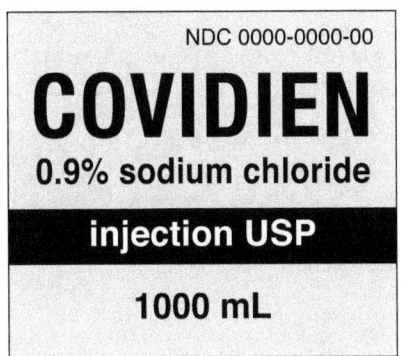

NDC 0000-0000-00

COVIDIEN

0.9% sodium chloride

injection USP

1000 mL

Remember that NS is 0.9% NaCl, or a concentration of 0.9 g/100 mL.

Using the ratio-proportion method:

Convert 1 L to 1,000 mL.

$$\frac{1{,}000 \text{ mL}}{x \text{ g}} = \frac{100 \text{ mL}}{0.9 \text{ g}}$$

$$x \text{ g } (100 \text{ mL}) = 0.9 \text{ g } (1{,}000 \text{ mL})$$

$$\frac{x \text{ g } (100 \text{ mL})}{100 \text{ mL}} = \frac{0.9 \text{ g } (1{,}000 \text{ mL})}{100 \text{ mL}}$$

$$x = 9 \text{ g}$$

Using the dimensional analysis method:

$$1 \text{ L} \times \frac{1{,}000 \text{ mL}}{1 \text{ L}} \times \frac{0.9 \text{ g}}{100 \text{ mL}} = 9 \text{ g}$$

When the amount of active ingredient and the total volume of the final solution are known, you can calculate the percentage strength of the concentration, as shown in the following examples.

Example 7.1.6

If there are 30 g of dextrose in a 500 mL IV bag, what is the percentage strength of the solution?

Using the w/v equation:

$$x\% \text{ w/v} = \frac{30 \text{ g}}{500 \text{ mL}} \times 100 = 0.06 \text{ g/mL} \times 100$$

$$x\% \text{ w/v} = 6\% \text{ w/v}$$

Using the ratio-proportion method:

$$\frac{100 \text{ mL}}{x \text{ g}} = \frac{500 \text{ mL}}{30 \text{ g}}$$

$$x \text{ g} (500 \text{ mL}) = 30 \text{ g} (100 \text{ mL})$$

$$\frac{x \text{ g} (\cancel{500 \text{ mL}})}{\cancel{500 \text{ mL}}} = \frac{30 \text{ g} (100 \cancel{\text{ mL}})}{500 \cancel{\text{ mL}}}$$

$$x = 6 \text{ g}$$

$$\frac{6 \text{ g}}{100 \text{ mL}} = 6\% \text{ w/v}$$

Example 7.1.7

 If there are 5 g of lipids in a 250 mL IV fat emulsion, what is the percentage strength of the solution?

Using the w/v equation:

$$x\% \text{ w/v} = \frac{5 \text{ g}}{250 \text{ mL}} \times 100 = 0.02 \text{ g/mL} \times 100$$

$$x\% \text{ w/v} = 2\% \text{ w/v}$$

Using the ratio-proportion method:

$$\frac{100 \text{ mL}}{x \text{ g}} = \frac{250 \text{ mL}}{5 \text{ g}}$$

$$x \text{ g} (250 \text{ mL}) = 5 \text{ g} (100 \text{ mL})$$

$$\frac{x \text{ g} (\cancel{250 \text{ mL}})}{\cancel{250 \text{ mL}}} = \frac{5 \text{ g} (100 \cancel{\text{ mL}})}{250 \cancel{\text{ mL}}}$$

$$x = 2 \text{ g}$$

$$\frac{2 \text{ g}}{100 \text{ mL}} = 2\% \text{ w/v}$$

Example 7.1.8

If there are 25 mL of medication in a 1,000 mL IV bag, what is the percentage strength of the solution?

Using the v/v equation:

$$\% \text{ v/v} = \frac{\text{mL of active ingredient}}{100 \text{ mL of solution}} \times 100$$

$$\% \text{ v/v} = \frac{25 \text{ mL}}{1,000 \text{ mL}} \times 100 = 0.025 \text{ mL/mL} \times 100$$

$$x = 2.5\% \text{ v/v}$$

Using the ratio-proportion method:

$$\frac{100 \text{ mL solution}}{x \text{ mL medication}} = \frac{1{,}000 \text{ mL solution}}{25 \text{ mL medication}}$$

$$x \text{ mL medication } (1{,}000 \text{ mL solution}) = 25 \text{ mL medication } (100 \text{ mL solution})$$

$$\frac{x \text{ mL medication } (\cancel{1{,}000 \text{ mL solution}})}{\cancel{1{,}000 \text{ mL solution}}} = \frac{25 \text{ mL medication } (100 \cancel{\text{ mL solution}})}{1{,}000 \cancel{\text{ mL solution}}}$$

$$x = 2.5 \text{ mL medication}$$

$$\frac{2.5 \text{ mL}}{100 \text{ mL}} = 2.5\% \text{ v/v}$$

Name Exchange

The generic medication furosemide is commonly known among pharmacy personnel by the brand name Lasix.

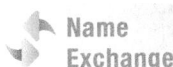

Example 7.1.9

Use the label provided to determine the percentage strength of the solution.

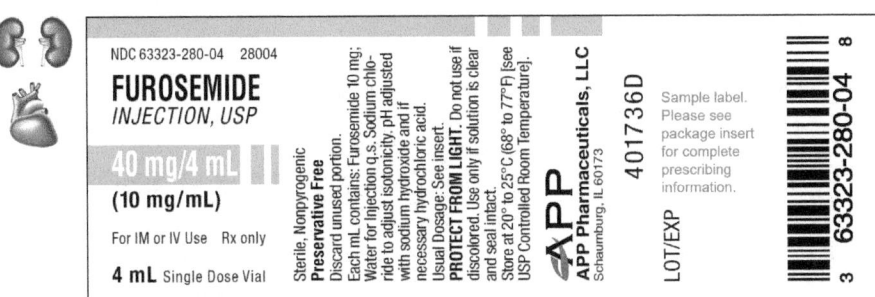

NDC 63323-280-04   28004

FUROSEMIDE
INJECTION, USP

40 mg/4 mL
(10 mg/mL)

For IM or IV Use   Rx only

4 mL Single Dose Vial

Sterile, Nonpyrogenic
Preservative Free
Discard unused portion.
Each mL contains: Furosemide 10 mg; Water for Injection q.s. Sodium chloride to adjust isotonicity. pH adjusted with sodium hydroxide and if necessary hydrochloric acid.
Usual Dosage: See insert.
PROTECT FROM LIGHT. Do not use if discolored. Use only if solution is clear and seal intact.
Store at 20° to 25°C (68° to 77°F) [see USP Controlled Room Temperature].

APP
APP Pharmaceuticals, LLC
Schaumburg, IL 60173

401736D

LOT/EXP

Sample label. Please see package insert for complete prescribing information.

63323-280-04

Convert 40 mg to 0.04 g.

Using the w/v equation:

$$x\% \text{ w/v} = \frac{0.04 \text{ g}}{4 \text{ mL}} \times 100 = 0.01 \text{ g/mL} \times 100$$

$$x\% \text{ w/v} = 1\% \text{ w/v}$$

Using the ratio-proportion method:

$$\frac{100 \text{ mL}}{x \text{ g}} = \frac{4 \text{ mL}}{0.04 \text{ g}}$$

$$x \text{ g } (4 \text{ mL}) = 0.04 \text{ g } (100 \text{ mL})$$

$$\frac{x \text{ g } (\cancel{4 \text{ mL}})}{\cancel{4 \text{ mL}}} = \frac{0.04 \text{ g } (100 \cancel{\text{ mL}})}{4 \cancel{\text{ mL}}}$$

$$x = 1 \text{ g}$$

$$\frac{1 \text{ g}}{100 \text{ mL}} = 1\% \text{ w/v}$$

7.1 Problem Set

Express the following items in questions 1–4 as weight-in-volume (w/v) or volume-in-volume (v/v) solutions.

1. the components of 10% dextrose as a w/v solution

2. the components of 0.45% NaCl as a w/v solution

3. the components of acetic acid 0.25% as a v/v solution

4. the components of Aminosyn 7% as a v/v solution

Perform calculations to answer questions 5–8.

5. If a patient receives an IV solution containing 500 mL of a 10% IV fat emulsion, how many grams of fat did the patient receive?

6. A patient receives an injection of 1.3 mL lidocaine 2%. How many milligrams of lidocaine are in this solution?

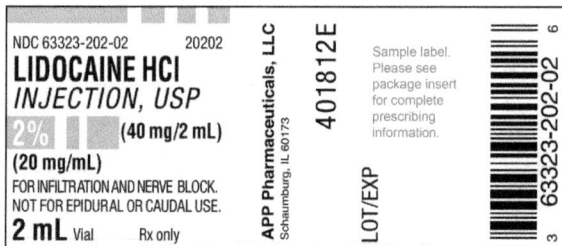

7. A total parenteral nutrition (TPN) order calls for 15 g of dextrose per 100 mL of solution. The total volume of the TPN solution is 2 L. What is the percentage strength of dextrose?

8. A patient receives NaCl 20 g in a 500 mL solution. What is the percentage strength of the solution?

Based on the labels provided in questions 9–14, determine the percentage strength of each medication.

9.

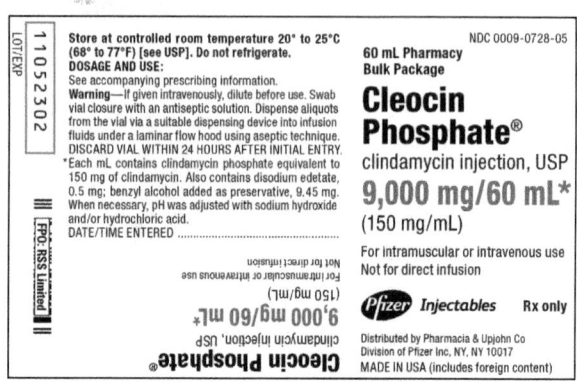

10.

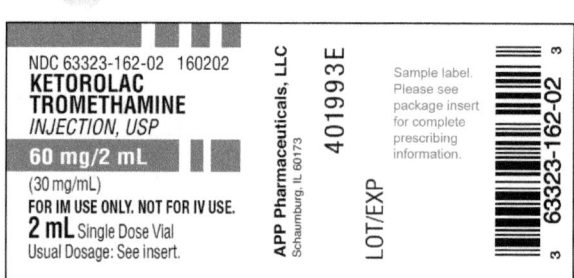

11.

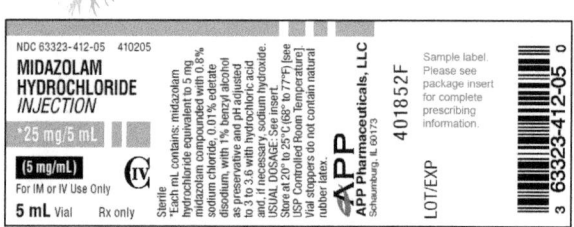

12.

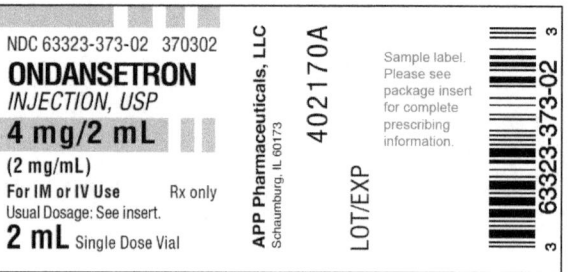

13.

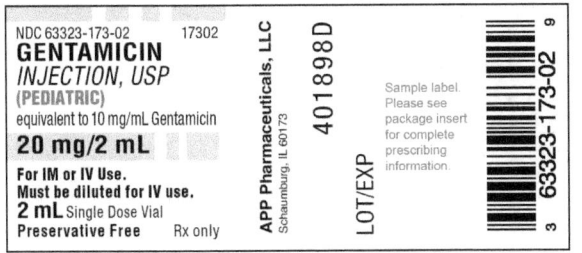

NDC 63323-173-02   17302
GENTAMICIN
INJECTION, USP
(PEDIATRIC)
equivalent to 10 mg/mL Gentamicin
20 mg/2 mL
For IM or IV Use.
Must be diluted for IV use.
2 mL Single Dose Vial
Preservative Free   Rx only

APP Pharmaceuticals, LLC
Schaumburg, IL 60173

401898D

LOT/EXP

Sample label.
Please see
package insert
for complete
prescribing
information.

63323-173-02

14.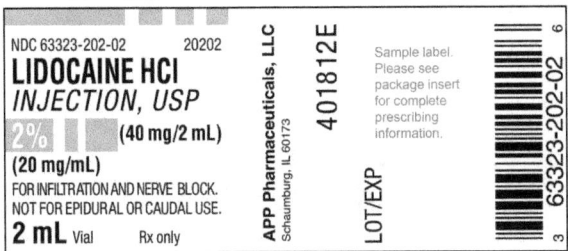

NDC 63323-202-02   20202
LIDOCAINE HCl
INJECTION, USP
2%   **(40 mg/2 mL)**
(20 mg/mL)
FOR INFILTRATION AND NERVE BLOCK.
NOT FOR EPIDURAL OR CAUDAL USE.
2 mL Vial   Rx only

APP Pharmaceuticals, LLC
Schaumburg, IL 60173

401812E

LOT/EXP

Sample label.
Please see
package insert
for complete
prescribing
information.

63323-202-02

Calculate the amount of medication or active ingredient (in grams) for each of the following solutions in questions 15–24.

15. amino acid 3.5%, 2.5 L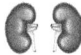

16. dextrose 10%, 1,000 mL

17. acetic acid 0.25%, 1,000 mL

18. sodium chloride 0.9%, 100 mL

19. NaCl 4%, 500 mL

20. NaCl 0.45%, 1 L

21. D_5W, 1,000 mL

22. aminophylline 0.4%, 500 mL

23. lidocaine 4%, 0.5 L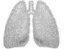

24. dopamine 2%, 250 mL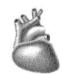

For questions 25–29, calculate the amount of medication or active ingredient (in milligrams) in the following doses.

25. How many milligrams of medication are in 5 mL of a 7.5% dextrose solution?

26. How many milligrams of medication are in 50 mL of a 0.5% solution?

27. How many milligrams are in 0.5 mL of a 1% solution?

28. How many milligrams of epinephrine are in 1 mL of a 1:1,000 solution?

NDC 0517-1071-25
EPINEPHRINE
INJECTION, USP
1:1000 (1 mg/mL)

1 mL AMPULE
FOR SC AND IM USE. FOR IV
AND IC USE AFTER DILUTION.
Rx Only
CONTAINS NO SULFITES.
PRESERVATIVE FREE.
Store below 23°C (73°F). Do not freeze.
AMERICAN REGENT, INC.
SHIRLEY, NY 11967 Rev. 5/05

Lot / Exp.

29. You have a 1:5,000 solution on hand. If the dose is 5 mL, how many milligrams are in one dose?

 Use the medication order below to answer questions 30 and 31.

ID#: L0382201			Memorial Hospital
Name: Luke, Tamika			
DOB: 03/04/67			
Room: 299			Physician's Medication Order
Dr: Dr. Ahmed Vincelette			

ALLERGY OR SENSITIVITY			DIAGNOSIS	
NKA			diverticulitis	
DATE	TIME	ORDERS		PHYSICIAN'S SIG.
10/21/2018	3:16 PM	Change TPN base solution to		
		deliver 100 grams of		
		dextrose per liter of TPN fluid		
			Dr. Ahmed Vincelette	

30. What is the final percentage strength of dextrose?

31. If the patient receives 3,000 mL/24 hours of the TPN solution described above, how many grams of dextrose will she receive in one day?

Using the medication order below to answer questions 32 and 33.

ID#: L0382201			Memorial Hospital
Name: Ransom, Harold G.			
DOB: 12/01/39			Rx
Room: 454			
Dr: Bettina Kelly, M.D.			Physician's Medication Order
ALLERGY OR SENSITIVITY		DIAGNOSIS	
PCN		dehydration	
DATE	TIME	ORDERS	PHYSICIAN'S SIG.
04/26/2017	0220	IVF: NS w/20 mEq	
		potassium chloride @ 150 mL/hour	
			Bettina Kelly, M.D.

32.   What is the percentage strength of NS?

33.   How many grams of NaCl will the patient receive in a 24-hour period?

For questions 34–37, use the label provided below to determine how many grams of NaCl are in the following volumes of NS (0.9% NaCl).

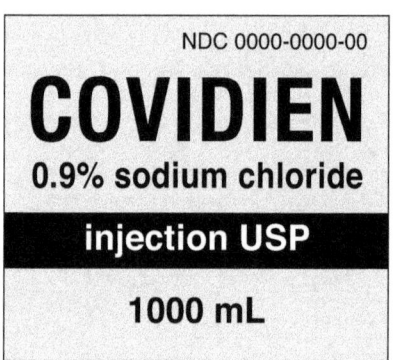

NDC 0000-0000-00

COVIDIEN

0.9% sodium chloride

injection USP

1000 mL

34.   250 mL

35.   500 mL

36.   1,000 mL

37.   2,225 mL

For questions 38–42, determine how many grams of NaCl are in the following volumes of ½ NS (0.45% NaCl).

38.   125 mL

39.   250 mL

40.   750 mL

41.   1,800 mL

42.   2,600 mL

For questions 43–46, use the label provided below to determine how many grams of dextrose are in the following volumes of D_5W (5%).

⊙	⊙	2B0064 NDC 0338-0017-04

5% Dextrose Injection USP

1000 mL

EACH 100 mL CONTAINS 5 g DEXTROSE HYDROUS USP pH 4.0 (3.2 TO 6.5) OSMOLARITY 252 mOsmol/L (CALC) STERILE NONPYROGENIC SINGLE DOSE CONTAINER ADDITIVES MAY BE INCOMPATIBLE CONSULT WITH PHARMACIST IF AVAILABLE WHEN INTRODUCING ADDITIVES USE ASEPTIC TECHNIQUE MIX THOROUGHLY DO NOT STORE DOSAGE INTRAVENOUSLY AS DIRECTED BY A PHYSICIAN SEE DIRECTIONS CAUTIONS SQUEEZE AND INSPECT INNER BAG WHICH MAINTAINS PRODUCT STERILITY DISCARD IF LEAKS ARE FOUND MUST NOT BE USED IN SERIES CONNECTIONS DO NOT ADMINISTER SIMULTANEOUSLY WITH BLOOD DO NOT USE UNLESS SOLUTION IS CLEAR Rx ONLY STORE UNIT IN MOISTURE BARRIER OVERWRAP AT ROOM TEMPERATURE (25°C/77°F) UNTIL READY TO USE AVOID EXCESSIVE HEAT SEE INSERT

VIAFLEX CONTAINER   PL 146 PLASTIC

BAXTER VIAFLEX AND PL 146 ARE TRADEMARKS OF BAXTER INTERNATIONAL INC

FOR PRODUCT INFORMATION 1-800-933-0303

Baxter
BAXTER HEALTHCARE CORPORATION
DEERFIELD IL 60015 USA
MADE IN USA

(scale markings: 1 2 3 4 5 6 7 8 9)

43.   75 mL

44.   385 mL

45.   525 mL

46.   1,350 mL

For questions 47–50, determine how many grams of dextrose are in the following volumes of $D_{10}W$ (10%).

47.   100 mL

48.   325 mL

49.   450 mL

50.   875 mL

Self-check your work in Appendix A.

7.2 IV Flow Rates

℞ **Put Down Roots**

The abbreviation *gtt* comes from the Latin word *gutta*, which means "drop."

Pharmacy staff members use the **flow rate** (also called the *administration rate*) of an IV solution to determine the answers to various questions encountered in daily practice. These questions may address the days' supply of a patient's IV solution or the administration of a particular parenteral dose. The IV flow rate typically refers to the number of milliliters of medication a patient should receive in one hour. Depending on the particular medication, the physician may also order the IV flow rate in units per hour (units/hr), or by the drops per minute (gtts/min) a patient should receive. The flow rate may be expressed in terms of how much IV fluid should be administered per dose or per day. The IV flow rate is often referred to as the *infusion rate* or *rate of infusion*.

The physician typically orders the type of IV fluid to be given (called the *base solution*) and any additives (such as a medication or an electrolyte) that are required. The physician also indicates the rate at which the IV solution should be administered in milliliters per hour (mL/hr). The nursing staff closely monitors IV fluid administration to ensure that an appropriate volume of fluid—and the corresponding amount or dosage of any additive—is given over the specified period to achieve the intended therapeutic response.

The days' supply of an IV preparation may be calculated using the following formula:

$$\frac{\text{total volume (mL)}}{\text{flow rate (mL/hr)}} = \text{number of hours one IV bag will last}$$

Be sure that the units for volume and flow rate correspond. For example, use mL and mL/hr, respectively. When calculating the duration of therapy, always round your answer down to the whole hour.

Example 7.2.1

A 1 L IV is administered at a flow rate of 125 mL/hr. How long will the IV bag last?

Using the volume/flow rate equation:

$$\frac{\text{total volume}}{\text{flow rate}} = x \text{ number of hours one IV bag will last}$$

$$\text{total volume} = 1 \text{ L} = 1{,}000 \text{ mL}$$

$$\text{flow rate} = 125 \text{ mL/hr}$$

$$\frac{1{,}000 \text{ mL}}{125 \text{ mL/hr}} = x \text{ hr}$$

$$x = 8 \text{ hr}$$

Using the ratio-proportion method:

$$\frac{1{,}000 \text{ mL}}{x \text{ hr}} = \frac{125 \text{ mL}}{1 \text{ hr}}$$

$$x \text{ hr } (125 \text{ mL}) = 1 \text{ hr } (1{,}000 \text{ mL})$$

$$\frac{x \text{ hr } (\cancel{125 \text{ mL}})}{\cancel{125 \text{ mL}}} = \frac{1 \text{ hr } (1{,}000 \cancel{\text{ mL}})}{125 \cancel{\text{ mL}}}$$

$$x \text{ hr} = 8 \text{ hr}$$

Using the dimensional analysis method:

$$\cancel{1 \text{ L}} \times \frac{1{,}000 \ \cancel{\text{mL}}}{\cancel{1 \text{ L}}} \times \frac{1 \text{ hr}}{125 \ \cancel{\text{mL}}} = 8 \text{ hr}$$

Example 7.2.2

The prescriber has ordered a 1 L bag of D$_5$NS to run at 150 mL/hr. How many bags will be needed in a 24-hour period?

Using the volume/flow rate equation:

First, determine how long a single bag will last:

$$\frac{\text{total volume}}{\text{flow rate}} = x \text{ hr}$$

$$\text{total volume} = 1 \text{ L} = 1{,}000 \text{ mL}$$

$$\text{flow rate} = 150 \text{ mL/hr}$$

$$\frac{1{,}000 \text{ mL}}{150 \text{ mL/hr}} = x \text{ hr}$$

$$x = 6.67 \text{ hr per bag}$$

Then determine how many bags will be needed for 24 hours:

$$\frac{24 \text{ hr}}{\text{time one bag lasts (hr)}} = \text{number of bags}$$

$$\frac{24 \text{ hr}}{6.67 \text{ hr per bag}} = 3.6 \text{ bags (rounded up to 4 bags because only whole bags are supplied)}$$

Using the ratio-proportion method:

$$\frac{1{,}000 \text{ mL}}{x \text{ hr}} = \frac{150 \text{ mL}}{1 \text{ hr}}$$

$$x \text{ hr } (150 \text{ mL}) = 1 \text{ hr } (1{,}000 \text{ mL})$$

$$\frac{x \text{ hr } (150 \ \cancel{\text{mL}})}{150 \ \cancel{\text{mL}}} = \frac{1 \text{ hr } (1{,}000 \ \cancel{\text{mL}})}{150 \ \cancel{\text{mL}}}$$

$$x = 6.67 \text{ hr}$$

$$\frac{24 \text{ hr}}{6.67 \text{ hr per bag}} = 3.6 \text{ bags (rounded to 4 bags)}$$

Using the dimensional analysis method:

$$\frac{1 \text{ bag}}{\cancel{1 \text{ L}}} \times \frac{\cancel{1 \text{ L}}}{1{,}000 \ \cancel{\text{mL}}} \times \frac{150 \ \cancel{\text{mL}}}{1 \ \cancel{\text{hr}}} \times \frac{24 \ \cancel{\text{hr}}}{\text{day}} = 3.6 \text{ bag/day (rounded to 4 bags/day)}$$

For Good Measure

When determining days' supply for an IV bag, technicians should always round up to the nearest 1 L.

When an order specifies a certain volume to be infused over a specific period (also known as the *duration of therapy*), the IV flow rate can be calculated using the following formula:

$$\text{IV flow rate (mL/hr)} = \frac{\text{total volume of fluid or amount to be infused (mL)}}{\text{duration of therapy (hr)}}$$

Example 7.2.3

The physician has ordered a 1 L IV bag to be infused over 10 hours. What is the IV flow rate in milliliters per hour (mL/hr)?

Using the volume/duration equation:

$$\text{IV flow rate} = \frac{\text{total volume of fluid or amount to be infused}}{\text{duration of therapy}}$$

$$\text{volume} = 1\text{ L} = 1{,}000\text{ mL}$$

$$\text{duration of therapy} = 10\text{ hr}$$

$$\frac{1{,}000\text{ mL}}{10\text{ hr}} = 100\text{ mL/hr}$$

Using the ratio-proportion method:

Convert 1 L to 1,000 mL.

$$\frac{1\text{ hr}}{x\text{ mL}} = \frac{10\text{ hr}}{1{,}000\text{ mL}}$$

$$x\text{ mL (10 hr)} = 1{,}000\text{ mL (1 hr)}$$

$$\frac{x\text{ mL (10 hr)}}{10\text{ hr}} = \frac{1{,}000\text{ mL (1 hr)}}{10\text{ hr}}$$

$$x = 100\text{ mL/hour}$$

When a medication order specifies an amount or a dosage of a medication that is to be infused over a specific period, the amount of medication administered per hour (expressed as milligrams/hour or mg/hr) can be calculated using the following formula:

$$\text{amount of medication infused (mg/hr)} = \frac{\text{total amount of medication (mg)}}{\text{duration of therapy (hr)}}$$

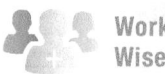

An intravenous piggyback is a secondary IV medication or fluid that is connected to the IV tubing of a primary medication or fluid.

Example 7.2.4

 The physician has ordered a 250 mL intravenous piggyback (IVPB) with 500 mg of Solu-Cortef to be infused over 4 hours. What is the dose of medication in milligrams being administered per hour?

Using the total medication/duration equation:

$$\text{amount of medication infused} = \frac{\text{total amount of medication}}{\text{duration of therapy}}$$

$$\text{total amount of medication} = 500 \text{ mg}$$

$$\text{duration of therapy} = 4 \text{ hr}$$

$$\frac{500 \text{ mg}}{4 \text{ hr}} = 125 \text{ mg/hr}$$

Using the ratio-proportion method:

$$\frac{1 \text{ hr}}{x \text{ mg}} = \frac{4 \text{ hr}}{500 \text{ mg}}$$

$$x \text{ mg} (4 \text{ hr}) = 500 \text{ mg} (1 \text{ hr})$$

$$\frac{x \text{ mg} (4 \text{ hr})}{4 \text{ hr}} = \frac{500 \text{ mg} (1 \text{ hr})}{4 \text{ hr}}$$

$$x = 125 \text{ mg/hour}$$

Example 7.2.5

 A patient receives 8,100 units of heparin over 6 hours at a constant rate. How many units of heparin does the patient receive each hour?

Using the medication/duration equation:

$$\text{amount of medication administered} = \frac{\text{total amount of medication}}{\text{duration of therapy}}$$

$$\text{total amount of medication} = 8,100 \text{ units}$$

$$\text{duration of therapy} = 6 \text{ hours}$$

$$\frac{8,100 \text{ units}}{6 \text{ hr}} = 1,350 \text{ units/hr}$$

Using the ratio-proportion method:

$$\frac{1 \text{ hr}}{x \text{ units}} = \frac{6 \text{ hr}}{8,100 \text{ units}}$$

$$x \text{ units} (6 \text{ hr}) = 8,100 \text{ units} (1 \text{ hr})$$

$$\frac{x \text{ units} (6 \text{ hr})}{6 \text{ hr}} = \frac{8,100 \text{ units} (1 \text{ hr})}{6 \text{ hr}}$$

$$x = 1,350 \text{ units/hour}$$

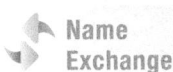 **Name Exchange**

The anti-infective generic drug cefazolin is also known as the brand name Ancef.

Example 7.2.6

The following order is received in the IV room.

℞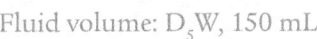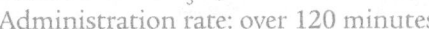
Medication: cefazolin, 1 g
Fluid volume: D₅W, 150 mL
Administration rate: over 120 minutes

What volume of fluid is administered per hour, and what amount of medication is given per hour?

First, determine the volume of fluid given per hour (in mL/hr).
Note that 120 minutes = 2 hours.

Using the volume/duration equation:

$$\text{IV flow rate} = \frac{\text{total volume of fluid or amount to be infused}}{\text{duration of therapy}}$$

$$\frac{150 \text{ mL}}{2 \text{ hr}} = 75 \text{ mL/hr}$$

Using the ratio-proportion method:

$$\frac{1 \text{ hr}}{x \text{ mL}} = \frac{2 \text{ hr}}{150 \text{ mL}}$$

$$x \text{ mL} (2 \text{ hr}) = 150 \text{ mL} (1 \text{ hr})$$

$$\frac{x \text{ mL} (2 \text{ hr})}{2 \text{ hr}} = \frac{150 \text{ mL} (1 \text{ hr})}{2 \text{ hr}}$$

$$x = 75 \text{ mL/hour}$$

Then calculate the amount of medication given per hour (in mg/hr).
Note that 1 g = 1,000 mg.

Using the total medication/duration equation:

$$\text{amount of medication infused} = \frac{\text{total amount of medication}}{\text{duration of therapy}}$$

$$\frac{1,000 \text{ mg}}{2 \text{ hr}} = 500 \text{ mg/hr}$$

Using the ratio-proportion method:

Convert 1 g to 1,000 mg.

$$\frac{1 \text{ hr}}{x \text{ mg}} = \frac{2 \text{ hr}}{1,000 \text{ mg}}$$

$$x \text{ mg} (2 \text{ hr}) = 1,000 \text{ mg} (1 \text{ hr})$$

$$\frac{x \text{ mg} (2 \text{ hr})}{2 \text{ hr}} = \frac{1,000 \text{ mg} (1 \text{ hr})}{2 \text{ hr}}$$

$$x = 500 \text{ mg/hour}$$

7.2 Problem Set

Perform calculations to answer questions 1–5.

1. A 1 L IV bag is running at 50 mL/hour. How long will it last?

2. A 1 L bag of IV fluid is hung at 7 PM and has a flow rate of 100 mL/hr. What time will the next bag be needed?

3. A 500 mL bag of IV fluid has a flow rate of 30 mL/hr. How long will it last?

4. If a patient is given 60 mg of medication in 75 mL over 45 minutes, what is the flow rate in milliliters per hour?

5. A patient receives 20,000 units of heparin in an IV of 100 mL over 45 minutes. What is the flow rate in milliliters per hour?

Use the IVPB label below to answer questions 6 and 7.

> *****IV Piggyback*****
> Memorial Hospital
> **Name:** Washington, Deandra   **Room:** ICU-4
> **Pt. ID#:** 776263663   **Rx#:** 77283993
> ___
> **Vancomycin 1,500 mg**
> **Dextrose 5% in water (D$_5$W) 250 mL**
> **Rate: over 5 hr**
>
> Expires _____
> RPh _____
> Tech _____
>
> Keep refrigerated – warm to room temperature
> before use.

6. What is the flow rate in milliliters per hour?

7. What is the vancomycin dosage in milligrams per hour?

Use the IVPB label below to answer questions 8 and 9.

> *****IV Piggyback*****
> Memorial Hospital
> **Name:** Parker, Shirley   **Room:** 345
> **Pt. ID#:** 88273000   **Rx#:** 8827730
> ___
> **Cefazolin 500 mg**
> **Sodium chloride 0.9% (NS) 50 mL**
> **Rate: over 60 min**
>
> Expires _____
> RPh _____
> Tech _____
>
> Keep refrigerated – warm to room temperature
> before use.

8. What is the flow rate in milliliters per hour?

9. What is the cefazolin dosage in milligrams per hour?

Use the IV label below to answer questions 10–15.

> *****Large-Volume Parenteral*****
> Memorial Hospital
> **Name:** Le, Thu   **Room:** OB-14
> **Pt. ID#:** 449009288   **Rx#:** 7200182
> ___
> **Potassium chloride 20 mEq**
> **D$_5$NS 1,000 mL**
> **Rate: 100 mL/hr**
>
> Expires _____
> RPh _____
> Tech _____
>
> Keep refrigerated – warm to room temperature
> before use.

10. What is the flow rate in milliliters per hour?

11. How many hours will this IV bag last?

12. How many IV bags will be needed in a 24-hour period? (Round up to the nearest 1 L bag.)

13. What is the potassium dosage in milliequivalents per hour?

14. How many grams of dextrose are in this IV bag?

15. How many grams of NaCl are in this IV bag?

For each rate in questions 16–25, determine the quantity of 1 L bags needed for 24 hours. (Round up to the nearest 1 L bag.)

16. 50 mL/hr _____

17. 75 mL/hr _____

18. 100 mL/hr _____

19. 120 mL/hr _____

20. 125 mL/hr _____

21. 130 mL/hr _____

22. 150 mL/hr _____

23. 175 mL/hr _____

24. 200 mL/hr _____

25. 225 mL/hr _____

Using what you have learned, interpret the prescriptions and perform the necessary calculations to answer questions 26–32.

26. Medication: Solu-Cortef (hydrocortisone) 250 mg
    Fluid volume: 250 mL
    Time of infusion: 4 hr

    a. What is the flow rate in milliliters per hour?

    b. How many milligrams will be administered per hour?

27. Medication: penicillin G 12 million units
    Fluid volume: 500 mL
    Time of infusion: 12 hr

    a. What is the flow rate in milliliters per hour?

    b. How many units will be administered per hour?

28. Medication: lidocaine 4%
    Fluid volume: 500 mL
    Rate: 800 mg/hr

    a. What is the flow rate in milliliters per hour?

    b. How many hours will it take until the entire IV bag has been administered?

29. Medication: Solu-Medrol (methylprednisolone) 250 mg
    Fluid volume: 500 mL
    Rate: 20 mg/hr

    a. What is the flow rate in milliliters per hour?

    b. How many hours will it take until the entire dose has been administered?

30. Medication: dopamine 1,600 mcg in D_5W
    Fluid volume: 500 mL
    Dose: 4 mcg/min

    a. What is the flow rate in milliliters per hour?

    b. How many micrograms will be administered per hour?

31. A physician has ordered an IV infusion of dopamine hydrochloride (Intropin) 800 mg in 250 mL of D_5W to run at 5 mg/hr. Dopamine is available in a 20 mL vial at a concentration of 200 mg/5 mL.

    a. How many milliliters of dopamine must be drawn up to prepare this dose?

    b. What is the IV flow rate in milliliters per hour?

32. A physician has ordered an IVPB of gentamicin 2 mg/kg q8h for a patient who weighs 176 lb. The IVPB will be prepared in a base solution of D$_5$W 100 mL and will be administered over 60 min. Gentamicin is available in a 20 mL vial at a concentration of 40 mg/mL.

a. How many milliliters of gentamicin must be drawn up to prepare a single dose?

b. What is the administration rate in milliliters per hour?

Self-check your work in Appendix A.

7.3 Drop Factor and Infusion Rates

Nursing staff—and, occasionally, pharmacy staff—are required to calculate the rate of administration for an IV fluid in *drops per minute* (expressed as gtts/min). Most inpatient facilities now use electronic infusion pumps to regulate both the volume and the rate of a patient's IV medication. Nursing personnel program the prescribed rate into the electronic infusion pump at the patient's bedside to administer the prescribed number of drops per minute. The rate can be digitally adjusted, which causes the pump's internal clamp to slow or quicken the rate at which the fluid flows through tubing routed through a chamber in the pump. Pumps can be set to give IV fluids in milliliters per hour or drops per minute.

Occasionally, nursing staff must manually adjust the IV flow rate using the tubing's roll clamp, which controls the rate of the fluid volume being administered to the patient. The rate in drops per minute can be calculated manually by counting the number of drops of fluid that fall into the drip chamber in one minute. The nurse can then manually adjust the rate up or down by using the roll clamp.

Calculating the flow rate in drops per minute is complicated by the variety of IV tubing—sometimes called *IV tubing sets*, or simply *IV sets*—that is available. Manufacturers produce calibrated IV sets that result in different size drops. An IV set is identified by the number of drops it takes to make 1 mL. This calibration may be referred to as a *drop set* or a *drip set* but is most commonly called the IV set's **drop factor**. The most common IV sets have drop set factors of 10, 15, 20, and 60, meaning 10 gtts/mL, 15 gtts/mL, 20 gtts/mL, and 60 gtts/mL, respectively. The 10, 15, and 20 drop factors produce large drops called *macrodrops*, and IV tubing with these drop factors is called *macrodrip IV tubing* or a **macro-drip set**. The 60 drop factor tubing produces *microdrops* and is called *microdrip IV tubing* or a **mini-drip set**. Figure 7.1 illustrates these different drop sizes.

The drop factor for an IV set is prominently displayed on the outside of the package. The 10 drop and 15 drop sets are commonly used for adult patients, whereas the 60 drop set is used for pediatric patients or patients who are critically ill and are being given medications that have a narrow therapeutic window, meaning that there is only a small difference between toxic and therapeutic doses.

To determine the IV flow rate in drops per minute when the total volume and infusion time are known, use the following formula:

$$\frac{\text{total volume (TV)}}{\text{infusion time (IT) in minutes}} \times \text{drop factor (DF)} = \text{drops/minute}$$

$$\frac{\text{TV}}{\text{IT}} \times \text{DF} = \text{gtts/min}$$

> **For Good Measure**
>
> When performing drop factor calculations, pharmacy technicians must examine the IV set or tubing package to determine the drop size in gtts/mL.

> **For Good Measure**
>
> If remembering the gtts/min formula is difficult, think of the calculation in terms of the dimensional analysis method instead. The dimensional analysis method produces a similar equation.

FIGURE 7.1
IV Drop Sets

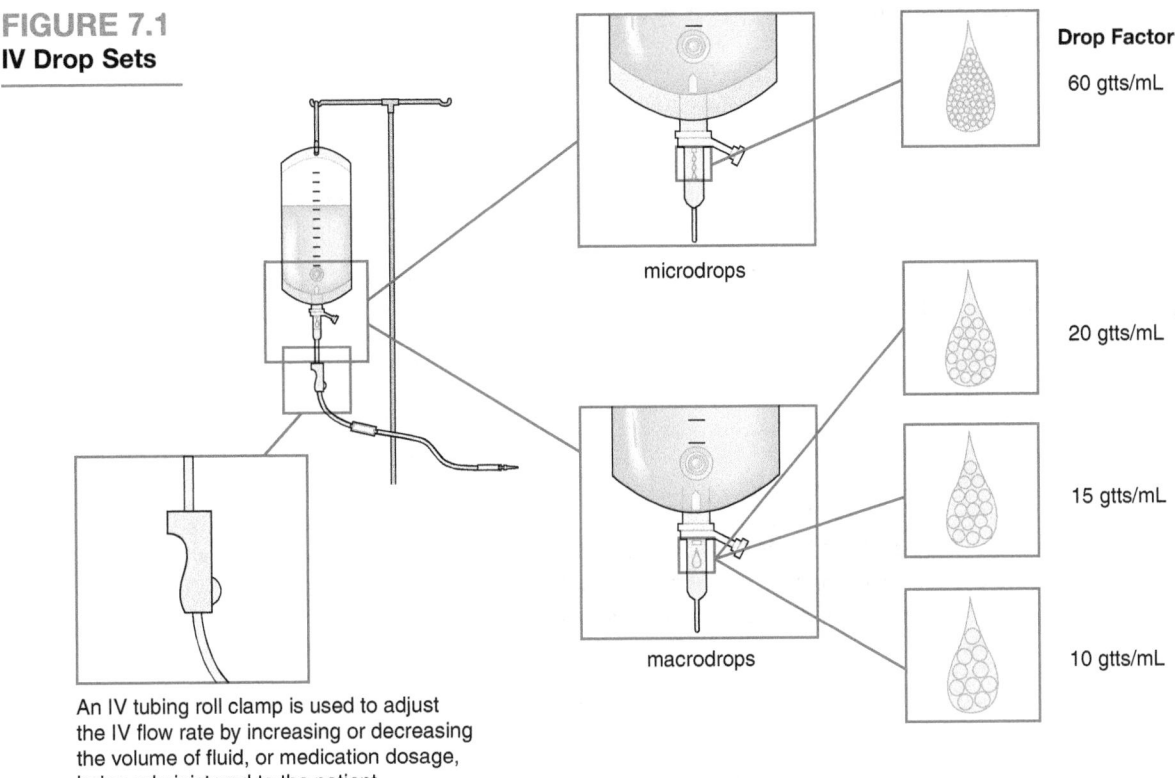

Drop Factor

60 gtts/mL

microdrops

20 gtts/mL

15 gtts/mL

macrodrops

10 gtts/mL

An IV tubing roll clamp is used to adjust the IV flow rate by increasing or decreasing the volume of fluid, or medication dosage, being administered to the patient.

To better understand this equation, consider the units that may be used.

$$\frac{\cancel{mL}}{min} \times \frac{drops}{\cancel{mL}} = drops/min$$

Dimensional analysis may also be used to solve this type of equation. The following examples demonstrate how to use this formula in various scenarios. It is common practice to round down to the nearest whole drop in the event a partial drop per minute is calculated. For example, 20.6 gtts/min would be rounded down to 20 gtts/min.

For Good Measure

When a drop per minute calculation results in a partial drop, pharmacy technicians should round down to the nearest whole drop.

Example 7.3.1

An IV has a total volume of 250 mL and is being administered over 60 minutes using macrodrip tubing with a drop factor of 15 gtts/mL. What is the rate in drops per minute?

$$\frac{TV}{IT} \times DF = drops/minute$$

$$\frac{250 \cancel{mL}}{60 \, min} \times \frac{15 \, gtts}{\cancel{mL}} = 62.5 \, gtts/min, \text{ rounded to } 62 \, gtts/min$$

To determine the rate in drops per minute when the IV flow rate (in milliliters per hour) and the drop factor are known, use the following formula:

$$\frac{\text{IV flow rate (IVFR)}}{60 \text{ min/hr}} \times \text{drop factor (DF)} = \text{drops/minute}$$

$$\frac{\text{IVFR}}{60 \text{ min/hr}} \times \text{DF} = \text{gtts/min}$$

As before, consider how the units in the formula cancel to better understand how it was derived.

$$\frac{\cancel{\text{mL}}/\cancel{\text{hr}}}{60 \text{ min}/\cancel{\text{hr}}} \times \frac{\text{drops}}{\cancel{\text{mL}}} = \text{drops/min}$$

Example 7.3.2

An IV of D$_5$W with 20,000 units of heparin is being administered at a rate of 40 mL/hr using macrodrip tubing with a drop factor of 20 gtts/mL. How many drops per minute are being administered?

Using the gtts/min formula:

Begin by identifying the amounts to insert into the formula.

$$\frac{\text{IV flow rate (IVFR)}}{60 \text{ min/hr}} \times \text{drop factor (DF)} = \text{drops/min}$$

$$\text{IVFR} = 40 \text{ mL/hr}$$

$$\text{drop factor} = 20 \text{ gtts/mL}$$

Insert the values from the problem statement into the formula to determine the drops per minute rate.

$$\frac{40 \cancel{\text{mL}}/\cancel{\text{hr}}}{60 \text{ min}/\cancel{\text{hr}}} \times \frac{20 \text{ gtts}}{\cancel{\text{mL}}} = 13.33 \text{ gtts/min, rounded to 13 gtts/min}$$

Using the dimensional analysis method:

$$\frac{40 \cancel{\text{mL}}}{\cancel{\text{hr}}} \times \frac{20 \text{ drops}}{1 \cancel{\text{mL}}} \times \frac{1 \cancel{\text{hr}}}{60 \text{ mins}} = 13.33 \text{ drops/min, rounded to 13 drops/min}$$

Occasionally, pharmacy personnel use drop factor calculations to determine the amount of a medication that will be infused over a specific period. These types of problems are sometimes referred to as *IV drip rate calculations* and can be solved by using the following formula:

Step 1 Determine the concentration of the solution in mg/mL by dividing the total number of milligrams in the solution by the total volume in the solution (in mL).

$$\frac{\text{total milligrams}}{\text{total volume (TV)}} = \text{concentration in mg/mL}$$

Step 2 Determine the number of milligrams in each drop, using the given drop factor.

$$\frac{\text{concentration (mg/mL)}}{\text{drop factor (DF; drops/mL)}} = \text{mg/drop}$$

The following examples demonstrate this type of calculation.

Example 7.3.3

 The prescriber has ordered a dopamine drip of 800 mg in 250 mL D$_5$W. The IV will be administered at 10 mL/hr through tubing that has a drop factor of 10 gtts/mL. How many milligrams of dopamine are in each drop?

Using the IV drip rate calculation formula:

Step 1 Determine the concentration of the solution in mg/mL.

total milligrams = 800 mg
total volume (TV) = 250 mL
800/250 = 3.2 mg/mL

Step 2 Determine the number of milligrams of dopamine per drop (mg/gtt).

concentration = 3.2 mg/mL (determined in Step 1 above)
drop factor (DF) = 10 gtts/mL
3.2/10 = 0.32 mg/gtt

There are 0.32 mg of dopamine in each drop.

Using the dimensional analysis method:

$$\frac{800 \text{ mg}}{250 \text{ mL}} \times \frac{1 \text{ mL}}{10 \text{ gtts}} = 0.32 \text{ mg/gtt}$$

Example 7.3.4

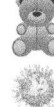 **A physician has ordered vancomycin 250 mg in 100 mL NS every six hours for a pediatric patient. The IV will be administered at 50 mL/hr through 20 gtts/mL macrodrip tubing. How many milligrams of vancomycin are in each drop?**

Using the IV drip rate calculation formula:

Step 1 Determine the concentration of the solution in mg/mL.

total milligrams = 250 mg
total volume (TV) = 100 mL
250/100 = 2.5 mg/mL

Step 2 Determine the number of milligrams of vancomycin per drop.

concentration = 2.5 mg/mL (determined in Step 1 above)

drop factor (DF) = 20 gtts/mL

2.5/20 = 0.125 mg/gtt

There are 0.125 mg of vancomycin in each drop.

Using the dimensional analysis method:

$$\frac{250\ \text{mg}}{100\ \cancel{\text{mL}}} \times \frac{1\ \cancel{\text{mL}}}{20\ \text{gtts}} = 0.125\ \text{mg/gtt}$$

7.3 Problem Set

Perform calculations to answer the following questions.

1. An IV rate is 10 mL/hr. Using an IV tubing set with a drop factor of 10 gtts/mL, what is the rate in drops per minute?

2. What is the IV flow rate in drops per minute for an IV that is administered at 35 mL/hr using a 60 drop set?

3. A patient is to receive 1 g of cefazolin in 100 mL of ½ NS over one hour using a 10 drop set. What is the rate in drops per minute?

4. A nurse will be administering 500 mg of medication in 50 mL over 30 minutes using microdrip tubing. What is the flow rate in drops per minute?

5. A physician orders 20,000 units of heparin in an IV of D_5NS 500 mL to be administered continuously over 24 hours. Using a 15 drop set, what is the rate in drops per minute?

6. A physician orders 750 mg of vancomycin in 250 mL IVPB over one hour using a 15 drop set. How many drops per minute will be administered?

7. A patient is to be given 1,000 mL of Lactated Ringer's (LR) solution at 50 mL/hr. If tubing with a drop factor of 15 is used, what is the rate in drops per minute?

8. A patient is to be given TPN at 95 mL/hr. What will the drip rate be if a 20 drop set is used?

9. A physician orders 40 mEq of potassium chloride in 100 mL of D_5W to be administered over 4 hours. If a 10 drop set is used, how many milliequivalents of potassium will be in each drop?

10. A patient is to receive 20,000 units of heparin in 500 mL of D_5 ½ NS at a flow rate of 25 mL/hr. If tubing with a drop factor of 15 is used, what will the rate be in drops per minute?

11. The pharmacy receives the order below. What is the rate in drops per minute if microdrip tubing is used?

ID#: Y7HH7992			Memorial Hospital
Name: Baldwin, Flora			
DOB: 11/22/90			Rx
Room: 514			
Dr: Dr. Ahmed Vincelette			Physician's Medication Order
ALLERGY OR SENSITIVITY		DIAGNOSIS	
ASA, latex		pancreatitis	
DATE	TIME	ORDERS	PHYSICIAN'S SIG.
10/28/2019	2316	IVF — D5NS 1L w/20 mEq	
		potassium chloride, 1 mg folic acid,	
		and 1 amp MVI @ 50 mL/hr	
			Ahmed Vincelette, M.D.

12. A pharmacy receives the order below. What is the rate in drops per minute if tubing with a drop factor of 20 is used?

ID#: MBYUU97II			Memorial Hospital
Name: Mosier, Bud			
DOB: 02/22/59			
Room: 716			Physician's Medication Order
Dr: Jeremiah King, M.D.			

ALLERGY OR SENSITIVITY			DIAGNOSIS	
PCN, sulfa, shellfish, tape			asthmatic bronchitis	
DATE	TIME	ORDERS		PHYSICIAN'S SIG.
5/15/2017	3:27 PM	Aminophylline 1 g in 250 mL D5W		
		@ 10 mL/hr		
				Jeremiah King, M.D.

13. A pharmacy receives the order below. If microdrip tubing is used, how many milligrams of amiodarone will be in each drop?

ID#: 9927739992			Memorial Hospital
Name: Brzyznski, Martha			
DOB: 01/09/48			
Room: ICU-24			Physician's Medication Order
Dr: Amarite Gaya, M.D.			

ALLERGY OR SENSITIVITY			DIAGNOSIS	
NKDA			myocardial infarction	
DATE	TIME	ORDERS		PHYSICIAN'S SIG.
5/15/2017		Administer amiodarone drip		
		450 mg in 250 mL NS at 8 mL/hr		
				Amarite Gaya, M.D.

14. A pharmacy receives the order below. Using tubing with a drop factor of 10, how many milligrams per drop will be administered?

ID#: UHy08llieX			Memorial Hospital
Name: Lazaar, Howard			
DOB: 07/20/50			
Room: CCU -03			Physician's Medication Order
Dr: Thu Singh, M.D.			

ALLERGY OR SENSITIVITY			DIAGNOSIS	
NSAIDs, ASA, sulfa, PCN, milk			CHF	
DATE	TIME	ORDERS		PHYSICIAN'S SIG.
10/30/2017		Norepinephrine 8 mg/250 mL		
		D5W over 24 hours		
				Thu Singh, M.D.

15. The label below is received in the IV room. If the nurse administers this IVPB using tubing with a drop factor of 10, how many drops per minute will be administered?

IV Piggyback

Memorial Hospital

Name: Geist, Polly	Room: PICU
Pt. ID#: KKU882799	Rx#: 66729937

Tobramycin 40 mg
Dextrose 5% in water (D$_5$W) 25 mL
Rate: over 60 min

Expires _____
RPh _____
Tech _____

Keep refrigerated – warm to room temperature before use.

16. The following label is received in the IV room. If the nurse administers it using microdrip tubing, how many milliequivalents will be administered with each drop?

Large-Volume Parenteral

Memorial Hospital

Name: Briggs, Jennifer   **Room:** NICU

Pt. ID#: H68YY7   **Rx#:** 6638927

D$_{10}$W 500 mL
Potassium acetate 10 mEq
Rate: 5 mL/hr

Expires _____
RPh _____
Tech _____

Keep refrigerated – warm to room temperature
before use.

Self-check your work in Appendix A.

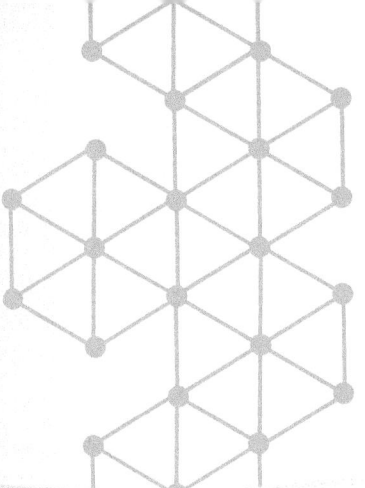

- A solution is a mixture of two or more substances, each of which may be in the form of a gas, liquid, or solid.

- A solution comprises a solute (the substance dissolved in a liquid) and a solvent (the liquid).

- The concentration of one substance dissolved in another substance may be expressed as either a percentage strength or a ratio strength.

- The percentage strength of a solution refers to the number of grams/100 mL and can be classified as a solid in a liquid (weight in volume) or two liquids (volume in volume).

- The IV flow rate, also called the IV rate or administration rate, is the number of milliliters of fluid the patient will receive in one hour.

- Pharmacy technicians can determine how long an IV bag will last by dividing the total volume by the IV flow rate.

- Technicians can determine how many milliliters will be administered to a patient by dividing the total volume by the number of hours over which it will be administered.

- An IV set is identified by the number of drops it takes to make 1 mL.

- Macrodrip IV tubing—also known as a macro-drip set—is typically used for adult patients and comes in the following drop factors: 10, 15, and 20.

- Microdrip IV tubing—also known as a mini-drip set—is typically used for pediatric patients and patients who are critically ill and has a drop factor of 60 gtts/mL.

- Pharmacy technicians sometimes use the drop factor of tubing to calculate the amount of medication that will be administered over a certain period.

To determine the percentage strength of a w/v solution:

$$\text{percentage strength of w/v solution} = \frac{\text{g of active ingredient}}{100 \text{ mL of solution}} \times 100$$

To determine the percentage strength of a v/v solution:

$$\text{percentage strength of v/v solution} = \frac{\text{mL of active ingredient}}{100 \text{ mL of solution}} \times 100$$

To determine the number of grams in a solution using the ratio-proportion method:

$$\frac{\text{number of grams}}{100 \text{ mL}} = \frac{x \text{ g}}{\text{total volume of solution}}$$

To determine how long an IV bag will last:

$$\frac{\text{total volume (mL)}}{\text{flow rate (mL/hr)}} = \text{number of hours a single IV bag will last}$$

To determine IV drip rate:

$$\text{IV drip rate (gtts/min)} = \frac{\text{IV flow rate (mL/hr)}}{60 \text{ min/hr}} \times \text{drop factor (gtts/mL)}$$

To determine IV flow rate:

$$\text{IV flow rate (mL/hr)} = \frac{\text{total volume of fluid or amount to be infused (mL)}}{\text{duration of therapy (hr)}}$$

To determine the amount of drug administered:

$$\text{amount of drug administered} = \frac{\text{total amount of drug}}{\text{duration of therapy}}$$

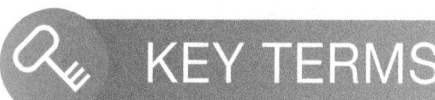 KEY TERMS

concentrated when comparing two solutions that contain the same components, the solution containing the larger amount of solute

dilute when comparing two solutions that contain the same components, the solution containing the smaller amount of solute

drop factor the number of drops an IV set takes to make 1 mL; also called *drip set*

flow rate the rate, expressed in milliliters per hour or drops per minute, at which medication is flowing through an IV line; also called *infusion rate* and *rate of infusion*

macro-drip set a drop set at a rate of 10, 15, or 20 gtts/mL

microdrip a drop set at a rate of 60 gtts/mL that uses microdrip tubing

solute the substance dissolved in the liquid
solvent in a solution

solution a mixture of two or more substances

solvent the liquid that dissolves the solute in
a solution

volume in volume (v/v) the number of milliliters of a drug (solute) in 100 mL of the
final product (solution)

weight in volume (w/v) the number of grams
of a drug (solute) in 100 mL of the final
product (solution)

CHAPTER REVIEW

Finding Solutions

*To gain practice in handling challenging situations in the workplace, consider the following real-world scenarios,
and then use the guiding questions to help you formulate your responses.*

 Scenario A: You have just received the
following medication order in the pharmacy. Answer the questions below based
on this medication order.

ID#: KU88399			Memorial Hospital
Name: Barker, Wally			
DOB: 10/09/45			
Room: 1018			Physician's
Dr: Marshall Rutz, M.D.			Medication Order
ALLERGY OR SENSITIVITY		DIAGNOSIS	
Bactrim, EES		*hypokalemia*	
DATE	TIME	ORDERS	PHYSICIAN'S SIG.
5/22/2017	3:51 PM	*Potassium chloride 20 mEq/L DSNS*	
		@ 125 mL/hr	
		Marshall Rutz, M.D.	

1. How many milliequivalents of KCl will the patient receive in 24 hours?

2. How many grams of dextrose will the patient receive in 24 hours?

3. How many grams of sodium chloride will the patient receive in 24 hours?

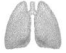 **Scenario B:** The following IV label is
received in the IV room. Answer the ques-
tions below based on this IV label.

Large-Volume Parenteral

Memorial Hospital

Name: Vaughn, Perry   **Room:** TCU
Pt. ID#: YHYTELLL **Rx#:** 2299388

Aminophylline 1 g
D$_5$W 500 mL
Rate: 20 mL/hr

Expires _____
RPh _____
Tech _____

Keep refrigerated—warm to room temperature
before use.

4. How many grams of dextrose will the patient receive in 24 hours?

5. How many milligrams of aminophylline will the patient receive in 24 hours?

6. How many milliliters of fluid will the patient receive in 24 hours?

Scenario C: A physician has prescribed the following order. Answer the questions below based on this medication order.

ID#: LK9968811687			Memorial Hospital
Name: Brzyznski, Martha			
DOB: 01/09/48			
Room: 588			Physician's
Dr: Amarite Gaya, M.D.			Medication Order

ALLERGY OR SENSITIVITY			DIAGNOSIS	
penicillins			*cellulitis*	

DATE	TIME	ORDERS	PHYSICIAN'S SIG.
5/20/2017	3:51 PM	*Vancomycin 1500 mg in 500 mL*	
		D5W IV q12h	
			Amarite Gaya, M.D.

7. A reconstituted vial of vancomycin contains 500 mg/5 mL. How many vials will be needed to prepare the order?

8. What is the percentage strength of vancomycin?

9. The maximum concentration of vancomycin should not exceed 5 mg/mL. Is the ordered concentration appropriate?

10. The recommended infusion time for vancomycin is at least 30 minutes for every 500 mg administered to prevent infusion-related reactions. What is the minimum infusion time for this order?

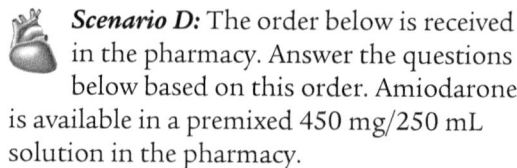 **Scenario D:** The order below is received in the pharmacy. Answer the questions below based on this order. Amiodarone is available in a premixed 450 mg/250 mL solution in the pharmacy.

ID#: SU8447864494			Memorial Hospital
Name: Lazaar, Howard			
DOB: 10/20/50			
Room: 1547			Physician's
Dr: Jeremiah King, M.D.			Medication Order

ALLERGY OR SENSITIVITY			DIAGNOSIS	
NKA			*atrial fibrillation*	

DATE	TIME	ORDERS	PHYSICIAN'S SIG.
5/22/2017	3:51 PM	*Amiodarone 0.5 mg/min IV*	
		to be given over 18 hours	
			Jeremiah King, M.D.

11. What is the IV rate in mL/hr?

12. If a 15 drop set is being used, what is the IV flow rate in drops/minute?

13. How many IV bags will be needed to fulfill the order?

14. If the order was started at 1800, when will the patient need a new IV bag?

Navigator ✚

Access interactive chapter review exercises, practice activities, flash cards, and study games.

8

Using Special Calculations in Compounding

Lisa McCartney, M.Ed, CPhT, PhTR

Learning Objectives

1 Calculate the amount of each ingredient needed to enlarge a formula or recipe.

2 Calculate the amount of each ingredient needed to reduce a formula or recipe.

3 Compute the amount of two strengths of active ingredient needed to prepare a product whose concentration lies between the two strengths.

4 Determine the amount of two ingredients using the weight-in-weight formula.

5 Determine the amount of concentrate and diluent needed to prepare a special dilution.

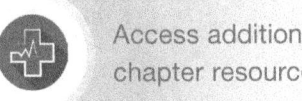 Access additional chapter resources.

8.1 Compound Formulas

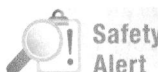
Safety Alert

Pharmacies that produce mass quantities of compounded medications have come under scrutiny due to contaminated products that resulted in serious illness and death. The FDA has since become more aggressive in its inspections and enforcement methods.

Compounding is the process of using raw ingredients and/or prepared ingredients to create a medication for a patient. Compounding usually involves both **active ingredients** (components that provide pharmacologic activity) and **inactive ingredients** (components that do not affect pharmacologic activity). The process of compounding is similar to making a cake from scratch by using ingredients such as butter, sugar, eggs, flour, and baking powder. Compounding is regularly done at special compounding pharmacies (pharmacies that primarily compound medications) but is also done in institutional pharmacies. Some community pharmacies also engage in medication compounding.

A compounded medication is prepared using a **formula** or *recipe*. The formula is a written document prepared by a pharmacist that lists the ingredients and instructions needed to prepare a specific compound. Some formulas are intended to prepare a single prescription, whereas others are intended to prepare a **compounded stock preparation**, or a larger amount to be divided and dispensed for individual prescription orders later. Commonly ordered compounds can be made in advance to have on hand as needed. A **compounded sterile preparation** (CSP) is a product made by mixing one or more sterile products using aseptic technique (a method designed to prevent or minimize the risk of contamination).

Work Wise

If you are interested in a career as a compounding pharmacy technician, you may find it helpful to complete specialized training. Several professional organizations offer compounding certifications. You can list certifications on your resume to help distinguish yourself from other candidates.

Some pharmacies routinely compound preparations for physicians who prescribe these special preparations on a regular basis. A pharmacy that prepares these compounds will often have a recipe for making a large amount to have on hand. It is not uncommon to prepare a compound that can be divided and dispensed to as many as 20 patients. Preparing larger batches is sometimes referred to as *batch compounding*. Preparing compounds in advance can result in cost savings by reducing the labor needed to make the product and can also save time in providing the compound to the patient. Although the Food and Drug Administration (FDA) prohibits retail pharmacies from mass manufacturing compounded medications, anticipatory compounding is permitted in small quantities when a particular pharmacy is located near a physician's office that routinely orders certain compounded prescriptions.

Pharmacies store formulas in many ways. They may be maintained using a computerized file system or informally in a card file or binder. A pharmacy's set of formulas is often called the pharmacy recipe book. Some pharmacies also have different formulas for different prescribers, as each prescriber may prefer a slightly different version of a particular compound.

Enlarging or reducing formulas involves taking the recipe for a particular compounded medication and adjusting the amount of the ingredients to meet the needs of the pharmacy's order. This practice is similar to doubling the ingredients in a recipe for cookies to make twice as many cookies. Retaining the correct proportion of each ingredient in this process is critical. A cookie made from a doubled batch should have the same ratio of ingredients as a cookie made from a single batch. The same must be true when a formula is doubled in the compounding pharmacy.

It is essential for a pharmacy to maintain accurate records and documentation of the mathematical calculations used in reducing or enlarging a formula. All amounts should be calculated and recorded before weighing, measuring, or mixing. The final prepared product must match the concentration (also referred to as the *strength* or *percent*) and amount ordered by the prescriber.

To accurately compound a prescription, pharmacy technicians must locate the **current formula**, which is the formula that is kept on hand in the pharmacy recipe book. In addition, technicians will need to know the **desired formula**, which is a specialized pharmaceutical recipe ordered by a prescriber that alters various components of a current formula.

Compound formulas often include the abbreviation QSAD. QSAD is an abbreviation for the Latin term *quantum sufficiat ad* which means "a quantity sufficient to make." QSAD almost always refers to an inactive ingredient in a formula. It instructs the preparer to use an ingredient up to the specified quantity. For example, suppose you are preparing 100 mL of a compounded medication that contains two ingredients (one active and one inactive). The formula calls for 5 g of the powder form of the active ingredient. The formula also instructs QSAD 240 mL of the inactive ingredient (which is a liquid).

To prepare the formula you would first measure the 5 g of the active ingredient. You would then add a sufficient amount of the inactive ingredient until the total volume of the compounded medication was 240 mL. The volume of the inactive ingredient you would add is actually less than 240 mL, because the formula makes 240 mL total, and the active ingredient takes up volume.

For Good Measure

The abbreviation QSAD means "quantity sufficient" or "a sufficient quantity to make." Pharmacy technicians may either see this abbreviation written on prescriptions or in formulas as "QSAD to ___ mL" or—more commonly—as "QSAD ___ mL."

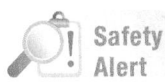

Safety Alert

When enlarging or reducing a formula for compounding, pharmacy technicians must always retain the correct proportion of ingredients from the original formula.

The following examples demonstrate the calculations for reducing or enlarging formulas.

Example 8.1.1

 A prescriber has ordered a patient to receive 100 mL of a commonly used topical iodine solution. The pharmacy's recipe book lists a formula to prepare 1,000 mL of the solution. Determine how much of each ingredient will be needed to prepare 100 mL of the solution.

Step 1 Determine the ratio to compare the desired formula with the current formula.

Desired formula requires you to provide 100 mL of the solution.

Current formula provides 1,000 mL of the solution.

$$\frac{100}{1,000} = \frac{1}{10}$$

Therefore, you will need ¹⁄₁₀ (i.e., 100 mL desired/1,000 mL formula) of the amount of each ingredient listed in the current recipe. To find the amount of each ingredient, you will divide each amount by 10, as shown in Step 2.

Step 2 Calculate the amount of each ingredient.

Current Formula (for 1,000 mL):

Iodine   30 g
Sodium iodide   25 g
Purified water   QSAD to 1,000 mL

Desired Formula (for 100 mL):

Iodine $\frac{30\text{ g}}{10} = 3$ g

Sodium iodide $\frac{25\text{ g}}{10} = 2.5$ g

Purified water   QSAD to $\frac{1,000\text{ mL}}{10} = 100$ mL

You will need 3 g of iodine and 2.5 g of sodium iodide. You will also need enough purified water so that the final volume is 100 mL, because the desired formula indicates QSAD to 100 mL.

Example 8.1.2

 You need to prepare 16 oz of coal tar ointment, a compounded medication, for a patient. The pharmacy's recipe book lists a formula to prepare 4 oz of the ointment. Determine how much of each ingredient you will need to prepare 16 oz of the ointment.

Step 1 Determine the ratio to compare the desired formula with the current formula.

Desired formula requires you to provide 16 oz of the ointment.

Current formula provides 4 oz of the ointment.

$$\frac{16}{4} = \frac{4}{1}$$

Therefore, you will need four times (i.e., 16 desired/4 current = 4) the amount of each ingredient listed in the current formula. To find the amount of each ingredient, you will multiply each amount by 4, as shown in Step 2.

Step 2 Calculate the amount of each ingredient.

Current Formula (for 4 oz):

Coal tar	4 g
Salicylic acid	1 g
Triamcinolone 0.1%	15 g
Aqua-base ointment	100 g

Desired Formula (for 16 oz):

Coal tar	4 g × 4 = 16 g
Salicylic acid	1 g × 4 = 4 g
Triamcinolone 0.1%	15 g × 4 = 60 g
Aqua-base ointment	100 g × 4 = 400 g

You will need 16 g of coal tar, 4 g of salicylic acid, 60 g of triamcinolone 0.1%, and 400 g of aqua-base ointment.

8.1 Problem Set

1. The following pharmacy recipe provides a formula that yields 120 g of coal tar ointment. You are asked to prepare a 30 g jar of coal tar ointment. By what number do you need to divide each ingredient to make the desired formula? State how much of each ingredient you will need. Round to the nearest hundredth of a gram.

Coal tar	4 g
Salicylic acid	1 g
Triamcinolone 0.1% ung	15 g
Aqua-base ointment	100 g

2. The following pharmacy recipe provides a formula that yields 30 vaginal suppositories. You are to prepare 150 vaginal suppositories. By what number do you need to multiply each ingredient to make the desired formula? State how much of each ingredient you will need. Round to the nearest gram.

Progesterone	2.4 g
Polyethylene glycol 3350	30 g
Polyethylene glycol 1000	90 g

3. The following pharmacy recipe provides a formula that yields 20 mL of solution. You are to prepare 120 mL of the solution. State how much of each ingredient you will need. Round to the nearest milliliter.

| Podophyllum resin | 25% |
| Benzoin tincture | QSAD 20 mL |

4. The following pharmacy recipe provides a formula that yields 8 oz of solution. You are to prepare 120 mL of the solution. State how much of each ingredient you will need. Round to the nearest tenth of a milliliter.

Pharmacy Stock Formula (yields 8 oz)

Tetracycline 500 mg capsules	16 capsules
Hydrocortisone suspension	15 mL
Lidocaine oral suspension	30 mL
Mylanta suspension	QSAD 240 mL

5. The following pharmacy recipe provides a formula to prepare one 30 mL dropper bottle of Oticaine. You are to prepare four 15 mL dropper bottles of Oticaine. State how much of each ingredient you will need to prepare the entire batch. Round to the nearest tenth of gram.

Pharmacy Stock Formula (yields 30 mL)

Antipyrine	1.8 g
Benzocaine	0.5 g
Glycerin	QSAD 30 mL

Self-check your work in Appendix A.

8.2 Alligations

Occasionally, a prescriber will write a prescription for a medication strength that is not commercially available, or a medication strength that is not kept on hand in the pharmacy. In these instances, the pharmacy may be required to mix two different strengths of the same active ingredient of a drug or solution to make the desired strength. A higher-percent strength (i.e., the more concentrated ingredient) of a drug or solution is mixed with a lower-percent strength (i.e., the less concentrated ingredient) of a drug or solution to make the desired strength, which falls somewhere between the two extremes. This scenario requires you to employ a calculation called the **alligation method**, or simply *alligation*. Alligations are rarely performed by pharmacy technicians, but you may need to carry out this kind of calculation from time to time. To understand how to set up an alligation problem, refer to Figure 8.1. Use this grid as your template for the scenario that follows.

Safety Alert

As a means of checking to see that you have set up your grid properly, your desired percent should always be a value in between the two concentrations you are combining.

FIGURE 8.1 Tic-Tac-Toe Alligation Grid

A (higher %)		D (parts of higher %; the difference of B − C)
	B (desired %)	
C (lower %)		E (parts of lower %; the difference of A − B)

KEY
A = higher concentration or strength (stated as a percent [%])
B = desired concentration or strength (stated as a percent [%])
C = lower concentration or strength (stated as a percent [%])

Example 8.2.1

The compounded sterile preparation (CSP) label shown below indicates that the prescriber has ordered 250 mL of dextrose 7% in water (D7W). In your pharmacy, you have both dextrose 5% in water (D5W) and dextrose 70% in water (D70W). Because 7 falls between 5 and 70, you can use these two strengths to make the 7% you need. How much D5% and D70% do you combine to make an intravenous (IV) solution with a dextrose concentration of 7% (D7W) and a total volume of 250 mL for infusion?

IV Solution – LVP

Mercy Hospital

Pt. Name: Werekela, Francis   **Room:** PICU-4

ID#: 543678   **Rx#:** 420883

Dextrose 7% in Water (D7W) 250 mL
Rate: 10 mL/hr

Keep refrigerated – warm to room temperature
before administration.

Expiration Day/Time: _____ Tech _____ RPh _____

Step 1   Identify the variables by determining the component concentrations. The desired concentration (B%) is what the prescriber has written on the medication order and, therefore, is indicated on the CSP label. The higher concentration (A%) and lower concentration (C%) are determined by the stock IV base solution strengths on hand in your pharmacy. In this case, the desired concentration is 7%, the higher concentration is 70%, and the lower concentration is 5%.

Step 2   Using the alligation template from Figure 8.1, fill in the concentration strengths (given as percentages) in the Key section below the tic-tac-toe grid. Place the same strengths in their designated squares on the grid.

A (higher %) 70		D (parts of higher %; the difference of B – C)
	B (desired %) 7	
C (lower %) 5		E (parts of lower %; the difference of A – B)

For Good Measure

When using the tic-tac-toe alligation grid, pharmacy technicians should be sure to place the desired percent in the center square, the higher percent in the upper left-hand square, and the lower percent in the bottom left-hand square. It is also important to remember that subtraction is performed diagonally but that the "parts" are read horizontally, or across the grid.

Key:
A% = 70
B% = 7
C% = 5
D (parts of 70% solution) =
E (parts of 5% solution) =

Step 3 Determine the number of parts of each component (higher % and lower %).

a. To find the value of D in the upper right-hand square, set up the equation B − C = D.

Then fill in the values for B and C (found in Step 2) in the equation, as shown below:

7 − 5 = D
D = 2 (or the number of parts of 70% dextrose)

Record the number 2 in the key and in the upper right-hand square.

b. To find the value of E in the lower right-hand square, set up the equation A − B = E.

Then fill in the values for A and B (found in Step 2) in the equation, as shown below:

70 − 7 = E
E = 63 (or the number of parts of 5% dextrose)

Record the number 63 in the key and in the lower right-hand square.

Check that your completed grid now matches the grid shown below:

A (higher %) 70		D (parts of higher %) 2
	B (desired %) 7	
C (lower %) 5		E (parts of lower %) 63

Key:
A% = 70
B% = 7
C% = 5
D (parts of 70% solution) = 2
E (parts of 5% solution) = 63

Step 4 Set up a ratio using the values of D and E as shown in the right-hand column of your completed grid:

$$\frac{D}{E} = \frac{2}{63}$$

This ratio indicates that to prepare the desired concentration (in this case, a D7% solution), dextrose 70% (D70W) and dextrose 5% (D5W) must be mixed in a 2:63 ratio: 2 parts of D70% and 63 parts of D5%.

Step 5   Using the ratio from Step 4, add D and E to obtain the total number of parts (TP):

$$D + E = TP$$

$$2 + 63 = TP$$

$$65 = TP$$

Step 6   Now you need to determine the exact volume of each component needed to prepare 250 mL of D7W. Because you already know the ratio in which the parts must be combined and the total number of parts, you can set up a ratio-proportion problem.

a. To find the volume of D70W needed for the CSP, use the following formula:

$$\frac{D}{TP} = \frac{x}{TV}$$

D = parts of the higher % solution
TP = total number of parts
TV = total volume of desired concentration

$$\frac{2}{65} = \frac{x}{250 \text{ mL}}$$

$$x = 7.69 \text{ mL (rounded to 7.7 mL) of D70W}$$

For Good Measure

Technicians must add the parts of both strengths (determined in Step 5) to find the total number of parts. This number is then used as the divisor in Step 6.

b. To find the volume of D5W needed for the CSP, use the following formula:

$$\frac{E}{TP} = \frac{x}{TV}$$

E = parts of the lower % solution
TP = total number of parts
TV = total volume of desired concentration

$$\frac{63}{65} = \frac{x}{250 \text{ mL}}$$

$$x = 242.31 \text{ mL (rounded to 242.3 mL) of D5W}$$

Step 7   To verify the volume of each component (determined in Step 6), add the volumes of the two components. Your answer should equal the total volume of the desired concentration.

7.7 mL (D70W) + 242.3 mL (D5W) = 250 mL (total volume of desired concentration)

Example 8.2.2

The prescriber has ordered an IV infusion of 500 mL of dextrose 7%. You have stock concentrations of 5% dextrose and 70% dextrose on hand in the pharmacy. How much D70W% and D5W% must be combined to make an IV solution with a dextrose concentration of 7% (D7W) and a total volume of 500 mL for infusion?

Step 1 Identify the variables. Determine the component concentrations by identifying the desired concentration (in this case, 7%); the higher concentration (in this case, 70%); and the lower concentration (in this case, 5%):

A (higher %) = 70
B (desired %) = 7
C (lower %) = 5

Reminder: The desired concentration (B%) is what the prescriber has written on the medication order, and it is also listed on the CSP label. The higher concentration (A%) and lower concentration (C%) are determined by the stock IV base solution strengths that you have on hand in your pharmacy.

Step 2 Set up a tic-tac-toe grid.

A (higher %) 70		D (parts of higher %; the difference of B − C)
	B (desired %) 7	
C (lower %) 5		E (parts of lower %; the difference of A − B)

Step 3 Determine the number of parts of each component (higher % and lower %).

a. Subtract the center number in the tic-tac-toe grid from the number in the upper left-hand square of the tic-tac-toe grid (A − B); place this number in the lower right-hand square of the grid (E).

$$A - B = E; 70 - 7 = 63$$

b. Subtract the number in the lower left-hand square of the tic-tac-toe grid from the number in the center of the grid (B − C); place this number in the upper right-hand square of the grid (D).

$$B - C = D; 7 - 5 = 2$$

D = 2 (parts of 70% dextrose)
E = 63 (parts of 5% dextrose)

Step 4 Set up a ratio using the information you determined in Step 3.

$$\frac{D}{E} = \frac{2}{63}$$

This ratio indicates that to prepare the desired concentration (in this case, a D7% solution), dextrose 70% (D70W) and dextrose 5% (D5W) must be mixed in a 2:63 ratio; in other words, 2 parts of D70% and 63 parts of D5%.

Step 5 Determine the total number of parts in the ratio.

$$D + E = \text{total number of parts}$$

$$2 + 63 = 65 \text{ (total number of parts)}$$

Step 6 Determine the volume of each component.

a. Determine the volume of dextrose 70% (D70W) needed for the CSP:

total volume (TV) of desired concentration = 500 mL
parts of D70W (D) = 2
total number of parts (TP) = 65

$$\frac{D}{TP} = \frac{x}{TV}$$

$$\frac{2}{65} = \frac{x}{500 \text{ mL}}$$

$$x = 15.4 \text{ mL of D70W}$$

b. Determine the volume of dextrose 5% (D5W) needed for the CSP:

total volume (TV) of desired concentration = 500 mL
parts of D5W (D) = 63
total number of parts (TP) = 65

$$\frac{D}{TP} = \frac{x}{TV}$$

$$\frac{63}{65} = \frac{x}{500 \text{ mL}}$$

$$x = 484.6 \text{ mL of D}_5\text{W}$$

Therefore, to make D7% (D7W) 500 mL, mix 15.4 mL of dextrose 70% (D70W) with 484.6 mL of dextrose 5% (D5W).

Step 7 Verify your answer.

The volume of each component (determined in Steps 6a and 6b) added together should equal the total volume of the desired concentration:

volume of D70W = 15.4 mL
volume of D5W = 484.6 mL

15.4 mL + 484.6 mL = 500 mL

The alligation method may also be used in compounding situations that require you to mix two strengths of an active ingredient to compound a product whose desired strength lies between the two extremes.

Example 8.2.3

The prescriber has ordered a topical preparation of 1.25% hydrocortisone cream 120 g. The pharmacy carries hydrocortisone cream in the following concentrations: 2.5% and 1%. Determine how much of the 2.5% cream and how much of the 1% cream will be needed to prepare 120 g of the desired 1.25% concentration.

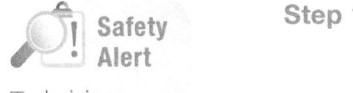

Safety Alert

Technicians should always document calculations before compounding.

Step 1 Identify the variables. Determine the component concentrations by identifying the desired concentration (in this case, 1.25%); the higher concentration (in this case, 2.5%); and the lower concentration (in this case, 1%):

A (higher %) = 2.5%
B (desired %) = 1.25%
C (lower %) = 1%

Step 2 Set up the tic-tac-toe grid.

A (higher %) 2.5		D (parts of higher %; the difference of B – C)
	B (desired %) 1.25	
C (lower %) 1		E (parts of lower %; the difference of A – B)

Step 3 Determine the number of parts of each component.

a. Subtract the center number in the tic-tac-toe grid from the number in the upper left-hand square of the tic-tac-toe grid (A − B); place this number in the lower right-hand square of the grid (E).

A − B = E; 2.5 − 1.25 = 1.25

b. Subtract the number in the lower left-hand square of the tic-tac-toe grid from the number in the center of the grid (B − C); place this number in the upper right-hand square of the grid (D).

B − C = D; 1.25 − 1 = 0.25

Fill in the values for D and E on the tic-tac-toe grid.

A (higher %) 2.5		D (parts of higher %; the difference of B − C) 0.25
	B (desired %) 1.25	
C (lower %) 1		E (parts of lower %; the difference of A − B) 1.25

Step 4 Set up a ratio using the parts you determined in Step 3.

$$\frac{D}{E} = \frac{0.25}{1.25}$$

This indicates that to prepare the desired concentration (in this case, 1.25% hydrocortisone cream), hydrocortisone 2.5% and hydrocortisone 1% must be mixed in a 0.25:1.25 ratio.

Step 5 Determine the total number of parts.

$$D + E = 0.25 + 1.25 = 1.5 \text{ (total number of parts)}$$

Step 6 Determine the amount of each component.

a. Determine the amount of hydrocortisone 2.5% needed.

$$\frac{D}{TP} = \frac{x}{TV}$$

D = parts of the higher % ingredient = 0.25
TP = total number of parts = 1.5
TV = total amount of desired concentration = 1.25

$$\frac{0.25}{1.5} = \frac{x}{120}$$

$x = 20$ g of 2.5% hydrocortisone cream

b. Determine the amount of hydrocortisone 1% cream is needed.

$$\frac{E}{TP} = \frac{x}{TV}$$

E = parts of the lower % ingredient = 1.25
TP = total number of parts = 1.5
TV = total amount of desired concentration = 1.25

$$\frac{1.25}{1.5} = \frac{x}{120}$$

$x = 100$ g of 1% hydrocortisone cream

Step 7   Verify your answer. The amount of each component (determined in Steps 7a and 7b) added together should equal the total amount of the desired cream.

amount of hyrdrocortisone 2.5% = 20 g

amount of hydrocortisone 1% = 100 g

$$20 \text{ g} + 100 \text{ g} = 120 \text{ g}$$

8.2 Problem Set

Use the alligation method to solve the following problems. Round to the nearest gram or milliliter.

1.   Prepare 200 mL of 7.5% dextrose solution using D5W and D10W. How many milliliters of each solution will you need?

2.   Prepare 400 mL of D8W using D5W and D20W. How many milliliters of each solution will you need?

3.   Prepare 500 mL of D12.5W. You have on hand D70W and D5W. How many milliliters of each solution will you need?

4.   You must prepare a 250 mL solution of 6% dextrose (D6W). You have D10W and D5W on hand. How many milliliters of each solution will you need?

5.   Prepare a total volume of 500 mL of D7.5W. You have D5W and D50W on hand. How many milliliters of each solution will you need?

6.   Prepare 250 mL of 8% dextrose from D5W and D20W. How many milliliters of each solution will you need?

7.   Prepare 300 mL of 7.5% dextrose using D5W and D20W. How many milliliters of each solution will you need?

8.   Prepare 500 mL of 12.5% dextrose using D10W and D20W. How many milliliters of each solution will you need?

9.   Prepare 150 mL of 7.5% dextrose from D5W and D10W. How many milliliters of each solution will you need?

10.   A physician has ordered 250 mL of D12.5W. You have D10W and D20W available. How many milliliters of each solution will you need?

11.   Prepare 60 g of a 3% cream from a 1% cream and a 10% cream. How many grams of each cream will you need?

12.   Prepare 30 g of a 7.5% cream from a 5% cream and a 15% cream. How many grams of each cream will you need?

13.   The pharmacy has received an order that requires the batch preparation of four 30 g jars of hydrocortisone 3% cream. The pharmacy has a 1% hydrocortisone cream and a 5% hydrocortisone cream on hand. How many grams of each cream will you need to prepare the entire batch?

14.   Prepare 45 g of 10% zinc oxide using a 5% zinc oxide ointment and a 20% zinc oxide ointment. How many grams of each ointment will you need?

15.   Prepare 100 g of an 8% cream from a 5% cream and a 10% cream. How many grams of each cream will you need?

Self-check your work in Appendix A.

8.3 Weight-in-Weight (w/w) Calculations

When compounding two solid ingredients—an active ingredient and an inactive ingredient—the weight-in-weight (w/w) formula is sometimes used to determine the amount of each ingredient needed for the preparation. The **weight-in-weight (w/w) formula** identifies the number of grams of medication per 100 g of the product. This concentration can be expressed as a fraction, as shown in the following equation:

$$\text{weight-in-weight (w/w)} = \frac{x \text{ g medication}}{100 \text{ g product}}$$

When determining percentage strength, the unknown (designated by an x) will always be placed over 100. The term *percentage strength* means "parts of 100" or "percent of the whole" (with the "whole" meaning 100%). Additionally, percentage strength signifies the number of grams of a drug per 100 g of the product. The following formula may be used to determine the percentage strength of w/w preparations:

$$\text{percentage strength of w/w preparation} = \frac{\text{g of active ingredient}}{100 \text{ g of product}} \times 100$$

Example 8.3.1

 You have a compound with a concentration of 5 g hydrocortisone powder in 100 g of petrolatum. Determine the percentage strength of this compound.

$$\frac{5 \text{ g medication}}{100 \text{ g product}} \times 100$$

$$\frac{5}{100} = 0.05$$

$$0.05 \times 100 = 5$$

The percentage strength of a compound with 5 g hydrocortisone powder in 100 g of petrolatum is 5%.

When the percentage strength of the product is known, the w/w formula may also be used to determine how many grams of an active ingredient are in a defined amount of an inactive ingredient. Apply the ratio-proportion method to determine the number of grams of active ingredient needed to compound the preparation.

Example 8.3.2

If a compounded preparation has a percentage strength of 3%, how many grams of medication are in 50 g of the preparation?

$$3\% = \frac{3 \text{ g}}{100 \text{ g}}$$

Using the ratio-proportion method:

$$\frac{3\text{ g}}{100\text{ g}} = \frac{x\text{ g}}{50\text{ g}}$$

$$x = 1.5\text{ g}$$

Using dimensional analysis:

$$50\text{ g total product} \times \frac{3\text{ g medication}}{100\text{ g total product}} = 1.5\text{ g medication}$$

There are 1.5 g of medication in 50 g of the preparation.

Example 8.3.3

A compounded preparation has a percentage strength of 0.5%. The final product contains 15 g of medication. How many total grams of medication are in the final product?

$$0.5\% = \frac{0.5\text{ g}}{100\text{ g}}$$

Using the ratio-proportion method:

$$\frac{0.5\text{ g}}{100\text{ g}} = \frac{x\text{ g}}{15\text{ g}}$$

$$x = 0.075\text{ g}$$

Using dimensional analysis:

$$\frac{15\text{ g total product}}{1} \times \frac{0.5\text{ g medication}}{100\text{ g total product}} = 0.075\text{ g}$$

8.3 Problem Set

Use the w/w method to solve the following problems.

1. Prepare a compound of hydrocortisone cream in petrolatum with a concentration of 2.0%. How many grams of hydrocortisone are contained in 75 g of the cream?

2. Prepare a compound of zinc oxide using 8.0 g of zinc oxide powder in 454 g of aqua-base ointment. What is the percentage strength of this compounded preparation? Round to the nearest tenth of a percent.

3. Prepare a compound of 100 g of acyclovir cream 2.5%. How many grams of acyclovir will you need for this preparation? Round to the nearest tenth of a milligram.

4. Prepare a compound that mixes 10.0 g of acyclovir with 50.0 g of petrolatum. What is the percentage strength of this compounded preparation? Round to the nearest tenth of a percent.

5. The pharmacy has received a prescription for 30 g of a 2% triamcinolone ointment. How many grams of triamcinolone will you need to prepare this prescription? Round to the nearest tenth of a gram.

6. The pharmacy has received the following prescription:

> Todd Jackson, MD
> Anita Johnson, MD
> Kunal Gupta, MSN, FCNP
> 5730 Congress Avenue
> Boise, ID 83702
> (208) 555-1212 fax (208) 555-1313

DOB _October 18, 1978_ DEA# _____

Pt. Name _Lily Nguyen_____ Date _02/12/2017_

Address _____2934 Anderson Lane_____
_____Boise, ID 83722_____

Elocon (mometasone fumarate) 0.05%
cream aaa tid prn
Disp. 15 g

Refill __5__ times (no refill unless indicated)
____Anita Johnson_____ MD
_____N0972_____ License #

How many grams of mometasone fumarate will you need to prepare this prescription? Round to the nearest ten thousandth of a gram.

7. The pharmacy has received an order to compound a batch preparation of progesterone suppositories. You will need to prepare 100 suppositories, each containing 200 mg of progesterone. The total weight of each suppository is 1 g. Round to the nearest gram and percent.

   a. How many grams of progesterone will you need for the entire batch of suppositories?

   b. What is the percentage strength of each suppository?

8. The pharmacy has received the following prescription:

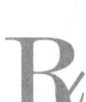

> Todd Jackson, MD
> Anita Johnson, MD
> Kunal Gupta, MSN, FCNP
> 5730 Congress Avenue
> Boise, ID 83702
> (208) 555-1212 fax (208) 555-1313

DOB _March 28, 1989_ DEA# _____

Pt. Name _Eeva Novak____ Date _07/14/2017_

Address _____4521 Birch Avenue_____
_____Boise, ID 83722_____

Metronidazole cream 0.75%
Compound without benzyl alcohol

Apply to facial rosacea flare qid prn
Dispense 30 g

Refill __2__ times (no refill unless indicated)
____Todd Jackson_____ MD
_____H0786_____ License #

You look at the patient's profile in the computer and realize she has an allergy to benzyl alcohol. Metronidazole 0.75% cream is commercially available, however all formulations have benzyl alcohol as an ingredient and you need to compound the medication. How many grams of metronidazole will you need to prepare this prescription? Round to the nearest hundredth of a gram.

9. The pharmacy has received the following medication order:

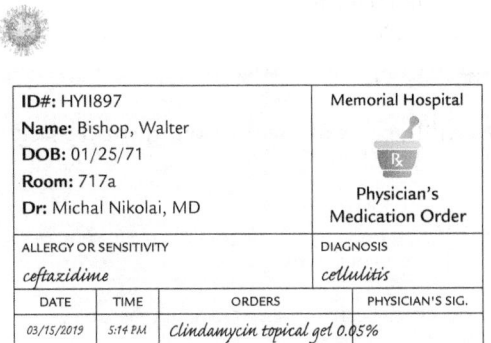

ID#: HYII897			Memorial Hospital
Name: Bishop, Walter			
DOB: 01/25/71			
Room: 717a			Physician's
Dr: Michal Nikolai, MD			Medication Order

| ALLERGY OR SENSITIVITY | | | DIAGNOSIS |
| ceftazidime | | | cellulitis |

DATE	TIME	ORDERS	PHYSICIAN'S SIG.
03/15/2019	5:14 PM	Clindamycin topical gel 0.05%	
		Apply 1 g to acne bid ut. dict.	
		Dispense 30 g tube	
			Michal Nikolai, MD

How many grams of clindamycin will you need to prepare this prescription? Round to the nearest hundredth of a gram.

10. The pharmacy has received the following medication order:

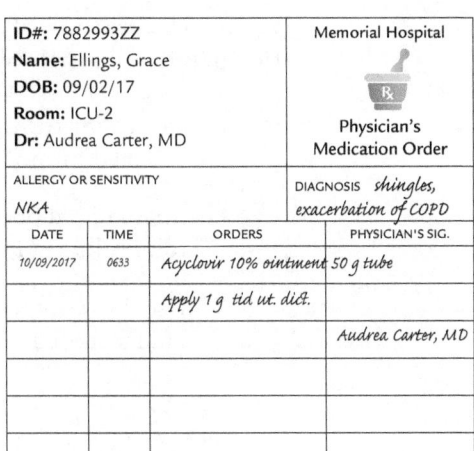

ID#: 7882993ZZ			Memorial Hospital
Name: Ellings, Grace			
DOB: 09/02/17			
Room: ICU-2			Physician's
Dr: Audrea Carter, MD			Medication Order

| ALLERGY OR SENSITIVITY | | DIAGNOSIS shingles, | |
| NKA | | exacerbation of COPD | |

DATE	TIME	ORDERS	PHYSICIAN'S SIG.
10/09/2017	0633	Acyclovir 10% ointment 50 g tube	
		Apply 1 g tid ut. dict.	
			Audrea Carter, MD

a. How many grams of acyclovir will you need to prepare this prescription? Round to the nearest gram.

b. How many doses are contained in this prescription?

Self-check your work in Appendix A.

8.4 Special Dilutions

For Good Measure

Typically, the ratio-proportion method is preferred over the dimensional analysis method to solve special dilution problems because it is easier to identify the parts of the equation.

Physicians often prescribe concentrations of medications that are not commercially available, and these prescriptions must be compounded in the pharmacy. Often compounding these prescriptions is accomplished by mixing a concentrated stock solution with a diluent. Calculations of this type were discussed in Chapters 6 and 7. However, there are times when pharmacy technicians are presented with more complex compounding scenarios, such as mixing pediatric CSPs. In general, pediatric CSPs are compounded by diluting adult formulations of medications with a diluent such as sterile water or sterile normal saline. However, there are times when the high concentrations of adult-strength medications make dilutions to child-sized doses difficult. In these situations, the pediatric doses are such small volumes that they are hard to draw up accurately in a syringe.

To provide accurate parenteral medication dosing for neonates or other particularly small patients, pharmacy technicians may be called upon to prepare a CSP with a diluted concentration. This is referred to as a **special dilution**. To prepare this type of CSP, technicians need to perform a series of calculations, as demonstrated in the following examples.

Example 8.4.1

 Prepare a special dilution of gentamicin with a total volume of 4 mL and a concentration of 5 mg/mL. Use a stock solution of gentamicin 10 mg/mL and sterile water to prepare this special dilution.

Step 1 Determine the total number of milligrams of medication in the desired special dilution.

desired final product = 5 mg/mL
total volume (TV) = 4 mL

Use the ratio-proportion method to determine the number of milligrams needed for the special dilution.

$$\frac{5 \text{ mg}}{1 \text{ mL}} = \frac{x \text{ mg}}{4 \text{ mL}}$$

$$x = 20 \text{ mg}$$

The total number of milligrams of gentamicin needed for the special dilution = 20 mg.

Note: Dimensional analysis could also be used to determine this step.

Step 2 Determine the number of milliliters of stock solution (10 mg/mL) needed to prepare the special dilution.

$$\frac{10 \text{ mg}}{1 \text{ mL}} = \frac{20 \text{ mg}}{x \text{ mL}}$$

$$x = 2 \text{ mL}$$

The total number of milliliters of gentamicin stock solution (10 mg/mL) needed to prepare the special dilution = 2 mL.

Note: Dimensional analysis could also be used to determine this step.

Step 3 Determine the number of milliliters of diluent (sterile water) needed to prepare the special dilution.

total volume (TV) − drug volume (DV) = volume of diluent

TV = 4 mL
DV = 2 mL
4 − 2 = 2
volume of diluent = 2 mL

The pharmacy technician must draw up 2 mL of the gentamicin 10 mg/mL stock solution and 2 mL of the sterile water diluent. Both syringes will be aseptically injected into a sterile, empty vial, and the resulting 4 mL special dilution will be gentamicin with a concentration of 5 mg/mL.

254   Chapter 8 *Using Special Calculations in Compounding*

There are times when a pharmacy technician needs to prepare a special dilution of an IV dextrose infusion with a percentage strength that is not commercially available. In most cases, this special dilution will be prepared by mixing a concentrated dextrose solution with sterile water to create the percentage strength ordered by the prescriber. The following example demonstrates the three-step process for solving this type of problem.

Example 8.4.2

Work Wise

Dextrose-containing solutions are often abbreviated when spoken aloud. Dextrose 10% in water is often called "D10" or "D10W."

Using a stock solution of dextrose 70% (D70W) and sterile water, prepare a 1,000 mL IV with a percentage strength of D10W.

Key:
TV = total volume of the IV solution ordered by prescriber
stock % = percentage strength of the solution that is stocked in the pharmacy
desired % = percentage strength of the solution ordered by the prescriber
mL = number of milliliters of the stock solution solution needed to prepare the IV solution

Step 1 Calculate the volume of concentrated dextrose solution.

Identify the variables:
TV = 1,000 mL
stock % = 70
desired % = 10

Formula used to calculate amount of concentrated dextrose solution needed:

$$\left(\frac{TV}{stock\ \%}\right) \times desired\ \% = number\ of\ milliliters$$

(1,000/70) × 10 = 142.86 mL, rounded to 142.9 mL

amount of dextrose needed = 142.9 mL

Step 2 Calculate the volume of sterile water by subtracting the amount determined in Step 1 from the total volume ordered by the prescriber.

1,000 − 142.9 = 857.1

amount of sterile water needed = 857.1 mL

Step 3 Verify the accuracy of your calculations. Add the volumes that you determined in Steps 1 and 2. If you have performed each of the calculations correctly, the sum should equal the total volume ordered by the physician—in this case, 1,000 mL.

TAKE NOTE

Sterile water for injection may be used to prepare intravenous solutions. While it may sound innocuous, sterile water for injection can be dangerous if used improperly because sterile water is a hypotonic solution (meaning it has a lower osmotic pressure than plasma). When too much of a hypotonic solution is administered intravenously to a patient, water moves from the outside of cells to the inside. This results in cell swelling and, in some cases, cell rupture, or *hemolysis*. Hemolysis can have negative health consequences and can even result in death. Be sure to always double check your calculations and measurements when using sterile water for injection.

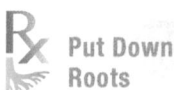

Work Wise

You may hear parenteral nutrition referred to as *hyperalimentation* in your practice setting.

Put Down Roots

The word *parenteral* comes from the Greek roots *para*, meaning "beside," and *enteron*, meaning "intestine." Therefore, a parenteral preparation refers to a product that bypasses—or goes "beside" rather than through— the gastrointestinal tract.

Occasionally, pharmacy technicians need to prepare a special dilution known as **total parenteral nutrition (TPN)**. TPN is an IV administration of total nutrient requirements to patients who require a long-term alternative to enteral feeding. TPN is generally a large-volume IV solution compounded from multiple solutions, such as dextrose, amino acids, fat emulsion, sterile water, electrolytes, vitamins, and minerals. The majority of volume from TPN (called the **TPN base solution**) comes from dextrose, amino acids, sterile water, and, in some cases, fat emulsion. The electrolytes, minerals, and vitamins are considered additives. **Additives** are substances such as medications, electrolytes, or other ingredients added to another product. The following examples demonstrate the five-part procedure for solving typical TPN problems.

Example 8.4.3

Prepare a 2,000 mL TPN with the base solution and additives shown below.

Base Solution
Dextrose 15%
Aminosyn (amino acid solution) 3.5%
Liposyn (fat emulsion) 5%
Sterile water QSAD to 2,000 mL

Additives
Sodium chloride 40 mEq
Potassium chloride 10 mEq
Potassium phosphate 6 mM
Multiple vitamin (MVI) 10 mL/day

*Prepared Using the Following Pharmacy Stock Solutions
(i.e., concentrations kept on hand in the pharmacy)*
Dextrose 70%
Aminosyn 10%
Liposyn 20%
Sodium chloride 4 mEq/mL
Potassium chloride 2 mEq/mL
Potassium phosphate 3 mM/mL
MVI 10 mL/day

Key:

TV = total volume of TPN ordered by prescriber

stock % = percentage strength of the solution that is stocked in the pharmacy

desired % = percentage strength of the solution ordered by the prescriber

mL = number of milliliters of stock solution needed to prepare the TPN solution

Formula used to calculate TPN base solution component:

$$\left(\frac{TV}{stock\ \%}\right) \times desired\ \% = number\ of\ milliliters$$

Note: The technician must perform this calculation to determine the volume for each component of the TPN.

Step 1 Calculate the volume of the TPN base components—dextrose, Aminosyn, and Liposyn. (*Note:* The sterile water volume will be calculated in Step 4.)

a. Start by determining the amount of dextrose needed. Identify the variables:

TV = 2,000 mL
stock % = 70
desired % = 15

$$\frac{TV}{stock\ \%} \times desired\ \% = number\ of\ milliliters$$

$$\left(\frac{2,000\ mL}{70\ \%}\right) \times 15\ \% = 428.57, rounded\ to\ 429$$

amount of dextrose needed = 429 mL

b. Next, determine the amount of Aminosyn needed.

Identify the variables:
TV = 2,000 mL
stock % = 10
desired % = 3.5

$$\left(\frac{2,000\ mL}{10\ \%}\right) \times 3.5\ \% = 700\ mL$$

amount of Aminosyn needed = 700 mL

c. Next, determine the amount of Liposyn needed.

Identify the variables:
TV = 2,000 mL
stock % = 20
desired % = 5

$$\left(\frac{2,000\ mL}{20\ \%}\right) \times 5\ \% = 500\ mL$$

amount of Liposyn needed = 500 mL

Step 2 Calculate the volume of each additive based on the following formula:

$$\frac{D}{H} = x$$

Key:

D = desired dose (the dose ordered by the prescriber)

H = concentration on hand (the concentration or strength of the drug *per milliliter*)

x = unknown volume of drug needed to be drawn up for the preparation of the additive

a. Start by determining the amount of sodium chloride needed.

Identify the variables:

D = 40 mEq

H = 4 mEq/mL

x = ? mL

$$\frac{40 \text{ mEq}}{4 \text{ mEq/mL}} = 10 \text{ mL}$$

amount of sodium chloride needed = 10 mL

b. Determine the amount of potassium chloride needed.

Identify the variables:

D = 10 mEq

H = 2 mEq/mL

x = ? mL

$$\frac{10 \text{ mEq}}{2 \text{ mEq/mL}} = 5 \text{ mL}$$

amount of potassium chloride needed = 5 mL

c. Determine the amount of potassium phosphate needed.

Identify the variables:

D = 6 mM

H = 3 mM/mL

x = ? mL

$$\frac{6 \text{ mM}}{3 \text{ mM/mL}} = 2 \text{ mL}$$

amount of potassium phosphate needed = 2 mL

d. Determine the amount of MVI needed. (*Note:* Because the prescriber has ordered a specific volume of MVI for the entire order, you will simply draw up the ordered volume.)

amount of MVI needed = 10 mL

Step 3 Add each of the volumes you determined in Steps 1 and 2 above.

$$
\begin{array}{r}
429 \text{ mL} \\
700 \text{ mL} \\
500 \text{ mL} \\
10 \text{ mL} \\
5 \text{ mL} \\
2 \text{ mL} \\
+ \ 10 \text{ mL} \\
\hline
1{,}656 \text{ mL}
\end{array}
$$

Step 4 Determine the amount of sterile water needed to QSAD to 2,000 mL. Subtract the total determined in Step 3 (the volume of base solution and additives) from the total volume of the TPN solution.

$$
\begin{array}{r}
2{,}000 \text{ mL} \\
-1{,}656 \text{ mL} \\
\hline
344 \text{ mL}
\end{array}
$$

amount of sterile water needed = 344 mL

Step 5 Verify the accuracy of your calculations by adding together all of the volumes. If you have performed each of the calculations correctly, they should equal the total volume ordered by the physician—in this case, 2,000 mL.

$$
\begin{array}{r}
429 \text{ mL} \\
700 \text{ mL} \\
500 \text{ mL} \\
10 \text{ mL} \\
5 \text{ mL} \\
2 \text{ mL} \\
10 \text{ mL} \\
+ \ 344 \text{ mL} \\
\hline
2{,}000 \text{ mL}
\end{array}
$$

8.4 Problem Set

1. Prepare a special dilution of acyclovir with a total volume of 10 mL and a concentration of 10 mg/mL. To create this special dilution, use a stock solution of acyclovir with a concentration of 100 mg/mL and sterile water. Round to the nearest milliliter.

   a. How many milligrams of acyclovir do you need for this special dilution?

   b. How many milliliters of the acyclovir stock solution do you need to draw up for this special dilution?

   c. How many milliliters of sterile water do you need to draw up for this special dilution?

2. Prepare a special dilution of tobramycin with a total volume of 5 mL and a concentration of 10 mg/mL. To create this special dilution, use a stock solution of tobramycin with a concentration of 40 mg/mL and sterile water. Round to the nearest milligram and hundredth of a milliliter.

a. How many milligrams of tobramycin do you need for this special dilution?

b. How many milliliters of the tobramycin stock solution do you need to draw up for this special dilution?

c. How many milliliters of sterile water do you need to draw up for this special dilution?

3. Prepare a special dilution of vancomycin with a total volume of 10 mL and a concentration of 10 mg/mL. To create this special dilution, use a stock solution of vancomycin with a concentration of 500 mg/5 mL and sterile water. Round to the nearest milligram and milliliter.

a. How many milligrams of vancomycin do you need for this special dilution?

b. How many milliliters of the vancomycin stock solution do you need to draw up for this special dilution?

c. How many milliliters of sterile water do you need to draw up for this special dilution?

4. Prepare a special dilution of dexamethasone with a total volume of 5 mL and a concentration of 1 mg/mL. To create this special dilution, use a stock solution of dexamethasone with a concentration of 4 mg/mL and sterile water. Round to the nearest milligram and hundredth of a milliliter.

a. How many milligrams of dexamethasone do you need for this special dilution?

b. How many milliliters of the dexamethasone stock solution do you need to draw up for this special dilution?

c. How many milliliters of sterile water do you need to draw up for this special dilution?

5. Prepare a special dilution of gentamicin with a total volume of 10 mL and a concentration of 1 mg/mL. To create this special dilution, use sterile water and the following gentamicin stock solution. Round to the nearest milligram and milliliter.

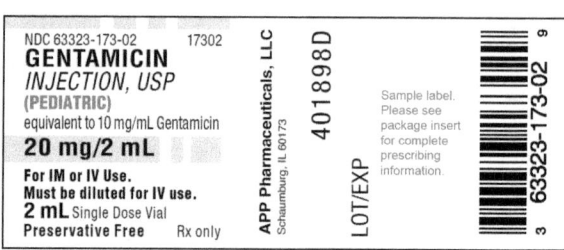

a. How many milligrams of gentamicin do you need for this special dilution?

b. How many milliliters of the gentamicin stock solution shown above do you need to draw up for this special dilution?

c. How many milliliters of sterile water do you need to up for this special dilution?

For questions 6–10, determine how much of each solution are needed to make the preparation. Round to the nearest milliliter.

6. Prepare 500 mL of D15W using dextrose 70% and sterile water.

7. Prepare 2,000 mL of D10W using dextrose 50% and sterile water.

8. Prepare 1,000 mL of D10W using D50W and sterile water.

9. Prepare 750 mL of D8W using D50W and sterile water.

10. Prepare 250 mL of D7.5% using D70W and sterile water.

11. The pharmacy has received the following TPN order:

TPN Standing Orders

Base Solution: Dextrose 17%
Aminosyn 3%
Liposyn 2.5%
Sterile water QSAD to 1500 mL

Additives: Sodium chloride 20 mEq/L
Potassium chloride 15 mEq/L
Potassium phosphate 10 mM/L
Sodium phosphate 3 mM/L
Magnesium sulfate 10 mEq/L
MVI 10 mL/day

Total volume: 1500 mL
Flow rate: 60 mL/hr
Physician: Dr. Serena Martinez
Signature: _Serena Martinez, M.D._

Patient: McGraw, Tilly
Room #: ICU-15
DOB: 03/26/41
Allergies: PCN
Pt. ID #: WWIKKD6773

Use the TPN order, along with the various pharmacy stock solutions carried by your pharmacy, to determine the volume of each base solution and additive. Round answers to the nearest hundredth of a milliliter.

The pharmacy carries the following stock solutions:

Dextrose 70%
Aminosyn 10%
Liposyn 20%
Sodium chloride 4 mEq/mL
Potassium chloride 2 mEq/mL
Potassium phosphate 3 mM/mL
Sodium phosphate 3 mM/mL
Magnesium sulfate 4.06 mEq/mL
MVI 10 mL/day

Determine the volume of each of the following:

a. Dextrose = _____ mL

b. Aminosyn = _____ mL

c. Liposyn = _____ mL

d. Sodium chloride = _____ mL

e. Potassium chloride = _____ mL

f. Potassium phosphate = _____ mL

g. Sodium phosphate = _____ mL

h. Magnesium sulfate = _____ mL

i. MVI = _____ mL

j. Sterile water = _____ mL

k. Total volume = _____ mL

12. The pharmacy receives the TPN order shown below. Use the TPN order, along with the various pharmacy stock solutions carried by your pharmacy, to determine the volume of each base solution and additive. Round answers to the nearest hundredth of a milliliter.

TPN Standing Orders

Base Solution: Dextrose 15%
Aminosyn 4%
Liposyn 3%
Sterile water QSAD to 1500 mL

Additives: Sodium chloride 25 mEq/L
Potassium chloride 12.5 mEq/L
Potassium phosphate 10 mM/L
Sodium phosphate 2 mM/L
Magnesium sulfate 10 mEq/L
MVI 10 mL/day

Total volume: 1500 mL
Flow rate: 60 mL/hr
Physician: Dr. Michael Flynn
Signature: _Michael Flynn_

Patient: Burda, Sara
Room #: ICU-3
Allergies: NKDA
Pt ID #: 1329890

The pharmacy carries the following stock solutions:

Dextrose 70%
Aminosyn 10%
Liposyn 20%
Sodium chloride 4 mEq/mL
Potassium chloride 2 mEq/mL
Potassium phosphate 3 mM/mL
Sodium phosphate 3 mM/mL
Magnesium sulfate 4.06 mEq/mL
MVI 10 mL/day

Determine the volume of each of the following:

a. Dextrose = _____ mL

b. Aminosyn = _____ mL

c. Liposyn = _____ mL

d. Sodium chloride = _____ mL

e. Potassium chloride = _____ mL

f. Potassium phosphate = _____ mL

g. Sodium phosphate = _____ mL

h. Magnesium sulfate = _____ mL

i. MVI = _____ mL

j. Sterile water = _____ mL

k. Total volume = _____ mL

Self-check your work in Appendix A.

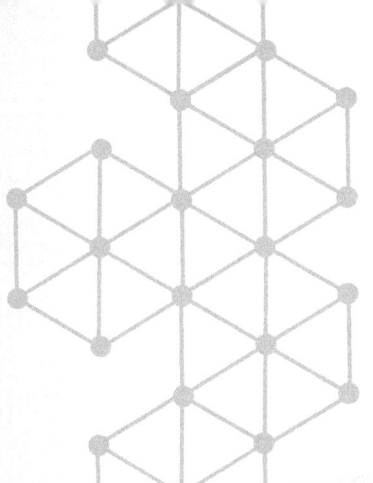

CHAPTER SUMMARY

- Compounding, the process of using raw ingredients and/or prepared ingredients to create a medication, is a task frequently performed by technicians in hospital and compounding pharmacies and, occasionally, in the community pharmacy setting.

- Compounding requires strict adherence to a recipe or formula.

- Technicians are often required to perform a series of calculations to reduce or enlarge an existing formula (known as the *current formula*) into a new, prescribed strength or amount (known as the *desired formula*).

- One way a technician can reduce or enlarge a formula is to compare the current formula with the desired formula by creating a ratio. The technician then either divides by that amount to reduce the formula, or multiplies by that amount to enlarge the formula.

- Occasionally, a technician may be required to mix two strengths of a particular ingredient to prepare a medication with a final strength whose concentration lies somewhere between the higher-strength and lower-strength ingredients. These situations require the technician to use the alligation method.

- When working with an alligation problem, the *desired strength* should be placed in the center of the tic-tac-toe grid; the *higher strength* (stronger concentration) should be placed in the upper-left corner of the tic-tac-toe grid; and the *lower strength* (weaker concentration) should be placed in the lower-left corner of the tic-tac-toe grid.

Tic-Tac-Toe Alligation Grid

A (higher %)		D (parts of higher %; the difference of B − C)
	B (desired %)	
C (lower %)		E (parts of lower %; the difference of A − B)

KEY
A = higher concentration or strength (stated as a percent [%])
B = desired concentration or strength (stated as a percent [%])
C = lower concentration or strength (stated as a percent [%])

- When using an alligation to determine the amount of each ingredient use the following formulas:

$$\frac{\text{D (higher \% solution)}}{\text{TP (total \# of parts)}} = \frac{x \text{ mL}}{\text{TV (total volume of desired concentration)}}$$

$$\frac{\text{E (lower \% solution)}}{\text{TP (total \# of parts)}} = \frac{x \text{ mL}}{\text{TV (total volume of desired concentration)}}$$

Cross multiply; then divide to solve for x.

- The weight-in-weight (w/w) formula identifies the number of grams per 100 g of product.

- A special dilution is a type of compounded sterile preparation that is prepared to provide a pediatric dosage of an injectable medication that is only commercially available in an adult-strength formulation.

Formulas for Success

Calculation for Percentage Strength of w/w Preparations

$$\text{percentage strength of w/w preparation} = \frac{\text{g of active ingredient}}{100 \text{ g of product}} \times 100$$

Formula used to calculate amount of concentrated solution needed:

$$\left(\frac{\text{TV}}{\text{stock \%}}\right) \times \text{desired \%} = \text{number of milliliters}$$

active ingredient the component of a pharmaceutical preparation or medication that exerts pharmacological activity designed to treat or prevent disease

additive a pharmaceutical substance, such as a medication, electrolyte, or other ingredient, that is added to another product, such as a compounded sterile preparation, in order to be easily administered to a patient

alligation method the mathematical calculation used to determine the amounts of two or more dilutions of differing strengths that will be mixed to prepare a product of a desired strength and quantity

compounded sterile preparation (CSP) a product made by mixing two or more sterile products using aseptic technique

compounded stock preparation a solution that is prepared in a large amount and kept in stock in the pharmacy to be divided for individual prescriptions

compounding the process of using raw ingredients and/or prepared ingredients to create a medication for a patient.

current formula a standard pharmaceutical recipe that is commonly used in pharmacy compounding; a recipe often used to prepare compounded stock preparations

desired formula a specialized pharmaceutical recipe ordered by a prescriber that alters various components of a current formula

formula a written document listing the ingredients and instructions needed to prepare a compound

inactive ingredient a component of a pharmaceutical preparation that does not affect pharmacologic activity

special dilution a custom-made diluted compounded sterile preparation (CSP)

total parenteral nutrition (TPN) IV administration of total nutrient requirements to patients who require a long-term alternative to enteral feeding

TPN base solution components of the TPN solution that provide the primary volumetric source, often comprised of a combination of dextrose, amino acids, sterile water, and, in some cases, fat emulsion

weight-in-weight (w/w) formula the number of grams of a medication (solid) in 100 g of the final product (solid)

Finding Solutions

To gain practice in handling challenging situations in the workplace, consider the following real-world scenarios, and then use the guiding questions to help you formulate your responses.

Scenario A: You have just received the following medication order in the pharmacy. Answer the accompanying questions based on this medication order. Round to the nearest milli-equivalent and milliliter.

ID#: PPIKIEI88929			Memorial Hospital
Name: Seaholm, Brinkley			
DOB: 07/04/81			
Room: 1124			Physician's
Dr: Sarai Gupta, M.D.			Medication Order

ALLERGY OR SENSITIVITY			DIAGNOSIS
NKA			dehydration

DATE	TIME	ORDERS	PHYSICIAN'S SIG.
5/5/2017	3:57 PM	Potassium chloride 20 mEq/L	
		in D12% 1000 mL	
		@ 125 mL/hr	
			Sarai Gupta, M.D.

Pharmacy Stock Solutions:

Dextrose 50%

Potassium chloride 2 mEq/mL

1. How many milliequivalents of KCl will you need for one IV bag?

2. How many IV bags will the patient need for 24 hours?

3. How many milliliters of dextrose will you need to prepare one IV bag?

4. How many milliliters of sterile water will you need to prepare one IV bag?

5. How many milliliters of IV fluid will the patient receive in 24 hours?

Scenario B: The following TPN label was received in the IV room. Answer the accompanying questions based on this label. Round to the nearest tenth of a milliliter.

TPN Solution

Memorial Hospital

Name: Burge, April   **Room:** 2284

Pt. ID#: HHUSY0068   **Rx#:** 7728829

Dextrose 15%
Aminosyn 5%
Liposyn 2.5%
SW QSAD
NaCl 10 mEq/L
KCl 10 mEq/L
MgSO$_4$ 2.5 mEq/L
Regular insulin 20 units/L
MVI 10 mL/day

Rate: 150 mL/hr

Expires _____
RPh _____
Tech _____

Keep refrigerated – warm to room temperature
before use.

Pharmacy Stock Solutions:

D70W

AA 10%

Liposyn 10%

NaCl 4 mEq/mL

KCl 2 mEq/mL

MgSO$_4$ 4.06 mEq/mL

Regular insulin 100 units/mL

MVI 10 mL/day

6. The TPN rate is 150 mL/hr. What is the total volume needed for 24 hours? (*Note:* This will be the TPN total volume—the QSAD amount that should be used to determine SW volume.)

7. How much dextrose will you need to make this compound?

8. How much Aminosyn (AA) will you need?

9. How much Liposyn will you need?

10. How much sodium chloride will you need?

11. How much potassium chloride will you need?

12. How much magnesium sulfate will you need?

13. How much regular insulin will you need?

14. How much MVI will you need?

15. How much sterile water will you need?

Scenario C: A prescriber has ordered a patient 8 ounces of your pharmacy's Magic Mouthwash with directions to swish, gargle, and spit one to two teaspoonsful every six hours as needed for irritation. The pharmacy's recipe book lists a formula to prepare 480 mL total.

Magic Mouthwash Recipe:
- 80 mL viscous lidocaine 2%
- 80 mL Mylanta
- 80 mL diphenhydramine 12.5 mg per 5 mL elixir
- 80 mL nystatin 100,000 units suspension
- 80 mL prednisolone 15 mg per 5 mL solution
- 80 mL distilled water

16. How many ounces does the pharmacy recipe book make?

17. How may ounces of each ingredient should you use to make 8 ounces? Round to the nearest tenth of an ounce.

18. How many milligrams of diphenhydramine are in 8 ounces of Magic Mouthwash?

19. How many milligrams of prednisolone are in 8 ounces of Magic Mouthwash?

20. Rewrite the administration instructions using the volume measurement of milliliters.

Navigator

Access interactive chapter review exercises, practice activities, flash cards, and study games.

9

Using Business Math in the Pharmacy

Shelina Hardwick-Moses, MBA, MSHCA, CPhT, PhTR

Learning Objectives

1 Define overhead and calculate overhead cost.

2 Explain the distinction between net profit and gross profit.

3 Calculate markup and the markup rate.

4 Calculate discounts.

5 Explain the concept of average wholesale price to profit calculations.

6 Calculate inventory turnover.

7 Define and calculate depreciation.

 Preview chapter terms and definitions.

9.1 Business-Related Calculations

Like other types of business, pharmacies must perform certain accounting operations on a regular basis. In the retail setting, it is important for the pharmacy to make a profit. A **profit** is the financial gain a business obtains when the income the business earns in a specified period is greater than the costs it incurs to run the business. In the hospital or institutional setting, pharmacy personnel must closely monitor the inventory of medication and supplies to determine if the facility is staying within its allotted budget. To make a profit and stay in business, retail pharmacies must effectively manage markup, discounts, sales, inventory, and overhead. The following sections explain these business concepts.

Overhead

A pharmacy's **overhead** is its costs related to doing business. This overall cost includes employee salaries, equipment, and operating expenses such as rent, taxes, utilities, and insurance. Overhead also includes the dollar value of the medications and supply items in the pharmacy inventory.

Income refers to the money or equivalent payments (such as those made with credit or debit cards) received from the sale of a medication, supply item, or equipment. In the simplest terms, a pharmacy's **base profit** is determined by subtracting total overhead expenses from total income.

Example 9.1.1

The River City Apothecary Shop has an annual income of $850,000.00. The pharmacy's annual overhead expenses are listed below.

salary of pharmacist	$120,000
salaries of two pharmacy technicians ($31,500 each)	63,000
rent	14,400
utilities	5,000
pharmacy software maintenance	2,200
liability insurance	3,500
business insurance	4,000
pharmacy inventory amount	550,000
total pharmacy overhead amount	$762,100

Using this information, determine the pharmacy's base profit by subtracting the total pharmacy overhead amount from the pharmacy's annual income.

income	$850,000
overhead	− 762,100
base profit	$87,900

Therefore, the base profit of the River City Apothecary Shop is $87,900.

Example 9.1.2

The Willington City Pharmacy has an annual income of $1,250,000. The pharmacy's annual overhead expenses are listed below.

salaries of two pharmacists ($120,000.00 each)	$240,000
salary of pharmacy technician	31,500
salary of pharmacy clerk	22,500
rent	16,200
utilities	7,000
pharmacy software maintenance	2,900
liability insurance	4,000
business insurance	5,000
pharmacy inventory amount	625,000
total pharmacy overhead amount	$954,100

Subtract the pharmacy's total annual overhead from its total annual income to determine the pharmacy's base profit.

income	$1,250,000
overhead	− 954,100
base profit	$295,900

Therefore, the base profit of the Willington City Pharmacy is $295,900.

A pharmacy manager often sets goals for the pharmacy's annual profit. To do this, the manager begins by finding the current percent of profit. The **current percentage of profit** is determined by dividing the base profit by income and then multiplying that quotient by 100.

Once the pharmacy manager knows the current percentage of profit, he or she can determine the desired percentage of profit. The **desired percentage of profit** is the percentage of profit the pharmacy intends to make after the overall cost is subtracted from the selling price. Establishing the desired percentage of profit can, in turn, help the pharmacy manager determine the amount of annual income needed to achieve this goal. These business calculations provide the manager with the necessary information to establish a pharmacy's budget and to set sales goals.

The following examples illustrate how to calculate percentage of profit and annual profit. Note that converting the desired percentage of profit to a decimal allows for easier calculation, but round to the nearest percentage for your final answer.

Example 9.1.3

Determine the River City Apothecary Shop's current percentage of profit based on the annual income and base profit information calculated in Example 9.1.1.

$$\frac{\text{base profit}}{\text{annual income}} \times 100 = \text{current percentage of profit}$$

$$\frac{\$87,900}{\$850,000} \times 100 = 10.34, \text{ rounded to } 10$$

The River City Apothecary Shop has a current percentage of profit of 10.

Example 9.1.4

Determine the Willington City Pharmacy's current percentage of profit based on the annual income and base profit information calculated in Example 9.1.2.

$$\frac{\text{base profit}}{\text{annual income}} \times 100 = \text{current percentage of profit}$$

$$\frac{\$295,900}{\$1,250,000} \times 100 = 23.67, \text{ rounded to } 24$$

The Willington City Pharmacy has a current percentage of profit of 24.

The River City Apothecary Shop has set a goal of a 25% profit. Based on the $762,100.00 overhead amount provided in Example 9.1.1, what annual income must the pharmacy have to meet this goal?

overhead × desired percentage of profit = desired amount of profit
$762,100 × 0.25 = $190,525

overhead + desired amount of profit = desired income goal
$762,100 + $190,525 = $952,625

Therefore, to meet the 25% profit goal (the desired percentage of profit), the pharmacy's must generate an annual income of $952,625.

The Willington City Pharmacy has set a goal of a 35% profit. Based on the overhead amount of $954,100.00 provided in Example 9.1.2, what annual income must the pharmacy have to meet this goal?

overhead × desired percentage of profit = desired amount of profit
$954,100 × 0.35 = $333,935

overhead + desired amount of profit = desired income goal
$954,100 + $333,935 = $1,288,035

Therefore, to meet the 35% profit goal (the desired percentage of profit), the pharmacy's generate an annual income of $1,288,035.

Net Profit

In the pharmacy, profit is influenced by the selling prices of medications. **Net profit** is the difference between the selling price of the medication and the overall cost. The selling price is the amount received when a pharmacy product is sold. The selling price is often called the *retail price* or *accounts receivable*. Simply put, the selling price determines the amount due from a customer to the pharmacy for the sale of drugs and other products and the overall cost of the medication. The **overall cost** is the sum of the cost to purchase the drug from the wholesaler or manufacturer (known as the pharmacy's **purchase price**) and the dispensing fee. The **dispensing fee** is the amount the pharmacy charges for a medication that is over and above the price it pays for the medication. The dispensing fee (also called the *cost to dispense a drug*) covers all costs beyond the drug's purchase price that are related to filling a prescription such as: pharmacy overhead, professional handling, prescription processing and recording, and patient consultation and counseling.

When calculating the net profit on an individual prescription, the overall cost of the medication (purchase price plus dispensing fee) is compared with the amount the pharmacy receives for the dispensed drug. In this situation, the term *profit* refers only to the pharmacy's purchase price of the drug and does not include the cost of materials, labor, or overhead. This includes any actual profit that is gained. **Actual profit** is the amount of profit the pharmacy receives after deducting the pharmacy's overhead, labor, materials and dispensing fees from the pharmacy's total income.

Based on its desired percentage of profit, a pharmacy will decide on a selling price for a medication or supply item. As mentioned earlier, the desired percentage of profit is the percentage of profit the pharmacy intends to make on the product after the overall cost is subtracted from the selling price. To easily calculate the selling price, convert the desired percentage of profit to a decimal. If the pharmacy has correctly set the selling price, the net profit should yield the desired percentage of profit.

pharmacy's purchase price + dispensing fee = overall cost

(overall cost × desired percentage of profit) + overall cost = selling price

selling price − overall cost = net profit

Example 9.1.7

The pharmacy purchase price of a pint bottle of Nystatin Oral Suspension is $20.25. After considering the various factors that influence pharmacy costs, the pharmacy determines that its cost to dispense this item is $5.10. Determine the overall cost for this item. If the pharmacy has a desired percentage of profit of 20% for this item, what should the selling price be?

pharmacy's purchase price + dispensing fee = overall cost
$20.25 + $5.10 = $25.35

(overall cost × desired percentage of profit) + overall cost = selling price
($25.35 × 0.20) + $25.35 = $30.42

selling price − overall cost = net profit
$30.42 − 25.35 = $5.07

The overall cost for a pint bottle of Nystatin Oral Suspension is $25.35. To yield a net profit of $5.07, or 20%, the selling price of the item must be $30.42.

For Good Measure

In pharmacy practice, the term *count* refers to the number of pills, doses, or units in a single container.

Example 9.1.8

The pharmacy purchased a 100-count bottle of propranolol 10 mg tablets at a price of $3.96. A customer presents a prescription that requires you to dispense a total of 30 tablets. The pharmacy charges a dispensing fee of $4.25 for each prescription it fills. The total charge to the customer for this prescription is $8.59. Calculate the net profit that the pharmacy made on the sale of this prescription.

Step 1. Pharmacy cost/count = cost per tablet (rounded to the nearest hundredth)

$$\frac{\$3.96}{100} = \$0.0396, \text{ rounded to } \$0.04 \text{ per tablet}$$

Step 2. Determine the pharmacy cost of the customer's prescription.

cost per tablet × amount dispensed = pharmacy cost of prescription

$0.04 × 30 = $1.20

Step 3. Calculate the overall cost.

Pharmacy cost of the prescription + dispensing fee = overall cost

$1.20 + $4.25 = $5.45

Step 4. Calculate the pharmacy's net profit for this prescription.

selling price − overall cost = net profit

$8.59 − $5.45 = $3.14

The pharmacy made a net profit of $3.14 on the sale of this prescription.

Gross Profit, Net Profit, and Markup

The difference between the selling price and the pharmacy's purchase price (the price that it costs for the pharmacy to purchase the drug from the manufacturer or drug wholesaler) is called **gross profit**. Gross profit is the difference between sales and cost of sales; however, this relationship between the purchase price and the selling price does not take into account the cost of preparing and dispensing the drug. Thus, the gross profit is always more than the net profit. Net profit is what remains after all expenses and taxes have been paid.

Gross profit and net profit are similar to gross pay and net pay. Gross pay is your pay before taxes and other deductions are taken out. Net pay is the amount you "take home." For example, you may earn $400.00 per week (gross pay), but your take-home pay (net pay) after all taxes and deductions are applied may be $325.00 per week.

Using the example of the Nystatin Oral Suspension from Example 9.1.7, the gross profit would be $10.17.

selling price − pharmacy's purchase price = gross profit

$30.42 − $20.25 = $10.17

The **profit margin** is the difference between the cost of doing business (the pharmacy's purchase price, overhead, and preparation costs) and the selling price of a drug or product. A loss—sometimes called a *negative profit*—occurs when the selling price of a product is less than the cost.

Like all businesses, pharmacies purchase their products (drugs or supply items) at one price from the manufacturer or **wholesaler**, and then sell them at a higher price. Although pharmacies are subject to governmental laws and regulations regarding the sale of drugs, markup plays a significant role in the pharmacies' pricing systems and, ultimately, their profit margins. The **markup rate**, also known as the *markup percent*, is calculated by dividing the **markup amount** by the pharmacy purchase price (cost), then multiplying by 100.

The markup rate is computed by first determining the markup amount:

selling price − pharmacy's purchase price = markup amount

The markup rate is expressed as a percentage and is computed as follows:

$$\frac{\text{markup amount}}{\text{pharmacy's purchase price}} \times 100 = \text{markup rate}$$

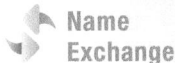

Name Exchange

The generic drug metformin is also known by the brand name Glucophage.

Example 9.1.9

A 30-day supply of the antidiabetic agent metformin has a selling price of $45.00. The pharmacy's purchase price is $30.00. What is the markup amount? What is the markup rate?

$$\text{selling price} - \text{pharmacy's purchase price} = \text{markup amount}$$

$$\$45.00 - \$30.00 = \$15.00$$

$$\frac{\text{markup amount}}{\text{pharmacy's purchase price}} \times 100 = \text{markup rate}$$

$$\frac{\$15.00}{\$30.00} = 0.5, 0.5 \times 100 = 50\%$$

The markup amount on a 30-day supply of metformin is $15.00. The markup rate is 50%.

Markup rates on brand name drug products are typically lower than markup rates on generic drugs. The markup rate for generic medications is typically much higher, but the selling prices of generic drugs are generally lower.

As a result of these markup practices, the percentage of profit from selling generic drugs is often higher than the percentage of profit for the corresponding brand name products. For example, a pharmacy may mark up a $15.00 generic drug by 33%, which would result in a selling price of $20.00, and a $5.00 profit for the pharmacy. The corresponding brand name drug may have a purchase price of $30.00 and a markup of 5%, which would result in a selling price of $31.50, and a $1.50 profit for the pharmacy.

In general, both the pharmacy and the patient benefit financially from using generic medications: The patient purchases the medication at a much lower cost, and the pharmacy receives a larger profit. Although the pharmacy's percentage of profit from selling a generic drug is generally higher than the percentage of profit for the corresponding brand name drug, the pharmacy may not make a huge profit from the sale of an individual drug due to a relatively low selling price of the generic drug.

A growing trend in retail pharmacies is to sell generic drugs to customers at a flat dollar rate, such as $4.00 or $7.00, regardless of the cost of the drug, which fluctuates over time. A **flat rate** is a low pharmacy selling price for a certain amount of medication, a supply designed to last a specific number of days—for example, a 30-day or 90-day supply. The types of medications that are available to customers at a flat rate are typically generic medications with low pharmacy purchase prices. Because the medications are inexpensive for the pharmacy to purchase, the pharmacy is still able to make a profit on the drugs while generating additional sales from nonpharmacy sales, over-the-counter (OTC) products, or other prescriptions that the patient may purchase at the same time. Table 9.1 lists examples of medications that are often sold at a flat rate.

TABLE 9.1 Flat-Rate Medications

Medication	Used to Treat...
amoxicillin	bacterial infections
atenolol	hypertension or heart conditions
estradiol	estrogen deficiency
fluoxetine	depression
levothyroxine	thyroid disorders
loratadine	allergies
metformin	diabetes
naproxen	pain and inflammation
triamcinolone	skin disorders

The following example applies the formulas for markup amount and markup rate to a flat-rate prescription to illustrate how profitable such sales can be for the pharmacy.

Example 9.1.10

 A retail pharmacy that has advertised a $4.00 flat-rate price for generic prescriptions receives a prescription for #30 amoxicillin 250 mg capsules. If the pharmacy's purchase price for these #30 capsules is $1.20, what is the percentage of profit on this prescription when it is sold for the flat-rate price?

First find the markup amount.

$$\text{selling price} - \text{pharmacy's purchase price} = \text{markup amount}$$
$$\$4.00 - \$1.20 = \$2.80$$

Then find the markup rate.

$$\frac{\text{markup amount}}{\text{pharmacy's purchase price}} \times 100 = \text{markup rate}$$

$$\frac{\$2.80}{\$1.20} \times 100 = 233$$

The percentage of profit on amoxicillin sold for the flat rate is 233%. Note that although the markup rate is high, the gross profit is still relatively low due to the drug's low cost.

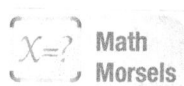

When working with percents, pharmacy technicians should change the discount rate from a percent to a decimal.

Discount

Sometimes, a manufacturer or supplier offers an item at a lower price to a pharmacy. The amount by which the price is reduced is the **discount**. Similarly, a pharmacy may offer consumers a discount, or a reduction from what is normally charged, as an incentive to purchase an item. The **discount rate** is the percent by which the price is reduced from the regular selling price. When working with percents, it is helpful to change the discount rate from a percent to a decimal.

$$\text{regular selling price} \times \text{discount rate} = \text{discount amount}$$

$$\text{regular selling price} - \text{discount amount} = \text{sale price}$$

Discounts are one of the easiest business-related math calculations, and you are already familiar with them because you use them nearly every time you buy something on sale. For example, a sale that offers 50% off means that a sale item may be purchased at one-half of the regular selling price. In such a scenario, the sale price (also known as *discounted selling price*) is calculated by multiplying the regular price by 0.50 (50% = 0.50). The sale price may also be calculated by dividing the regular price by two.

Example 9.1.11

A retail pharmacy has announced a 40%-off sale on all headache products during the two weeks leading up to the tax-filing deadline. The following products are on sale:

 Tylenol 325 mg tablets; 100 count; selling price $6.99

 Excedrin Migraine tablets; 100 count; selling price $7.89

 Advil 250 mg tablets; 100 count; selling price $7.29

If a customer purchases one bottle of each item at the sale price, how much will he or she pay for each drug? How much will the customer pay for the entire purchase?

Step 1. Calculate the discount amount on Tylenol.

$$\text{regular selling price} \times \text{discount rate} = \text{discount amount}$$
$$\$6.99 \times 0.40 = \$2.796, \text{ rounded to } \$2.80$$

Step 2. Determine the amount the customer will pay for Tylenol.

$$\text{regular selling price} - \text{discount amount} = \text{sale price}$$
$$\$6.99 - \$2.80 = \$4.19$$

Step 3. Calculate the discount amount on Excedrin Migraine.

$$\text{regular selling price} \times \text{discount rate} = \text{discount amount}$$
$$\$7.89 \times 0.40 = \$3.156, \text{ rounded to } \$3.16$$

Step 4. Determine the amount the customer will pay for Excedrin Migraine.

$$\text{regular selling price} - \text{discount amount} = \text{sale price}$$
$$\$7.89 - \$3.16 = \$4.73$$

Step 5. Calculate the discount amount on Advil.

regular selling price × discount rate = discount amount

$7.29 × 0.40 = $2.916, rounded to $2.92

Step 6. Determine the amount the customer will pay for Advil.

regular selling price − discount amount = sale price

$7.29 − $2.92 = $4.37

Step 7. Calculate the amount the customer will pay for the entire purchase by adding the sale price of each item.

$4.19 + $4.73 + $4.37 = $13.29

Therefore, the customer will pay $4.19 for Tylenol, $4.73 for Excedrin Migraine, and $4.37 for Advil. For the entire purchase, the customer will pay $13.29.

Example 9.1.12

 Assume the pharmacy purchases five cases of hydrocortisone cream at $100.00 per case. If the account is paid in full within 30 days, the wholesaler will give a 15% discount on the purchase. How much money will the pharmacy save if it pays the account in full within 30 days? What will be the sale price for the five cases?

Step 1. Calculate the regular selling price.

quantity of product × purchase price per unit = regular selling price

5 cases × $100.00 per case = $500.00

Step 2. Determine the discount amount.

regular selling price × discount rate = discount amount

$500.00 × 0.15 = $75.00

If the pharmacy pays the account in full within 30 days, it will save $75.00 off of the regular selling price.

Step 3. Calculate the discounted sales price.

regular selling price − discount amount = sale price

$500.00 − $75.00 = $425.00

Birch Lake Pharmacy has the following overhead expenses. Use this information to answer questions 1 through 3.

pharmacist salary	$135,000.00
technician salary	52,000.00
rent	23,000.00
utilities	6,000.00
computer maintenance	4,000.00
software subscriptions	2,000.00
liability insurance	4,000.00
business insurance	4,000.00
drug purchases	750,000.00

1. If an 18% profit is desirable, what must the pharmacy's income be to meet this goal?

2. If the pharmacy's income is $1,401,489.00, what is its percentage of profit?

3. If the pharmacy's income is $1,191,692.00, what is its percentage of profit?

Summit Avenue Pharmacy has the following overhead expenses. Use this information to answer questions 4 through 6.

pharmacist salary	$72,000.00
technician salary	52,000.00
rent	13,000.00
utilities	5,500.00
computer maintenance	2,000.00
software subscriptions	1,500.00
liability insurance	4,000.00
business insurance	3,500.00
drug purchases	50,000.00

4. If a 20% profit is desirable, what must the pharmacy's income be to meet this goal?

5. If the pharmacy's income is $991,982.00, what is its percentage of profit?

6. If the pharmacy's income is $1,248,301.00, what is its percentage of profit?

7. The pharmacy determines that its income for the week was $54,617.53 and that the net profit was $3,700.83. What was the overhead for the week?

8. Martelli's Pharmacy has a weekly overhead of $13,033.06. If this pharmacy is to make a 22% profit, what must its sales of goods and services amount to each week?

For items 9–15, calculate the dollar amount of net profit and the markup rate for the following prescription drug items (round to whole percents). The pharmacy charges a $4.25 dispensing fee for each prescription.

9. Medication: propranolol 10 mg
Pharmacy's purchase price: $3.96
Count: 100 tablets
Amount dispensed: 50 tablets
Pharmacy's selling price: $8.59

10. Medication: amoxicillin 250 mg
Pharmacy's purchase price: $8.50
Count: 500 capsules
Amount dispensed: 30 capsules
Pharmacy's selling price: $14.80

11. Medication: paroxetine 20 mg
Pharmacy's purchase price: $118.50
Count: 100 tablets
Amount dispensed: 30 tablets
Pharmacy's selling price: $45.50

12. Medication: furosemide 40 mg
Pharmacy's purchase price: $83.50
Count: 500 tablets
Amount dispensed: 100 tablets
Pharmacy's selling price: $23.16

13. Medication: levothyroxine 0.1 mg
Pharmacy's purchase price: $41.20
Count: 100 tablets
Amount dispensed: 90 tablets
Pharmacy's selling price: $41.70

14. Medication: promethazine cough syrup
Pharmacy's purchase price: $37.50
Count: one 16 oz bottle (480 mL)*
Amount dispensed: 8 oz
Pharmacy's selling price: $25.34
(*Use 480 mL for your calculation.)

15. Medication: Loestrin oral contraceptive
28-day pack
Pharmacy's purchase price: $62.30
Count: six 28-day packs
Amount dispensed: one 28-day pack
Pharmacy's selling price: $17.90

The pharmacy is selling the items listed in questions 16–23 at a discount this week. Calculate the sale price for each.

16. cough syrup: regular selling price, $5.89; discounted 20%

17. facial tissues: regular selling price, $1.19; discounted 15%

18. hair color kit: regular selling price, $7.29; discounted 30%

19. body lotion: regular selling price, $5.69; discounted 15%

20. baby shampoo: regular selling price, $3.89; discounted 25%

21. antacid liquid: regular selling price, $4.26; discounted 30%

22. acetaminophen tablets: regular selling price, $8.70; discounted 50%

23. toothpaste: regular selling price, $2.99; discounted 40%

For questions 24–29, perform the necessary calculations and state the answer in dollars or percentages as indicated.

24. Antiviral ointment costs a pharmacy $12.50 per tube. The standard markup is 30%. What is the total selling price of a box of 12 tubes?

25. Eyedrops with antihistamine are purchased from the manufacturer in cases of 36 drop-dispenser bottles. The pharmacy desires a markup of $1.75 per bottle. The pharmacy's purchase price is $111.60 per case. What is the selling price per bottle?

26. Identify the markup and the selling price of an oral antibiotic suspension that costs the pharmacist $15.60 per bottle if the markup rate is 25%.

27. An asthma tablet costs the pharmacy $24.80 for a month's supply, and the selling price is $30.75. Calculate the markup rate.

28. Calculate the gross profit from a medication that costs the pharmacy $520.00 for 1,000 tablets and sells for $650.00.

29. The cost of dispensing the medication in question 28 is $2.05 per 100 tablets. Calculate the net profit for selling one tablet.

The pharmacy where you work has received a shipment of medications and supplies from its wholesaler. Calculate the pharmacy's markup amount and selling price for each item listed in questions 30–36.

	Drug		Count/ Quantity	Pharmacy's Purchase Price	Markup Rate	Pharmacy's Markup Amount	Pharmacy's Selling Price
30.	Augmentin oral solution		1,200 mL	$120.50	25%		
31.	triamcinolone foot powder		12 containers	$24.00	15%		
32.	ibuprofen		2,000 tablets	$200.00	27%		
33.	Band-Aids		10 boxes	$27.50	21%		
34.	Neosporin antibiotic ointment		18 tubes	$67.50	18%		
35.	birth control 28-day packs		24 packs	$840.00	32%		
36.	DiaBeta		600 tablets	$550.00	30%		

37. Calculate the total amount that the pharmacy spent on the shipment above. Then determine the total amount the pharmacy made upon selling all of the items. Finally, calculate the overall markup rate for the entire shipment.

Self-check your work in Appendix A.

9.2 Insurance Reimbursements for Prescriptions

Reimbursement for prescription and pharmacy services is largely controlled by contracts with insurance companies and is often brokered through a large prescription processing service called a **pharmacy benefits manager (PBM)**. PBMs use a pharmacy benefits management system that determines the amount of money that will be paid to pharmacies in insurance reimbursement for prescriptions.

Prescription reimbursement may be calculated based on the pharmacy's purchase price, or the average wholesale price of a medication. Prescription reimbursement may also be established by a set contract for an approved list of preferred drugs. The amount of money paid by the PBM for a particular prescription is calculated and approved by the PBM's computer system, or by the pharmacy's computer system via an Internet connection with the PBM. Rarely is this cost calculated by personnel in the pharmacy. Nevertheless, it is helpful to understand the reimbursement process and the methods used to calculate the reimbursement amount for medications. Patients are likely to ask questions about charges and reimbursements, so having a basic understanding of this process, which is sometimes called *reconciliation*, is essential.

Some claims will be reconciled by an individual pharmacy, but most will pass electronically through a PBM or similar type of clearinghouse that is responsible for processing and settling insurance claims. These businesses bill the insurance companies under contract and then reimburse the pharmacy periodically for a batch of prescriptions. Batch reimbursements may be made daily, weekly, or monthly. Some large chain pharmacies may receive a single reimbursement payment that covers a large number of stores. In these instances, the individual store does not receive a check from the PBM, but rather an invoice or a memo indicating the amount of money that the company is being reimbursed.

One of the most challenging aspects of working in the retail pharmacy setting can occur when prescription drug charges are rejected or denied. In such instances, the customer must pay out-of-pocket for the prescriptions. Because of the cost of the prescriptions, some customers may be unable to pay for the medications and, therefore, become upset with pharmacy personnel.

Average Wholesale Price

A pharmacy may potentially receive payment from several different sources. Historically, patients were responsible for paying for their own medications. However, beginning in the mid-1970s, health maintenance organizations (HMOs) and health insurers began to assume a portion of the responsibility for healthcare costs, including patient medications. More recently, HMOs and health insurers have become major players in determining the cost of health care, including the cost of prescriptions. The very survival of a pharmacy depends on its ability to contain costs.

The **average wholesale price (AWP)** of a drug refers to an average price at which drugs are purchased at the wholesale level, or the average value at which wholesalers sell a particular drug to pharmacies. Usually, third parties, such as PBMs, reimburse a pharmacy based upon a percentage of the AWP. Therefore, the pharmacy has an incentive to purchase a drug below its AWP whenever possible. Wholesalers may sell drugs below AWP in some situations, such as when volume discounts, contract prices, or rebates from drug manufacturers are available.

Each third-party reimbursement system (insurance company or PBM) has a predetermined prescription reimbursement amount for each drug. The formula that determines the amount of prescription reimbursement varies depending on the current AWP for that drug, the percentage or markup rate (which may be either positive or negative depending on the agreement with the third party), and the individual pharmacy's dispensing fee. In practice, you will often hear phrases such as "AWP plus X or Y %" or "AWP less X or Y %." Note that when the phrase *AWP less* is used, it has the same meaning as *AWP minus* X or Y %.

$$\text{prescription reimbursement} = \text{AWP} \pm \text{percentage} + \text{dispensing fee}$$

The amount that an insurance company or patient is charged for a prescription is generally predetermined by PBMs and is done automatically through the pharmacy's computer system. Pricing information is preloaded into the PBM's computer system based on the insurance company contracts with the pharmacy. Pharmacy personnel access that pricing information via the Internet. The following examples illustrate one of the methods used to calculate the amount billed, which is similar to the calculation for prescription reimbursement shown above.

Example 9.2.1

A pharmacy has three drugs with the following AWPs:

Drug A, AWP $120.00

Drug B, AWP $80.00

Drug C, AWP $25.00

The pharmacy has a markup rate of 5% and a dispensing fee of $4.00 for each of these drugs. If a patient presents a prescription for each of these drugs, what will be the total billed?

Begin by calculating the amount billed to the patient for each of the individual drugs.

Drug A

$$AWP + markup\ amount + dispensing\ fee = amount\ billed$$
$$\$120.00 + (\$120.00 \times 0.05) + \$4.00 =$$
$$\$120.00 + \$6.00 + \$4.00 = \$130.00$$

Drug B

$$AWP + markup\ amount + dispensing\ fee = amount\ billed$$
$$\$80.00 + (\$80.00 \times 0.05) + \$4.00 =$$
$$\$80.00 + \$4.00 + \$4.00 = \$88.00$$

Drug C

$$AWP + markup\ amount + dispensing\ fee = amount\ billed$$
$$\$25.00 + (\$25.00 \times 0.05) + \$4.00 =$$
$$\$25.00 + \$1.25 + \$4.00 = \$30.25$$

Next, determine the total amount billed by adding the amounts billed for the three drugs.

$$\$130.00 + \$88.00 + \$30.25 = \$248.25$$

The total billed is $248.25.

Example 9.2.2

A certain tablet comes in a quantity of 60 and has an AWP of $100.00. The pharmacy has an agreement with the supplier to purchase the drug at the AWP minus 15%. The insurer is willing to pay AWP plus 5% plus a $2.00 dispensing fee. A patient on this insurer's plan purchases 30 tablets for $54.50. How much profit does the pharmacy make on this prescription?

Begin by calculating the amount of the discount.

$$\$100.00 \times 0.15 = \$15.00$$

Then calculate the pharmacy's purchase price of the drug.

$$\$100.00 - \$15.00 = \$85.00$$

Therefore, the pharmacy can purchase this drug at $85.00 per 60 tablets. The insurance company will pay the pharmacy AWP + 5%.

$$\$100.00 + (\$100.00 \times 0.05) =$$

$$\$100.00 + \$5.00 = \$105.00$$

Next find the amount the insurance company will pay to fill a prescription for 30 pills at that price.

$$(\$105.00 \div 2) + \$2.00 \text{ (dispensing fee)} =$$

$$\$52.50 + \$2.00 = \$54.50$$

Compare this amount with the pharmacy's cost of 30 tablets.

$$\$85.00 \div 2 = \$42.50$$

Finally, find the pharmacy's profit on 30 tablets.

$$\$54.50 - \$42.50 = \$12.00$$

The pharmacy will make a profit of $12.00 on 30 tablets.

Example 9.2.3

Two hundred capsules are purchased at AWP minus 20%, where AWP is $125. The insurer allows a charge of AWP plus 3% per 200 capsules. What is the highest charge per capsule allowed by the insurer? What will be the profit per capsule?

Begin by finding the pharmacy's discounted purchase price of 200 capsules.

$$\$125.00 - (\$125.00 \times 0.20) =$$

$$\$125.00 - \$25.00 = \$100.00$$

Then find the cost per capsule to the pharmacy.

$$\$100.00 \div 200 = \$0.50/\text{capsule}$$

The insurance company will pay the pharmacy AWP plus 3% per 200 capsules.

$$\$125.00 + (\$125.00 \times 0.03) =$$
$$\$125.00 + \$3.75 = \$128.75$$

Next, find the amount that the pharmacy should charge patients.

$$\$128.75 \div 200 \text{ capsules} = \$0.64375 \text{ rounded to } \$0.64/\text{capsule}$$

Finally, find the pharmacy's profit.

$$\text{selling price} - \text{pharmacy's purchase price} = \text{profit}$$
$$\$0.64/\text{capsule} - \$0.50/\text{capsule} = \$0.14/\text{capsule}$$

The pharmacy can charge $0.64/capsule and, therefore, earn a profit of $0.14/capsule.

Capitation Fee

Some insurers use a prescription reimbursement plan in which the pharmacy is paid a monthly fee, called a **capitation fee**, for some patients. The insurer pays the pharmacy the monthly fee whether or not the patients on the plan receive prescriptions during that month. Under this type of plan, the pharmacy must dispense the patients' prescriptions, even if the pharmacy's purchase price of the medications and the dispensing fees are more than the monthly reimbursement amount. Under plans that use capitation fees, pharmacies are not allowed to charge a dispensing fee unless the contract between the pharmacy and the third-party payer specifically states that a dispensing fee is allowed.

Example 9.2.4

O'Rourke's Drug Store receives a monthly capitation fee of $250.00 for Paul Arcand. During April, Paul fills three prescriptions totaling $198.75 which includes the dispensing fee. How much profit does the capitation fee provide?

In this case, the monthly fee exceeds the total of the pharmacy's purchase price, yielding a profit for the pharmacy.

$$\$250.00 - \$198.75 = \$51.25$$

The capitation fee provides O'Rourke's Drug Store with a profit of $51.25.

Example 9.2.5

Cindy Carver has the same insurance plan as Raoul Garcia, with the same capitation fee, $250 per month. During April, Cindy fills four prescriptions at the Willow Creek Pharmacy for a total of $301.25. What is the profit margin?

In this case, the pharmacy's purchase price of the prescriptions exceeds the monthly capitation fee. The pharmacy loses money, so the profit is expressed as a negative number.

$$\$250.00 - \$301.25 = -\$51.25$$

The Willow Creek Pharmacy has a negative profit.

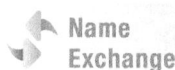 **Name Exchange**

The cardiovascular drug amlodipine is known by the trade name Norvasc.

Example 9.2.6

 The pharmacy purchased a 100-count bottle of amlodipine 10 mg tablets at the AWP of $118.00. A patient presents a prescription that requires you to dispense 30 tablets. The patient's insurance plan does not allow the pharmacy to charge a dispensing fee. If the plan calls for the pharmacy to be reimbursed at AWP less 10%, what is the pharmacy's reimbursement on this prescription?

Step 1. Calculate the pharmacy's cost of the prescription.

$$\frac{\text{pharmacy's purchase price}}{\text{count}} \times \frac{\text{amount}}{\text{dispensed}} = \frac{\text{pharmacy's cost}}{\text{of prescription}}$$

$$\frac{\$118.00}{100} \times 30 = \$35.40$$

Step 2. Determine the discount amount based on 10 percent.

$$\frac{\text{pharmacy's cost of}}{\text{prescription}} \times 10 \text{ percent} = \frac{\text{amount based}}{\text{on percent}}$$

$$\$35.40 \times 0.10 = \$3.54$$

Step 3. Calculate the pharmacy's reimbursement on this prescription. The instructions say "AWP less," so you must *subtract* the amount based on percent from the pharmacy's cost of the prescription.

$$\frac{\text{pharmacy's cost}}{\text{of prescription}} - \frac{\text{amount based}}{\text{on percent}} = \frac{\text{pharmacy's reimbursement}}{\text{amount}}$$

$$\$35.40 - \$3.54 = \$31.86$$

The pharmacy's reimbursement on this prescription is $31.86.

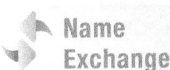
Name Exchange

The generic drug esomeprazole—also known as the brand name Nexium—is commonly prescribed to treat gastro-esophageal reflux disease (GERD).

Example 9.2.7

The pharmacy purchased a 250-count bottle of esomeprazole 40 mg capsules at AWP. The insurance plan reimburses at AWP plus 4% and allows a $5.00 dispensing fee on this prescription. If the AWP is $82.00 and the patient receives a prescription for 90 capsules, what is the amount that the pharmacy will submit for reimbursement? What is the pharmacy's profit?

Step 1. Calculate the pharmacy's cost of the prescription.

$$\frac{\text{pharmacy's purchase price}}{\text{count}} \times \frac{\text{amount}}{\text{dispensed}} = \frac{\text{pharmacy's cost}}{\text{of prescription}}$$

$$\frac{\$82.00}{250} \times 90 = \$29.52$$

Step 2. Determine the reimbursement amount based on 4 percent.

$$\frac{\text{pharmacy's cost of}}{\text{prescription}} \times 4 \text{ percent} = \frac{\text{reimbursement amount}}{\text{based on 4 percent}}$$

$$\$29.52 \times 0.04 = \$1.18$$

Step 3. Calculate the pharmacy's reimbursement on this prescription. The instructions say "AWP plus," so you must *add* the amount based on percent to the pharmacy's cost of the prescription.

$$\frac{\text{pharmacy's}}{\text{cost of}} + \frac{\text{reimbursement}}{\text{amount based}} + \frac{\text{dispensing}}{\text{fee}} = \frac{\text{pharmacy's total}}{\text{reimbursement}}$$
$$\text{prescription} \qquad \text{on percent} \qquad\qquad \text{amount}$$

$$\$29.52 + \$1.18 + \$5.00 = \$35.70$$

Step 4. Determine the pharmacy's profit.

$$\text{amount of reimbursement} - \text{pharmacy's cost of prescription} = \text{profit}$$

$$\$35.70 - \$29.52 = \$6.18$$

The pharmacy will submit $35.70 for reimbursement and will earn a $6.18 profit on this prescription.

9.2 Problem Set

For problems 1–3, calculate the amount that the pharmacy will submit for reimbursement on each prescription based on AWP less 13%. The pharmacy is not permitted to charge a dispensing fee on these prescriptions. Round to the nearest hundredth after finding the cost per tablet/item.

1. AWP $48.90 per 60 tablets and dispense 20 tablets

2. AWP $84.07 per 100 tablets and dispense 30 tablets

3. AWP $30.25 per 1,000 tablets and dispense 100 tablets

For problems 4–6, calculate the amount that the pharmacy will submit for reimbursement on each prescription based on AWP plus 4%. The pharmacy charges a $6.25 dispensing fee for each prescription. Round to the nearest hundredth after finding the cost per tablet/item.

4. AWP $120.68 per 500 tablets and dispense 30 tablets

5. AWP $39.78 per 100 capsules and dispense 60 capsules

6. AWP $317.50 per 30 tablets and dispense 20 tablets

For problems 7-10, round to the nearest hundredth after finding the cost per tablet/item.

7. The pharmacy purchased 100 tablets at $71.35. The insurer will pay AWP plus 3.5% and a $4.50 dispensing fee.

   a. If the pharmacy dispenses a prescription of 50 tablets, what is the pharmacy's cost of the prescription?

   b. What is the total amount that the pharmacy will submit to the insurance company for reimbursement on this prescription?

   c. How much profit will the pharmacy make on this prescription?

8. The pharmacy purchased five metered-dose inhalers (MDIs) at a cost of AWP less 3%. The third-party payer will reimburse at AWP plus 5% and does not allow a dispensing fee. The AWP is $36.35 per inhaler.

   a. If the pharmacy dispenses a single prescription of two MDIs, what is the pharmacy's cost of the prescription?

   b. What is the amount that the pharmacy will submit to the third-party payer for reimbursement on this prescription?

   c. How much profit will the pharmacy make on this prescription?

9. The pharmacy purchased a 30-count bottle of tadalafil (Cialis) tablets at an AWP of $302.35. The PBM will pay AWP less 3% and allows a $7.00 dispensing fee per prescription.

   a. If the pharmacy dispenses a prescription for 10 tablets, what is the pharmacy's cost of the prescription?

   b. What is the amount that the pharmacy will submit to the PBM for reimbursement on this prescription?

   c. How much profit will the pharmacy make on this prescription?

10. The pharmacy purchased 50 tablets of atorvastatin (Lipitor) for $117.35. The insurance company will reimburse at AWP plus 3% and a $4.00 dispensing fee.

    a. If the pharmacy dispenses 30 tablets, what is the pharmacy's cost of the prescription?

    b. What is the amount that the pharmacy will submit to the insurance company for this prescription?

    c. How much profit will the pharmacy make on this prescription?

11. The pharmacy purchased an 80 g bulk jar of triamcinolone (Kenalog) cream at a cost of $85.35. The PBM will reimburse at AWP plus 4.5% but does not allow a dispensing fee.

   a. If the pharmacy dispenses a prescription for 15 g of the cream, what is the pharmacy's cost of the prescription?

   b. What is the amount that the pharmacy will submit to the insurance company for this prescription?

   c. How much profit will the pharmacy make on this prescription?

12. Mountain HMO pays a per patient capitation fee of $310.00 per month. Six patients on this plan have prescriptions filled in July. The pharmacy's purchase price for the prescriptions are as follows:

   Patient #1: $15.75, $106.50, $27.80

   Patient #2: $210.00

   Patient #3: $47.50, $105.25, $160.00, $52.00

   Patient #4: $150.00, $210.00, $76.00

   Patient #5: $10.50, $28.00, $62.50

   Patient #6: $210.00, $210.00, $17.00

   a. What is the total amount that the HMO reimbursed the pharmacy for capitation fees?

   b. What is the pharmacy's purchase price for all of the prescriptions on this plan?

   c. Did the pharmacy make a profit or lose money?

   d. What is the amount of the pharmacy's profit or loss?

13. Valley HMO pays AWP plus 3% and a $2.00 dispensing fee for each prescription dispensed. Six patients on this plan have prescriptions filled in July. The pharmacy paid AWP purchase prices for the prescriptions as follows:

   Patient #1: $15.75, $106.50, $27.80

   Patient #2: $210.00

   Patient #3: $47.50, $105.25, $160.00, $52.00

   Patient #4: $150.00, $210.00, $76.00

   Patient #5: $10.50, $28.00, $62.50

   Patient #6: $210.00, $210.00, $17.00

   a. What is the pharmacy's purchase price for all of the prescriptions on this plan?

   b. What is the amount that the pharmacy will submit for insurance reimbursement on this plan?

   c. Did the pharmacy make a profit or lose money?

   d. What is the amount of the pharmacy's profit or loss?

   e. Compare your answers for question 13 with your answers for question 12. Did the pharmacy make more money under the Mountain HMO's capitation plan, or under the Valley HMO's plan?

   f. How much more or less?

14. Jackson HMO pays a per patient capitation fee of $275.00 per month to Healthy Pharmacy. Healthy Pharmacy contracts with Jackson HMO to serve 10 of Jackson's clients. Five of the Jackson HMO clients get prescriptions filled during the month of June; the other five patients do not get any prescriptions filled in June. The pharmacy's purchase prices for these prescriptions are as follows:

   Patient #1: $89.63

   Patient #2: $126.54 (total cost for two prescriptions)

   Patient #3: $420.45 (total cost for five prescriptions)

   Patient #4: $117.50

   Patient #5: $46.75

   a. What is the total amount that the HMO reimbursed the pharmacy for capitation fees?

   b. What is the pharmacy's purchase price for all of the prescriptions on this plan?

c. Did the pharmacy make a profit or lose money?

d. What is the amount of the pharmacy's profit or loss?

15. Baker HMO pays a per patient capitation fee of $275.00 per month to Healthy Pharmacy. Healthy Pharmacy contracts with Baker HMO to serve 12 of Baker's clients. Five of the Baker HMO clients get prescriptions filled during the month of May; the other seven clients did not get any prescriptions filled in May. The pharmacy's purchase prices for these prescriptions are as follows:

Patient #1: $78.26, $75.23, $25.48

Patient #2: $128.46, $21.86

Patient #3: $61.89, $41.20

Patient #4: $16.59, $5.80, $3.87, $21.67

Patient #5: $58.24

a. What is the total amount that the HMO reimbursed the pharmacy for capitation fees?

b. What is the pharmacy's purchase price for all of the prescriptions on this plan?

c. Did the pharmacy make a profit or lose money?

d. What is the amount of the pharmacy's profit or loss?

16. Blue Care HMO pays a per patient capitation fee of $225.00 per month to Key Pharmacy. Key Pharmacy contracts with Blue Care HMO to serve 40 of Blue Care's clients. Twelve of the Blue Care HMO clients get prescriptions filled during the month of August; the other 28 clients did not get any prescriptions filled in August. The pharmacy purchase price for all of the Blue Care prescriptions filled in August

are $1,867.50. The contract with Blue Care HMO allows the pharmacy to bill for a single charge of $60.00 for dispensing fees for the month.

a. Taking into consideration the allowable dispensing fees, what is the total amount that the HMO reimbursed the pharmacy for the month of August?

b. Did the pharmacy make a profit or lose money?

c. What is the amount of the pharmacy's profit or loss?

17. Wellness Insurance Company pays a per patient capitation fee of $210.00 per month to Apple Pharmacy. Apple Pharmacy contracts with Wellness to serve 42 of the Wellness Insurance Company's clients. During the month of September, 39 of the Wellness Insurance Company's clients had a total of 54 prescriptions filled. Apple Pharmacy's drug costs for all of the Wellness Insurance Company prescriptions filled in September are $9,634.73. The contract with Wellness Insurance Company allows the pharmacy to bill $4.25 in dispensing fees for each filled prescription.

a. Taking into consideration the allowable dispensing fees, what is the total amount that the insurance company reimbursed the pharmacy for the month of September?

b. Did the pharmacy make a profit or lose money?

c. What is the amount of the pharmacy's profit or loss?

Self-check your work in Appendix A.

9.3 Pharmacy Inventory

An **inventory** is a listing of all of the items that are available for sale in a business. A pharmacy's **inventory value** is the total value of all of the drugs and merchandise in stock on a given day. Pharmacies must maintain a record of all of the drugs, supplies, and merchandise purchased and sold to know when to reorder from the wholesaler to restock, or resupply, their shelves. Pharmacies continually adjust their inventory levels based on how quickly items are being sold.

Space must be properly allocated to maintain adequate inventory. Other considerations include shelving design and available refrigeration space. Keeping medications on the shelf is a cost to a pharmacy, and a large inventory can hinder cash flow. To minimize the shelf space needed and control inventory costs, pharmacy personnel need to manage their pharmacy's inventory so that medications are readily available when needed, but do not sit on the shelves for an extended period. Pharmacy personnel generally try to manage their inventory so that medications arrive from the wholesaler shortly before they are dispensed and sold. However, there are instances when a pharmacy may need to stock some slow-moving drugs as a service to a small number of customers who require those medications.

Managing Inventory

In the past, pharmacy personnel kept track of inventory by maintaining handwritten records of all pharmacy purchases and sales. Today, this labor- and time-intensive inventory system has been replaced by computerized inventory records. Each time drugs or other merchandise is purchased from the wholesaler and received in the pharmacy, the quantity and price are entered into the pharmacy's computer database. As customers make purchases from the pharmacy, the computer system automatically adjusts the inventory record for the items purchased. This method of updating the inventory based on purchases is known as **perpetual inventory**.

A pharmacy usually establishes an inventory range for each item, sometimes called a **par level**. The par level indicates the minimum and maximum number of units—packages, bottles, boxes, or containers—to have in pharmacy stock for each inventory item. When the inventory item drops to the predetermined minimum par level (sometimes called the *reorder point*), the item is purchased from the wholesaler to restock the pharmacy's supply. The reorder points and reorder quantity for each inventory item are predetermined based on the historical use of the item and the time it takes to get the reorder shipment from the pharmacy's wholesaler.

In general, reorder quantities are set to replenish the inventory item back up to at least the minimum par level. However, it may be more economical to order enough of the drug to bring the par level to the maximum level if ordering a larger package size saves the pharmacy money. In addition, there are circumstances that dictate a reorder quantity that exceeds the maximum par level. For example, during cold and flu season, an unusually high number of customers receive prescriptions for the same medications. Consequently, a pharmacy will typically keep a larger supply of anti-infective, antiviral, and OTC cold remedies in stock than it would at other times of the year.

Drug manufacturers typically supply medications in containers that hold various quantities, known as *package sizes*, or *counts*. For example, the anti-infective drug ampicillin, 250 mg capsules, is available in the following quantities: 50, 100, 250, 500, and 1,000. The package size that a pharmacy orders when replenishing inventory depends on how much of the drug the facility is using, how quickly the drug is being used, the package size that is typically ordered, and the price. Often, it is more economical to order a larger package size because both the drug manufacturer and the wholesaler usually offer lower prices on bulk package sizes.

These inventory reorder decisions are typically made by pharmacy personnel who have extensive experience in this area. However, pharmacy technicians should have a basic understanding of the calculations involved in inventory management. The following examples illustrate some of the scenarios encountered in inventory management and their possible solutions.

Example 9.3.1

The inventory of Zantac 150 mg is to be maintained at a minimum of 240 tablets and a maximum of 300 tablets. If 15 tablets are left on the shelf at the end of the day, how many bottles will be ordered to meet the inventory minimum? Zantac 150 mg is commercially available in a bottle containing 60 tablets.

Begin by determining the difference between the current inventory and the minimum inventory.

$$240 \text{ tablets} - 15 \text{ tablets} = 225 \text{ tablets}$$

Therefore, it will take at least 225 tablets to bring the inventory up to the minimum level for Zantac 150 mg. However, the tablets must be ordered in bottles of 60.

$$225 \text{ tablets} \div 60 \text{ tablets/bottle} = 3.75 \text{ bottles, rounded up to 4 bottles}$$

Therefore, four bottles of Zantac must be ordered to meet the inventory minimum.

Example 9.3.2

The inventory of propranolol 10 mg is to be maintained at a minimum of 300 tablets and a maximum of 1,500 tablets. If 212 tablets are left on the shelf at the end of the day, how many bottles will you order to meet the inventory minimum? Propranolol is available in bottles containing 100 tablets, 500 tablets, and 1,000 tablets. You typically order the largest-size bottle.

Begin by determining the minimum number of tablets that needs to be ordered.

$$300 \text{ tablets} - 212 \text{ tablets} = 88 \text{ tablets}$$

Although either of the smaller-sized bottles will work, it is common business practice to order the same package size. Therefore, even though it significantly surpasses the minimum, you will order one 1,000 count bottle of propranolol. The resulting inventory will still be within the acceptable range and will not exceed 1,500 tablets.

Example 9.3.3

You would like to replenish the lip balm that is kept on the pharmacy counter by the cash register, and you need 18 tubes to fill the container. When you look in the wholesale catalog, it states that the lip balm is $10.20/dozen. How much should you order?

You will order 2 dozen, or 24 tubes of lip balm.

As part of maintaining inventory, it is important to economize when purchasing stock medications. A pharmacy can often save money by buying in bulk, and it is usually more economical to buy a larger amount of a drug rather than a smaller amount because the per-tablet price is usually lower when the package size or quantity is larger. When purchasing drugs from the wholesaler, pharmacy personnel must balance the optimal inventory level with the replenishment costs of available bulk containers (such as bottles containing 100, 500, or 1,000 tablets). Because the largest containers typically have a lower cost per tablet (or other unit), it is usually cost-effective for a pharmacy to purchase these container sizes. However, this rationale may not be the case if the inventory item is used infrequently. If the item is used infrequently, a large bulk container may reach its expiration date before it is used. Because expired medications may not be dispensed, and must be destroyed, the pharmacy loses the cost of that inventory. The following examples illustrate calculations commonly performed when comparing bulk pricing and cost per unit.

Example 9.3.4

 An antibiotic is available in the following stock bottle sizes for the prices indicated.

> **100 capsules/bottle, $2.80**
>
> **500 capsules/bottle, $12.10**
>
> **1,000 capsules/bottle, $25.30**

Which container provides the best price per capsule, and what is the price per capsule?

Divide each amount by the number of capsules in the bulk container to determine the per capsule cost.

$$\$2.80/\text{bottle} \div 100 \text{ capsules/bottle} = \$0.028/\text{capsule}$$
$$\$12.10/\text{bottle} \div 500 \text{ capsules/bottle} = \$0.0242/\text{capsule}$$
$$\$25.30/\text{bottle} \div 1,000 \text{ capsules/bottle} = \$0.0253/\text{capsule}$$

The 500 count bottle is the best value purchase for this medication at 2.4 cents per capsule.

Example 9.3.5

 In your pharmacy, the maximum par level for ampicillin 250 mg capsules is 1,000; the minimum par level is 100. At the end of the day, the pharmacy computer prints a list of items that have fallen below the minimum par level and, therefore, need to be reordered. The printout shows that there are currently 75 ampicillin 250 mg capsules in the pharmacy stock. Due to a recent increase in the number of ampicillin prescriptions, the pharmacist has asked you to replenish to at least the maximum par level for this item. Given the following information, what scenario illustrates the most economical way to replenish the pharmacy's supply of ampicillin 250 mg capsules?

The wholesaler sells ampicillin 250 mg capsules in the following quantities and prices:

> Ampicillin 250 mg capsules; 1,000 count bottle; $12.55 per bottle
>
> Ampicillin 250 mg capsules; 500 count bottle; $8.75 per bottle
>
> Ampicillin 250 mg capsules; 250 count bottle; $4.65 per bottle
>
> Ampicillin 250 mg capsules; 100 count bottle; $3.60 per bottle
>
> Ampicillin 250 mg capsules; 50 count bottle; $2.50 per bottle
>
> Ampicillin 250 mg capsules; 25 count bottle; $1.85 per bottle

Step 1. Calculate how many capsules will be needed to replenish this item to at least the maximum par level.

$$\begin{matrix} \text{maximum} \\ \text{par level} \end{matrix} - \begin{matrix} \text{current} \\ \text{stock level} \end{matrix} = \begin{matrix} \text{amount needed to bring} \\ \text{to maximum par level} \end{matrix}$$

$$1{,}000 - 75 = 925 \text{ capsules}$$

Step 2. Determine the possible ways to replenish this item to the maximum par level.

Solution 1: Order exactly 925 capsules by purchasing one of each of the following:

> 500 count bottle at $8.75
>
> 250 count bottle at $4.65
>
> 100 count bottle at $3.60
>
> 50 count bottle at $2.50
>
> 25 count bottle at $1.85
> ─────────────────────
> 925 capsules $21.35

In this scenario, the cost to purchase the amount needed is $21.35.

Solution 2: Order enough stock to bring up the inventory to at least the maximum par level in the most cost-effective manner, by purchasing the following:

1,000 count bottle at $12.55

$\longrightarrow$

1,000 capsules $12.55

In this scenario, the cost to purchase the amount needed is $12.55.

Step 3. Determine which scenario is the most cost-effective way to replenish this item.

Solution 1 cost = $21.35

Solution 2 cost = $12.55

The most cost-effective way to replenish this item up to the maximum par level is to purchase a single, 1,000 count bottle of ampicillin 250 mg capsules for $12.55.

Inventory Goals

Today's retail pharmacies generally have at least $100,000.00 of inventory in the form of drugs, supplies, and other merchandise. If a large chain has 10 stores in a particular region, the amount of money in merchandise sitting on the shelves adds up quickly. Consequently, large companies often set goals for lowering the inventory to improve cash flow.

Setting inventory goals for a pharmacy requires pharmacy personnel to attempt to keep the approximate value of inventory on a pharmacy's shelves relatively equal to the cost of all of the drugs and merchandise sold in a specified period—usually either one week (7 days) or one month (30 days). For example, if a pharmacy manager establishes a goal of "30 days' supply," the pharmacy's goal is to keep the value of its inventory approximately equal to the total cost of the drugs and merchandise sold by the pharmacy in 30 days.

The pharmacy's computer system maintains a record of the value of the inventory currently on the pharmacy's shelves. In addition, most computer systems can provide an accurate record of the pharmacy's cost for all products sold by the pharmacy in a 24-hour period. Many of these systems can print off inventory and cost records, as well as average usage and costs for a specified period.

In rare instances, smaller independent pharmacies may not have ready access to this type of inventory and cost information. In these situations, a pharmacy manager may not know the best number of days to use as a goal in calculating costs. However, the manager likely has a good estimate of the current inventory value and can easily calculate average daily cost of items sold in the pharmacy (weekly costs/7 days). With this information, he or she can then determine how many days it will take (what is referred to as "inventory days' supply") for the average daily product costs to equal the value of the inventory on the shelves. The manager can use this information to revise the inventory goal as necessary.

$$\frac{\text{value of inventory on the shelves}}{\text{average daily cost of products sold}} = \text{number of days' supply}$$

Example 9.3.6

Toussaint's Pharmacy has a total inventory value of $103,699.00. It had sales last week of $37,546.00, and the cost to the pharmacy of the products sold was $28,837.00. What should the pharmacy's days' supply be to keep its inventory value stable?

First find Toussaint's Pharmacy average daily product costs.

$$\$28{,}837.00 \div 7 \text{ days} = \$4{,}120.00 \text{ (rounded)}$$

Now, according to the above formula, dividing the value of the inventory by the average daily product costs approximately equals the number of days' supply:

$$\text{number of days' supply} = \frac{\$103{,}699.00}{\$4{,}120.00} = 25 \text{ (rounded)}$$

Toussaint's Pharmacy will have sold products approximately equal to the value of its inventory in 25 days.

Example 9.3.7

Malaya's Pharmacy has a total inventory value of $176,989.00. Last week, it had sales of $45,813.00, and the cost to the pharmacy of the products sold came to $36,592.00. The pharmacy's goal for the number of days' supply is 29, but the facility is currently over that goal. How many days' supply is the pharmacy over, and how much inventory value does this represent?

First find the average daily product costs.

$$\$36{,}592.00 \div 7 \text{ days} = \$5{,}227.00 \text{ (rounded)}$$

Next, find the current number of days' supply for the pharmacy.

$$\frac{\$176{,}989.00}{\$5{,}227.00} = 34 \text{ (rounded)}$$

Therefore, it takes 34 days for costs to equal the inventory value. In other words, Malaya's Pharmacy is 5 days over its days' supply.

$$5 \times \$5{,}227.00 = \$26{,}135.00$$

If Malaya's Pharmacy can reduce its inventory by $26,135.00, the pharmacy will have met its goal of 29 days' supply.

Turnover Rate

If a pharmacy does not maintain computerized, or perpetual, inventory, it must perform a physical inventory—or actual count—at specified intervals, usually annually or semiannually. The physical inventory value is then used to determine the average inventory value as follows:

$$\frac{\text{value of initial inventory} + \text{value of current inventory}}{2} = \text{average annual inventory value}$$

Knowing the average inventory value allows a pharmacy to calculate the number of times its inventory was repurchased during a cycle (usually a year).

Dividing total annual inventory purchases by the average inventory value gives the **turnover rate**, or the number of times the amount of goods in inventory was sold during the year. Turnover rate can be calculated as follows:

$$\frac{\text{annual inventory purchases}}{\text{average inventory value}} = \text{turnover rate}$$

Turnover rate can be used to determine how quickly a particular item is being used. In addition, turnover rate can be applied more broadly to the entire pharmacy inventory, which helps the pharmacy manager know how well the pharmacy is meeting its cash flow goals. Knowing the turnover rate can help pharmacy personnel determine if the average inventory level should be increased or decreased, as extra costs may be associated with high or low inventories. Thus, if a pharmacy has an average inventory value of $25,250.00 and the cost of its annual inventory purchases is $75,000.00, the inventory will "turn over" 2.97 times, or approximately three times in a year.

$$\frac{\text{annual purchases of inventory}}{\text{average inventory value}} = \text{turnover rate}$$

$$\frac{\$75,000.00}{\$25,250.00} \approx 2.97$$

Example 9.3.8

A pharmacy does a quarterly inventory and has an average inventory value of $100,000.00. The pharmacy's annual inventory purchases are $500,000.00. What is the pharmacy's turnover rate?

$$\frac{\text{annual purchases of inventory}}{\text{average inventory value}} = \text{turnover rate}$$

$$\frac{\$500,000.00}{\$100,000.00} = 5$$

The pharmacy's inventory will "turn over" five times in a year.

Depreciation

Depreciation is an allowance made to account for the decreasing value of a fixed asset based on its age and estimated life as an asset. Properties, furnishings, and equipment (such as computers and cash registers) owned by the pharmacy are called *fixed assets*, or simply **assets**. Assets are generally put into two broad categories: current assets and long-term assets. The assets that can be consumed or converted into cash within one year—such as drugs and OTC products—are *current assets*; those that cannot be consumed or converted into cash within one year, such as buildings and very expensive equipment, are considered *long-term assets*. Depreciation and asset amounts are used by the pharmacy to prepare its annual taxes.

Most fixed assets gradually lose value due to use, obsolescence, and the passage of time. The straight-line method of calculating depreciation uses the total cost, the estimated life of the property (in years), and the **disposal value** of the item, the value of an item should it be sold or otherwise disposed of at the end of its useful life. Below is the depreciation formula:

$$\frac{\text{total cost} - \text{disposal value}}{\text{estimated life in years}} = \text{annual depreciation}$$

Example 9.3.9

Rafael's Pharmacy buys a used, compact car for drug deliveries to local customers. The cost of the car is $9,000.00. Its estimated useful life is five years, and the disposal value is $1,200.00. What is the annual depreciation?

$$\frac{\text{total cost} - \text{disposal value}}{\text{estimated life in years}} = \text{annual depreciation}$$

$$\frac{\$9,000 - \$1,200}{5} = \$1,560$$

The annual depreciation of the car is $1,560.

9.3 Problem Set

For items 1–9, calculate the number of units that need to be reordered for each item based on the current inventory and the number of units or packages needed to bring the drug up to at least the minimum par level.

	Drug	Count/ Package Size	Minimum Par Level	Maximum Par Level	Current Inventory	Reorder Amount
1.	tetracycline 250 mg cap	500	120	700	80	
2.	amoxicillin 500 mg cap	100	300	400	118	
3.	amoxicillin 250 mg cap	500	240	1,000	180	
4.	cefaclor 500 mg tab	60	20	120	35	
5.	cefprozil 250 mg tab	100	40	150	28	
6.	cefprozil 500 mg tab	50	20	75	24	
7.	metronidazole 500 mg tab	50	30	120	12	
8.	azithromycin 250 mg cap	30	18	60	36	
9.	doxycycline 50 mg cap	50	30	150	42	

The inventory of topical products, which are often dispensed as "partial containers" (e.g., 1 oz from a 16 oz jar), is checked frequently due to multiple compounding needs, manufacturer back orders, and poor computer tracking of dispensed partial containers of topical products. For this reason, reordering of topical products must be closely monitored, even with computer-generated orders.

Consider the following scenario: It is a Friday afternoon and Monday is a holiday; therefore, the pharmacy is expected to be very busy over the weekend. Because the pharmacy won't be able to get an order from its wholesaler until at least Tuesday, a pharmacy technician decides to order enough to bring the item up to at least the maximum par level. For questions 10–14, calculate the number of packages that need to be ordered to bring the item up to at least the maximum par level.

Drug	Count/ Package Size	Minimum Par Level	Maximum Par Level	Current Inventory	Reorder Amount
10. triamcinolone 0.25% cream	15 g	2	4	1	
	80 g	2	4	0	
11. triamcinolone 0.1% ung	15 g	1	2	1	
	60 g	1	2	1	
	80 g	1	2	0	
12. triamcinolone 0.1% lotion	60 mL	1	2	1	
13. fluocinolone 0.025% cream	15 g	1	2	1	
	60 g	1	2	1	
14. fluocinolone 0.025% ung	60 g	1	2	0 tubes and 1 order waiting	

For items 15–36, calculate the number of units that need to be reordered for each item based on the current inventory and the number of units or packages needed to bring the item up to at least the minimum par level.

Drug	Count/ Package Size	Minimum Par Level	Maximum Par Level	Current Inventory	Reorder Amount
15. desoximetasone 0.25% cream	15 g	1	2	0	
	60 g	1	2	0	
	4 oz	1	2	1	
16. desoximetasone 0.05% gel	15 g	1	1	0 on shelf and 1 order waiting	
	60 g	1	1	0	
17. halobetasol 0.05% cream	15 g	1	2	1	
	45 g	1	2	1	
18. fluocinonide 0.05% cream	15 g	1	2	1	
	30 g	2	4	1	
	60 g	2	4	2	
	120 g	1	2	0	

Drug	Count/ Package Size	Minimum Par Level	Maximum Par Level	Current Inventory	Reorder Amount
19. fluocinonide 0.05% gel	15 g	1	1	1	
	30 g	1	3	2	
	60 g	1	3	0	
20. fluocinonide 0.05% ung	15 g	1	2	1	
	30 g	1	2	1	
	60 g	1	2	1 partial	
	120 g	1	2	1	
21. fluocinonide 0.05% soln	20 mL	1	1	0	
	60 mL	1	3	1 partial	
22. ramipril 5 mg cap	100	120	240	64	
23. verapamil 120 mg SR	100	80	240	52	
24. verapamil 240 mg SR	100	120	360	30	
25. nicardipine 60 mg SR	60	120	240	20	
26. captopril 50 mg tab	100	150	300	76	
27. furosemide 40 mg tab	1,000	240	1,500	134	
28. doxazosin 2 mg tab	100	80	240	83	
29. atenolol 50 mg tab	1,000	240	1,500	107	
30. atenolol 100 mg tab	100	150	300	111	
31. nifedipine 60 mg tab	300	120	625	12, and two Rx for 60 pending	
32. nifedipine 90 mg tab	100	120	300	63	
33. lisinopril 5 mg tab	100	90	260	110	
34. lisinopril 10 mg tab	1,000	240	1,500	146	
35. lisinopril 20 mg tab	100	180	250	145	
36. lisinopril 40 mg tab	100	90	220	152	

37. Review John's Drug Shop inventory below and calculate the number of units that need to be reordered for each item based on the current inventory and the number of units or packages needed to bring the item up to at least the maximum par level.

Drug		Count/ Package Size	Minimum Par Level	Maximum Par Level	Current Inventory	Reorder Amount
a.	Eucerin cream	100 g jars	3 jars	10 jars	3 jars	
b.	ampicillin 250 mg caps	1,000 capsules	1,000 caps	5,000 caps	2,400 caps	
c.	NS Nasal Spray	30 mL spray bottle	12 bottles	24 bottles	4 bottles	
d.	Nystatin Oral Suspension	pint bottle (480 mL)	1 bottle	4 bottles	720 mL	
e.	NS Nasal Spray	100 mL bottle	3 bottles	12 bottles	1 bottle	

38. Grimm's Pharmacy has a total inventory value of $183,445.00. Last week, the pharmacy had sales of $47,293.00, and the cost to the pharmacy for the products sold came to $38,207.00. The pharmacy's goal is to have a days' supply of 28 days.

   a. How many days' supply does Grimm's Pharmacy have?

   b. How much is the pharmacy over or under its goal in dollars?

39. Corbin's Pharmacy has a total inventory value of $123,490.00. Last week, the pharmacy had sales of $34,829.00, and the cost to the pharmacy for the products sold came to $26,504.00. Corbin's goal is to have a days' supply of 26 days.

   a. How many days' supply does Corbin's Pharmacy have?

   b. How much is the pharmacy over or under its goal in dollars?

40. Singh's Pharmacy has $147,210.00 in inventory. The pharmacy is currently at its goal of 24 days' supply. What was the approximate cost of products sold last week?

41. Scott's Pharmacy had sales of $51,280.00 last week. What must the pharmacy's daily sales average be this week in order to make $5,000.00 more than last week?

42. If a pharmacy's average inventory for the past year was $132,936.00 and the annual cost total was $1,612,000.00, what was the turnover rate?

43. If a pharmacy's average inventory for the past year was $156,200.00 and the annual cost total was $1,768,000.00, what was the turnover rate?

For items 44–48, calculate the turnover rate for the following drugs sold at Ming's Pharmacy.

Drug		Average Inventory	Annual Purchases	Turnover Rate
44. metformin 500 mg		$520.00	$20,800.00	
45. divalproex 250 mg		$178.00	$5,760.00	
46. citalopram 40 mg		$360.00	$7,213.00	
47. raloxifene 60 mg		$320.00	$5,060.00	
48. montelukast chewtab 4 mg		$385.00	$6,000.00	

49. Nadia's Drug Shop purchases $52,500.00 of antibiotics annually. The pharmacy does an inventory count twice annually, and its average inventory of antibiotics is $5,000.00. What is the pharmacy's turnover rate for antibiotics?

50. A pharmacy has a new cash register system. The system costs $8,294.00 and should last six years. Its disposal value is $2,138.00. What is the annual depreciation?

51. A hospital pharmacy just purchased two new biological safety cabinets at $18,350.00 each. Each cabinet should last 12 years if maintained properly. The disposal value is $1,567.00 each. What is the annual depreciation amount for both cabinets?

Self-check your work in Appendix A.

9.4 Counting Change

 **Work Wise**

Always, always check the kind of bill offered to you by the customer before putting it into the change drawer so you don't assume a $20 bill is a $10 dollar bill or vice versa.

In any business, the collection of money will occur. In a retail pharmacy, the pharmacy technician is responsible for accepting payment for prescriptions or other pharmacy-related items. Basic math skills are essential in monetary transactions, such as calculating the correct costs and change. When a customer pays cash, the pharmacy technician should be able to count and present the customer with the correct change. Counting change is a key skill for excellent customer service and pharmacy accounting.

The cash register's screen will tell you the amount of change to give the customer if you have properly scanned and/or punched in all the numbers of the product price and properly entered in the money the customer has given to you. But you cannot just drop the change into the customer's hand. You need to count the cash as you hand it back to the customer to show that it is the correct amount. There are two ways you can count change. One method is to simply *count the amount listed on the register*, and the other is to *count from the purchase price*.

Counting the amount listed on the register is the easiest method. First, confirm the amount of change to be received based on the amount listed on the register. Second, count the money out (from biggest to smallest coins and biggest to smallest bills) as you place the money in the customer's hand.

Although counting change starting from the register total, it is the easiest for the technician, it is not the easiest for the customer to follow. Customers often do not know off the top of their heads how much change they should receive. The customer may feel most comfortable having the change counted back to them starting at the purchase price and ending with the amount of cash they gave you.

When *counting from the purchase price*, first take the amount of change needed, as noted on the register, from the cash drawer. Next, beginning at the purchase price, count out the coins needed to reach the next bill. Then, offer $1 bills to the point where you can use the next highest denomination, which would be a $5 bill. Continue to the next highest denomination until you reach the amount first given to you by the customer.

Example 9.4.1

A woman purchases a bottle of Tylenol and a bottle of Vitamin C for the total purchase price of $10.73. She offers you a $50 bill. How would you count out this customer's change?

Counting Out the Amount Listed on the Register:

Step 1. Confirm the amount of change to be received based on the amount listed on the register ($39.27). You can say, "You have *thirty-nine dollars and twenty-seven cents* in change coming." The customer can then tell you if there is a disagreement.

Step 2. Place the money into the customer's hand, from the biggest to smallest coins and biggest to smallest bills—first a quarter and two pennies, then a $20 bill, a $10, a $5, then four $1 bills, saying, "*Twenty-five, twenty-six, twenty-seven cents, twenty dollars, thirty, thirty-five, thirty-six, thirty-seven, thirty-eight, thirty-nine, thirty-nine twenty-seven.*"

Counting from the Purchase Price:

Step 1. Take the amount of change needed, as noted on the register, from the cash drawer ($39.27).

Step 2. Begin by stating the purchase price ($10.73) and counting out the coins needed to reach the next bill. Count into the customer's hand two pennies ($0.02 to reach $10.75), then a quarter ($0.25) to make $11.00, counting "*Ten-seventy-four, ten seventy-five, eleven dollars.*"

Step 3. Provide $1 bills until you can use the next highest denomination, which would be a $5 bill counting, "*Twelve, thirteen, fourteen, fifteen dollars.*"

Step 4. Use the next highest bill until you reach the amount first given to you by the customer. So you can use a $5 dollar bill to reach $20 dollars, then a then $10 bill to reach $30, and a $20 bill to reach $50, counting, "*Twenty, thirty, and fifty dollars.*"

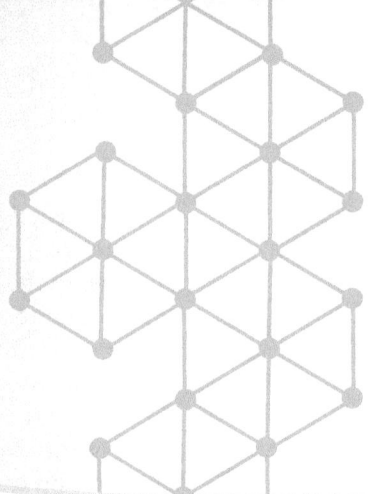

CHAPTER SUMMARY

- Pharmacies must consider both income and overhead when calculating actual profit and when setting goals for desired percentage of profit.

- The net profit of an item is based upon the percentage of profit that the pharmacy intends to make and is determined by subtracting the overall cost of an item from the item's selling price.

- Pharmacies have contracts with wholesalers who provide drugs and supply items from the manufacturer to the pharmacy.

- Pharmacies have contracts with pharmacy benefits managers (PBMs) who broker insurance reimbursement claims.

- Pharmacy personnel must be familiar with the average wholesale price and capitation fees that affect the profitability of the facility.

- Pharmacy technicians are actively involved in managing pharmacy inventory, determining days' supply, establishing the turnover rate, replenishing stock to the desired par level, and counting change.

KEY TERMS

assets properties, furnishings, inventory, supplies, and equipment owned by the pharmacy; may be put into two categories: current, or short-term, assets and long-term assets

average wholesale price (AWP) an average price at which drugs are purchased at the wholesale level, or the average value at which wholesalers sell a particular drug to pharmacies

base profit the amount of profit determined by subtracting the total pharmacy overhead amount from the pharmacy's income

capitation fee a monthly fee paid by some insurance plans to a pharmacy under a specific prescription reimbursement plan

current percentage of profit the amount of profit that is determined by dividing the base profit by income and then multiplying that quotient by 100; often used to determine the desired percentage of profit

depreciation an allowance made to account for the decreasing value of a fixed asset; properties, furnishings, and equipment owned by the pharmacy are called *fixed assets*, or simply *assets*

desired percentage of profit the percentage of profit the pharmacy intends to make on the product after the overall cost is subtracted from the selling price

discount a price that is reduced from what is typically charged

discount rate the percent that the discounted price is reduced from the regular selling price

dispensing fee the amount that is charged over and above the pharmacy's purchase price for a medication; this amount is meant to cover all costs related to filling a prescription, beyond the purchase price of the drug

disposal value the value of an item should it be sold or disposed of at the end of its useful life

flat rate a low pharmacy selling price for a certain amount of medication, a supply designed to last a specific number of days

gross profit the difference between the pharmacy's selling price and purchase price

income the money or equivalent received from the sale of medications, supply items, or equipment

inventory a listing of all of the items that are available for sale in a business

inventory value the total value of all of the drugs and merchandise in stock on a given day

markup amount the difference between the pharmacy's purchase price and the selling price

markup rate a percentage amount that is determined by subtracting the pharmacy's purchase price for an item from the pharmacy's selling price for that item

net profit the difference between the selling price and the overall cost

overall cost the sum of the cost to purchase the drug from the manufacturer (known as the pharmacy's purchase price) and the cost to dispense the drug

overhead the pharmacy's cost of doing business; this cost includes personnel salaries, equipment, and operating expenses such as rent, taxes, and utilities

par level an average inventory range for an item, which generally includes the minimum and maximum stock levels for the item

perpetual inventory method of accounting for inventory based on computerized point-of-sales

pharmacy benefits manager (PBM) a large prescription processing service that contracts with insurance companies and pharmacies to process insurance reimbursement

profit the financial gain made when the amount earned is greater than the amount spent during a specified period

profit margin the difference between the cost of doing business (the pharmacy's purchase price, overhead, and preparation costs) and the selling price of a drug or product

purchase price the cost to purchase a drug from the wholesaler or manufacturer

selling price the amount that the pharmacy charges for a particular drug or product; sometimes referred to as *accounts receivable*

turnover rate the number of times the amount of goods in inventory was sold during the year

wholesaler a company that sells and distributes a large number of goods such as medications and supply items to a pharmacy; a company that acts as a go-between for pharmacies and manufacturing companies such as drug manufacturers

CHAPTER REVIEW

Finding Solutions

To gain practice in handling challenging situations in the workplace, consider the following real-world scenarios and then use the guiding questions to help you formulate your responses.

Note: *To indicate your answers for Scenario A (Questions 1–3) and Scenario B (Questions 4–7), ask your instructor for the corresponding handouts.*

Scenario A: In your pharmacy, the minimum par level for ampicillin 250 mg capsules is 500; the maximum par level is 2,000. At the end of the day, the pharmacy computer prints a list of items that have fallen below the minimum par level and, therefore, need to be reordered. The printout shows that there are currently 350 ampicillin 250 mg capsules in the pharmacy stock. Given the information below, determine the most economical way to replenish the pharmacy's supply of ampicillin 250 mg capsules up to at least the minimum par level.

The wholesaler sells ampicillin 250 mg capsules in the following quantities and prices:

Ampicillin 250 mg capsules; 1,000 count bottle; $10.00 per bottle

Ampicillin 250 mg capsules; 500 count bottle; $8.75 per bottle

Ampicillin 250 mg capsules; 250 count bottle; $4.65 per bottle

Ampicillin 250 mg capsules; 100 count bottle; $3.60 per bottle

Ampicillin 250 mg capsules; 50 count bottle; $2.50 per bottle

Ampicillin 250 mg capsules; 25 count bottle; $1.85 per bottle

For Questions 1–3, record your answers on the handout that you obtained from your instructor.

1. What size/quantity bottle(s) will you order?
2. How many of each bottle will you order?
3. What will the final cost be for this order?

Scenario B: Beneficial HMO pays a per-client capitation fee of $149.00 per month to the Georgetown Pharmacy. The pharmacy is contracted to serve 127 of the HMO's clients and their families. During the month of December, 21 of these clients and/or their family members had a total of 52 prescriptions filled at the pharmacy. The pharmacy's total drug cost for these prescriptions was $6,283.24. The contract allows the pharmacy to bill a $3.50 dispensing fee for each filled prescription.

For Questions 4–7, record your answers on the handout that you obtained from your instructor.

4. What is the total amount that the HMO reimbursed the pharmacy for capitation fees?
5. What is the pharmacy's drug cost for all of the prescriptions on this plan?
6. Did the pharmacy make a profit or lose money?
7. What is the amount of the pharmacy's profit or loss?

Navigator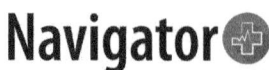

Access interactive chapter review exercises, practice activities, flash cards, and study games.

Problem Set and Finding Solutions Answers

Chapter 1

1.1 Problem Set

1. $\frac{1}{2}$
2. $\frac{3}{8}$
3. $\frac{2}{1}$
4. $\frac{2}{6}$
5. $\frac{1}{10}$
6. $1\frac{14}{15}$

Work

Solution 1.

Create common denominators:

$\frac{5}{6} \times \frac{10}{10} = \frac{50}{60}, \frac{7}{10} \times \frac{6}{6} = \frac{42}{60}, \frac{2}{5} \times \frac{12}{12} = \frac{24}{60}$

Add the numerators:

$\frac{50}{60} + \frac{42}{60} + \frac{24}{60} = \frac{116}{60}$

Simplify:

$\frac{116}{60} = \frac{156}{60} = 1\frac{14}{15}$

Solution 2.

Create common denominators:

$\frac{5}{6} \times \frac{5}{5} = \frac{25}{30}, \frac{7}{10} \times \frac{3}{3} = \frac{21}{30}, \frac{2}{5} \times \frac{6}{6} = \frac{12}{30}$

Add the numerators:

$\frac{25}{30} + \frac{21}{30} + \frac{12}{30} = \frac{58}{30}$

Simplify:

$\frac{58}{30} = \frac{29}{15} = 1\frac{14}{15}$

7. $1\frac{37}{96}$

Work

Create common denominators:

$\frac{21}{32} \times \frac{3}{3} = \frac{63}{96}, \frac{1}{12} \times \frac{8}{8} = \frac{8}{96}, \frac{31}{48} \times \frac{2}{2} = \frac{62}{96}$

Add the numerators:

$\frac{63}{96} + \frac{8}{96} + \frac{62}{96} = \frac{133}{96}$

Simplify:

$\frac{133}{96} = 1\frac{37}{96}$

8. $\frac{1}{4}$
9. $6\frac{7}{10}$
10. $2\frac{1}{5}$
11. $\frac{9}{10}$
12. $\frac{2}{5}$
13. $\frac{9}{10}$

Work

$126 = 12 \div 6 = 12 \times 16 = 112$

14. 3 tablets

Work

Create common denominators:

$\frac{1}{4}, \frac{1}{2} \times \frac{2}{2} = \frac{2}{4}, 1\frac{1}{2} = \frac{3}{2} \times \frac{2}{2} = \frac{6}{4}, \frac{3}{4}$

Add the numerators:

$\frac{1}{4} + \frac{2}{4} + \frac{6}{4} + \frac{3}{4} = \frac{12}{4}$

Simplify:

$\frac{12}{4} = 3$

15. 2 tablets containing $\frac{1}{100}$ grain in each tablet

Work

$2 \times \frac{1}{100} = \frac{2}{100} = \frac{1}{50}$

Because the denominator is smaller, $\frac{1}{50} > \frac{1}{150}$

16. $\dfrac{375 \text{ grains} \times 1 \text{ unit dose}}{\frac{1}{4} \text{ grain}} = 375 \times 4 = 1,500$ containers

17. 3 bags

Work

Create common denominators:

$\frac{1}{2} \times \frac{10}{10} = \frac{10}{20}$, $\frac{4}{5} \times \frac{4}{4} = \frac{16}{20}$, $\frac{1}{4} \times \frac{5}{5} = \frac{5}{20}$,
$2\frac{1}{2} = \frac{5}{2} \times \frac{10}{10} = \frac{50}{20}$

Add the numerators:

$\frac{10}{20} + \frac{16}{20} + \frac{5}{20} + \frac{50}{20} = \frac{81}{20}$

Simplify:

$\frac{81}{20} = 4\frac{1}{20}$ lb sugar needed

Sugar is sold in bags of 2 lb/bag; 2 bags would = 4 lb sugar (2 × 2 lb = 4 lb), and we need $\frac{1}{20}$ lb more than that, so 3 bags are needed.

18. 1 bag

Work

Since we need $4\frac{1}{20}$ lb sugar (problem 24), one 5 lb bag will provide the sugar needed.

1.2 Problem Set

1. 784.36
2. 0.9
3. 0.2
4. 0.05
5. 4.5
6. 0.3
7. 0.005
8. 0.002
9. 1.8
10. 0.04
11. 0.008
12. 1.88
13. 2.729
14. 14.373
15. 3.0983
16. 11.998
17. 467.42
18. 450
19. 1.846
20. 1.333
21. 3.87
22. 0.14
23. 0.08
24. 0.196
25. 0.049
26. 34.9
27. 1.4
28. a. 3 tablet/dose × 0.25 mg/tablet = 0.75 mg/dose

   b. 0.75 mg/dose × 3 doses/day = 2.25 mg

   c. 3 tablets/dose × 3 doses/day × 14 days = 126 tablets

   d. no; 126 tablets − 100 tablets = 26 tablets; the patient will need 26 more tablets

   e. alprazolam 0.25 mg #100/$14.95 + $7.59 = $22.54

29. a. 0.25 mg/tablet × 4 tablets /dose = 1 mg/dose

   b. $17.46 × 1.25 × $21.825, rounded to $21.83

   c. $23.87 × 0.5 = $11.935, rounded to $11.94

   d. 50 tablets × 1 day/3 tablets = 16.7 = 16 full days

30. a. 1,000 mL × 1 bottle/120 mL = 8.33 bottles, rounded to 8 bottles

    b. 120 mL/bottle × 8 bottles = 960 mL; 1,000 mL − 960 mL = 40 mL

31. 8.5 mL/dose × 2 doses/day × 2 days = 34 mL

    5.75 mL/dose × 2 doses/day × 5 days × 57.5 mL

    34 mL + 57.5 mL = 91.5 mL , rounded to 92 mL

32. a. $47

    b. $15

    c. $4

33. a. $70.08

    b. $111.64

34. a. 0.89

    b. 0.85

    c. 0.92

36. a. 5 tablets daily

    b. 150 tablets

    c. 20 days

1.3 Problem Set

1. 10

2. 5

3. 624

4. 2050

5. 48

6. XVII

7. LXVII

8. MCMXCV or MVM

9. 4.1

10. 0.6

11. 2.02

12. 0.017

13. 0

14. 6

15. 3

16. hundreds

17. hundredths

18. thousandths

19. ones

20. tenths

21. 68,000 (move decimal to the right 4 places)

22. 1,870,000 (move decimal to the right 6 places)

23. 10,300,000 (move decimal to the right 7 places)

24. 0.00084 (move decimal to the left 4 places)

25. 0.00768 (move decimal to the left 3 places)

26. 0.00006239 (move decimal to the left 5 places)

27. 3.29×10^{-9}

28. 3.9×10^{11}

29. 3.8×10^{-3}

30. 5.2×10^{16}

31. 3.779×10^{6}

32. 2.02×10^{-10}

33. 157.5 tablets (158 tablets, to the next whole tablet)

34. a. 10 grain

    b. 1 daily

    c. 100 tablets

35. a. 27 tablets

    b. 9 days

1.4 Problem Set

1. $7 estimate, $6.38 actual

2. $12 estimate, $12.25 actual

3. $5 estimate, $5.19 actual

4. $82 estimate, $81.71 actual

5. $50 estimate, $50.58 actual

6. 56,000 estimate, 52,060.8 actual

7. 1,400 estimate, 1,407.3 actual

8. 1) Round to 600 and 15, ignoring the 3 decimals. 2) 600 × 15 = 9,000. 3) Put 3 decimals back, so answer is 9. Actual is 8.976.

9. 1) Round to 5,000 and 1, ignoring 1 decimal. 2) 5,000 × 1 × 5,000. 3) Put decimal back, or 500. Actual is 444.1068.

10. 120,000 estimate, 111,294 actual

11. 9,000 estimate, 11,402.3 actual

12. 10 estimate, 10.28 actual

13. 300 estimate, 321.70 actual

14. 75 estimate, 73 actual

15. 200 estimate, 191.87 actual

16. $^{100}/_{10}$ = 10 estimate, 8.79 actual

17. food dye $2 estimate + sugar $8 estimate + soda $1 estimate + cherry $2 estimate + bleach $2 estimate + water $4 estimate = $19 estimate, $19.10 actual

18. 3 mL + 8 mL + 2 mL + 4 mL = 17 mL estimate; therefore, use 30 mL vial

19. 1,720 mL IV fluids + 150 mL juice + 130 mL coffee = 2,000 mL estimate

20. 800 mL + 100 mL + 300 mL + 1,000 mL = 2,200 mL estimate

1.5 Problem Set

1. 6

2. 2

3. 2

4. 3

5. 1

6. 4

7. 2

8. 1

9. 8

10. 1

11. 42.8

12. 100.0

13. 0.0427

14. 18.4

15. 0.00392

16. 0.35, 2 significant figures

17. 0.06, 1 significant figure

18. 1.99, 3 significant figures

19. 0.01, 1 significant figure

20. 1.03, 3 significant figures

21. 64

22. 30 (2 significant figures)

23. 200

24. a. 1.784 g to 1.78 g

b. 3.2 g

c. 3.2 g + 1.78 g + 2.46 g + 5.87 g = 13.31 g; 13.31 g/0.125 g = 106.48 capsules; 0.48 of a capsule × 0.125 g = 0.06 g

25. a. 21.65 mg × 45 doses = 974.25 mg

b. 5 significant figures

1.6 Problem Set

1. 0730

2. 1628

3. 0045

4. 2120

5. 0224

6. 2258

7. 2350

8. 0120

9. 0003

10. 1220

11. 5:30 PM

12. 11:49 PM

13. 3:22 PM

14. 12:34 AM

15. 12:04 PM

16. 3:55 AM

17. 10:45 PM

18. 5:19 PM

19. 1:00 PM

20. 1:45 AM

21. 0815; 1315; 1900

22. 0500

23. 10:00 PM

24. 6:00–7:00 PM

25. 1500; 1505; 1510

Finding Solutions

1. 1 tablet

2. Possible estimate: 44 tablets

3. 47 tablets

4. 2,000 mg

5. 250 mg

6. 2,250 mg

7. $3^1/_2$ tablets

8. 11:30 AM

9. The dosing spoon should be filled to $^3/_4$ tsp or 3.75 mL.

10. $^1/_2$

11. 1

12. 5 mg $\times$ $^1/_2$ = 2.5 mg

13. 20 tablets

14. 4 (1 tablet/ dose $\times$ 4 doses/ week)

15. 500 mcg = 0.500 mg

16. 50 tablets

17. 17

Chapter 2

2.1 Problem Set

1. $^3/_7$

2. $^8/_6$ = $^4/_3$ = $1^1/_3$

3. $^3/_4$

4. $^4/_6$ = $^2/_3$

5. $^1/_7$

6. 2:3

7. 6:8 = 3:4

8. 5:10 = 1:2

9. 1:9

10. 1:10,000

11. 30 mg:1 tablet or 1 tablet:30 mg

12. 100 mg: 1 capsule or 1 capsule:100 mg

13. 250 mg: 5 mL or 5 mL:250 mg

14. 90 mg/3 capsules

15. 200 mg/2 capsules

16. 750 mg/15 mL

17. 10 g, 1000 mL, 1 g (or x g/100 mL = 10 g/1000 mL; x g = 1 g)

18. 1 g, 100 mL, 5 g (or x g/500 mL = 1 g/100 mL; x g = 5 g)

19. 1 g, 250 mL, 4 g (or x g/1000 mL = 1 g/250 mL; x g = 4 g)

20. 1 g, 1000 mL, 0.05 g (or x g/50 mL = 1 g/1000 mL; x g = 0.05 g)

2.2 Problem Set

1. $^6/_7$ = 0.857, rounded to 0.86; 0.86 $\times$ 100 = 86%

2. $^5/_{12}$ = 0.416, rounded to 0.42; 0.42 × 100 = 42%

3. $^1/_4$ = 0.25; 0.25 × 100 = 25%

4. $^2/_3$ = 0.666, rounded to 0.67; 0.67 × 100 = 67%

5. $^{0.5}/_{10}$ = 0.05; 0.05 × 100 = 5%

6. $^2/_3$ = 0.666, rounded to 0.667; 0.667 × 100 = 66.7%

7. $^{1.5}/_{4.65}$ = 0.3225, rounded to 0.323; 0.323 × 100 = 32.3%

8. $^1/_{250}$ = 0.004; 0.004 × 100 = 0.4%

9. $^1/_{10,000}$ = 0.0001; 0.0001 × 100 = 0.01%, rounded to 0%

10. $^1/_6$ = 0.1666, rounded to 0.167; 0.167 × 100 = 16.7%

11. 50% = $^{50}/_{100}$ = $^5/_{10}$ = $^1/_2$

12. 2% = $^2/_{100}$ = $^1/_{50}$

13. 6% = $^6/_{100}$ = 0.06

14. 12.5% = $^{12.5}/_{100}$ = 0.125

15. 126% = $^{126}/_{100}$ = 1.26

16. 20 × 0.05 = 1

17. 60 × 0.20 = 12

18. 63 × 0.19 = 11.97

19. 70 × 1.10 = 77

20. 50 × 0.002 = 0.1

21. 1:3, 0.33

22. $^1/_{40}$, 0.025

23. 50%, 1:2

24. 1%, $^1/_{100}$

25. $^9/_{10}$, 9:10

26. $^2/_3$ or $^{67}/_{100}$; 2:3 or 67:100

27. 0.2%, 0.002

28. $^9/_{2000}$, 9:2000

29. $^1/_{20}$, 0.05

30. 1:5, 0.2

31. $^1/_{10,000}$ = 0.0001 × 100 = 0.01% solution

32. $^1/_{20}$ = 0.05 × 100 = 5% solution

33. $^1/_{25}$ = 0.04 × 100 = 4% solution

34. $^1/_{800}$ = 0.00125 × 100 = 0.125% solution

35. $^1/_{10}$ = 0.1 × 100 = 10% solution

2.3 Problem Set

1. 5

2. 0.07843, rounded to 0.08

3. 4.5

4. 0.1

5. 0.16

6. 5.7692, rounded to 5.77

7. 54.4

8. 242.6666, rounded to 242.67

9. 25.9411, rounded to 25.94

10. 16

11. 44.3571, rounded to 44.36

12. 21.3870, rounded to 21.39

13. 78.3333, rounded to 78.33

14. 10.7307, rounded to 10.73

15. 77.3636, rounded to 77.36

16. x%/100 = 72%/254; x% = 28.3464%, rounded to 28.35%

17. x/100% = 44/90%; x = 48.8888, rounded to 48.89

18. x/100% = 100/44%; x = 227.2727, rounded to 227.27

19. x/100% = 34/28%; x = 121.4285, rounded to 121.43

20. x%/100 = 24.5%/45; x% = 54.4444%, rounded to 54.44%

21. x g/100 mg = 1 g/1000 mg; x g = 0.1 g

22. x g/247 mg = 1 g/1000 mg; x g = 0.247 g

23. x g/1420 mg = 1 g/1000 mg; x g = 1.42 g

24. x g/495 mg = 1 g/1000 mg; x g = 0.495 g

25. x g/3781 mg = 1 g/1000 mg; x g = 3.781 g

26. x mg/0.349 g = 1000 mg/1 g; x mg = 349 mg

27. x mg/1.5 g = 1000 mg/1 g; x mg = 1500 mg

28. x mg/0.083 g = 1000 mg/1 g; x mg = 83 mg

29. x mg/0.01 g = 1000 mg/1 g; x mg = 10 mg

30. x mg/2.1 g = 1000 mg/1 g; x mg = 2100 mg

31. x kg/6.3 lb = 1 kg/2.2 lb; x kg = 2.863 kg, rounded to 2.9 kg

32. x kg/15 lb = 1 kg/2.2 lb; x kg = 6.818 kg, rounded to 6.8 kg

33. x kg/97 lb = 1 kg/2.2 lb; x kg = 44.090 kg, rounded to 44.1 kg

34. x kg/115 lb = 1 kg/2.2 lb; x kg = 52.272 kg, rounded to 52.3 kg

35. x kg/186 lb = 1 kg/2.2 lb; x kg = 84.545 kg, rounded to 84.5 kg

36. x lb/7.5 kg = 2.2 lb/1 kg; x lb = 16.5 lb

37. x lb/3.6 kg = 2.2 lb/1 kg; x lb = 7.92 lb, rounded to 7.9 lb

38. x lb/79.2 kg = 2.2 lb/1 kg; x lb = 174.24 lb, rounded to 174.2 lb

39. x lb/90 kg = 2.2 lb/1 kg; x lb = 198 lb

40. x lb/0.5 kg = 2.2 lb/1 kg; x lb = 1.1 lb

41. x mL/100 mg = 1 mL/50 mg; x mL = 2 mL

42. x tablets/375 mg = 1 tablet/125 mg; x tablets = 3 tablets

43. x mL/300 mg = 1 mL/20 mg; x mL = 15 mL

44. x folders/$15.00 = 100 folders/$7.40; x folders = 202.7 folders; 200 folders can be purchased (2 boxes of 100 folders)

45. x mL/10,000 units = 15 mL/250,000 units; x mL = 0.6 mL

46. x mL/60 mg = 2 mL/20 mg; x mL = 6 mL

47. x mL/60 mg = 4 mL/40 mg; x mL = 6 mL

48. x mL/300 mg = 10 mL/500 mg; x mL = 6 mL

49. x mL/30 mg = 1 mL/5 mg; x mL = 6 mL

50. x mL/30 mg = 1 mL/20 mg; x mL = 1.5 mL

51. x mg/5 mL = 20 mg/2 mL; x mg = 50 mg

52. x mL/80 mg = 2 mL/20 mg; x mL = 8 mL

53. x mL/50 mg = 2 mL/20 mg; x mL = 5 mL

54. x mL/12.5 mg = 2 mL/20 mg; x mL = 1.25 mL

55. x mg/3.5 mL = 20 mg/2 mL; x mg = 35 mg

2.4 Problem Set

1. 189 mg − 185 mg = 4 mg; (4 mg/185 mg) × 100 = 2.162%, rounded to 2.16%

2. 500 mg − 476 mg = 24 mg; (24 mg/500 mg) × 100 = 4.8%

3. 1507 mg − 1200 mg = 307 mg; (307 mg/1200 mg) × 100 = 25.583%, rounded to 25.58%

4. 15 mg − 12.5 mg = 2.5 mg; (2.5 mg/15 mg) × 100 = 16.666%, rounded to 16.67%

5. 415 mcg − 400 mcg = 15 mcg; (15 mcg/400 mcg) × 100 = 3.75%

6. 6.3 mL − 5 mL = 1.3 mL; (1.3 mL/5 mL) × 100 = 26%

7. 15 mL − 13 mL = 2 mL; (2 mL/15 mL) × 100 = 13.333%, rounded to 13.33%

8. 20 mL − 15 mL = 5 mL; (5 mL/15 mL) × 100 = 33.333%, rounded to 33.33%

9. 1.5 L − 1.45 L = 0.05 L; (0.05 L/1.5 L) × 100 = 3.333%, rounded to 3.33%

10. 726 mL − 700 mL = 26 mL; (26 mL/700 mL) × 100 = 3.714%, rounded to 3.71%

11. No. 0.4/3 = 13.3%

12. No. 0.4/12.5 = 3.2%

13. No. 0.3/1.8 = 16.7%

14. Yes. 0.09/3.2 = 2.8%

15. Yes. 1/150 = 0.7%

16. Yes. 8/200 = 4%

17. Yes. 1.5/30 = 5%

18. Yes. 4/454 = 0.9%

19. 200 mL × 0.005 = 1 mL; 200 mL − 1 mL = 199 mL; 200 mL + 1 mL = 201 mL; the acceptable range is 199 mL to 201 mL

20. 10.3 mL × 0.0075 = 0.07725 mL, rounded to 0.08 mL; 10.3 mL − 0.08 mL = 10.22 mL; 10.3 mL + 0.08 mL = 10.38 mL; the acceptable range is 10.22 mL to 10.38 mL

21. 830 mL × 0.02 = 16.6 mL; 830 mL − 16.6 mL = 813.4 mL; 830 mL + 16.6 mL = 846.6 mL; the acceptable range is 813.4 mL to 846.6 mL

22. 18 g × 0.0015 = 0.027 g, rounded to 0.03 g; 18 g − 0.03 g = 17.97 g; 18 g + 0.03 g = 18.03 g; the acceptable range is 17.97 g to 18.03 g

23. 750 mg × 0.004 = 3 mg; 750 mg − 3 mg = 747 mg; 750 mg + 3 mg = 753 mg; the acceptable range is 747 mg to 753 mg

24. 100 mg × 0.2 = 20 mg; so the range of accuracy is 80 mg (100 mg − 20 mg) to 120 mg (100 mg + 20 mg)

25. 500 mg × 0.12 = 60 mg; so the range of vitamin C contained in the tablet is 440 mg (500 mg − 60 mg) to 560 mg (500 mg + 60 mg)

Finding Solutions

1. The dosing cup is the correct measuring device and should be filled to the 20 mL graduation mark.

2. 180 mL

3. two bottles

4. 4.3 kg

5. four cartons

6. $86.00

7. 96 tubes

8. $14.00

9. $3.44

10. 1 mL

11. 2 mL

12. 20 mL

13. 250 mg/10 mL

14. 96%

15. 10 questions

Chapter 3

3.1 Problem Set

1. Number does not meet standard validity tests. J is not an appropriate initial letter for the DEA number of a medical doctor. Checksum calculation: 2 + 6 + 8 = 16; (1 + 9 + 7) × 2 = 34; 16 + 34 = 50; last digit of checksum matches last digit (0).

2. The number meets standard validity tests. M is an appropriate initial letter for the DEA number of a mid-level practitioner; G is the first letter of the prescriber's last name. Checksum calculation: 3 + 8 + 6 = 17; (0 + 1 + 5) × 2 = 12; 17 + 12 = 29; last digit of checksum matches last digit (9).

3. Number does not meet standard validity tests. B is an appropriate initial letter for the DEA number of a primary practitioner; H is not the first letter of the prescriber's last name. Checksum calculation: 9 + 9 + 0 = 18; (9 + 8 + 7) × 2 = 48; 18 + 48 = 66; last digit of sum (6) does not match checksum digit (0).

4. Number does not meet standard validity tests. A is an appropriate initial letter for the DEA number of a primary practitioner; L is the first letter of the prescriber's last name. Checksum calculation: 6 + 3 + 6 = 15; (2 + 0 + 1) × 2 = 6; 15 + 6 = 21; Last digit of sum (1) does not match checksum digit (8).

5. Number does not meet standard validity tests. The second letter (D) of the DEA number does not match the first letter of the physician's last name (C). Checksum calculation: 7 + 3 + 2 = 12; (6 + 8 + 2) × 2 = 32; 12 + 32 = 44; last digit of checksum matches last digit (4).

6. Number meets standard validity tests. B is an appropriate initial letter for the DEA number of a primary practitioner; P is the first letter of the prescriber's last name. Checksum calculation: $4 + 1 + 2 = 7$; $(4 + 2 + 0) \times 2 = 12$; $7 + 12 = 19$; last digit of checksum matches last digit (9).

7. Number meets standard validity tests. A is an appropriate initial letter for the DEA number of a primary practitioner; K is the first letter of the prescriber's last name. Checksum calculation: $3 + 5 + 4 = 12$; $(0 + 1 + 9) \times 2 = 20$; $12 + 20 = 32$; last digit of checksum matches last digit (2).

8. Number meets standard validity tests. M is an appropriate initial letter for the DEA number of a mid-level practitioner; S is the first letter of the prescriber's last name. Checksum calculation: $2 + 6 + 2 = 10$; $(8 + 4 + 2) \times 2 = 28$; $10 + 28 = 38$; last digit of checksum matches last digit (8).

9. b. 0.25% acetic acid is correct answer. Calculation: x g/100 mL = 1 g/400 mL; x g = 0.25 g

10. c. isoproterenol 1:200 solution is correct answer. Calculation: x g/100 mL = 0.005 g/mL; x g = 0.5 g, or 0.5%, a 1:200 solution

11. Brand/trade name: Macrobid
Generic name: nitrofurantoin monohydrate
Dosage form: capsules
Strength: 100 mg
Total quantity: 100 capsules
Storage requirements: Store at controlled room temperature (59–86 °F)
Manufacturer: Norwich Pharmaceuticals, Inc and distributed by Almitica Pharma
NDC number: 52427-285-01

12. Brand/trade name: Prozac
Generic name: fluoxetine
Dosage form: pulvules or capsules
Strength: 20 mg
Total quantity: 100 capsules
Storage requirement(s): room temperature (59–86 °F)
Manufacturer: Eli Lilly & Company (Dista)
NDC number: 0777-3105-02

13. Brand/trade name: Strattera
Generic name: atomoxetine HCl

Dosage form: capsules
Strength: 18 mg
Total quantity: 30 capsules
Storage requirements: Store at 25 °C (77 °F) excursions permitted 15–30 °C (59–86 °F)
Manufacturer: Lilly
NDC number: 0002-3238-30

14. Brand/trade name: none
Generic name: spironolactone
Dosage form: tablets
Strength: 50 mg
Total quantity: 100 tablets
Storage requirements: 20° to 25 °C (68° to 77 °F). (See USP Controlled Room Temp.) Room Temperature (68–77 °F)
Manufacturer: Mylan
NDC number: 0378-0243-01

15. Brand/trade name: Vistaril
Generic name: hydroxyzine pamoate
Dosage form: capsules
Strength: 50 mg
Total quantity: 100 capsules
Storage requirements: Store below 86 °F (30 °C)
Manufacturer: Pfizer Labs
NDC number: 0069-5420-66

16. Brand/trade name: Restoril
Generic name: temazepam
Dosage form: capsule
Strength: 7.5 mg
Total quantity: 100 capsules
Storage requirement(s): 20 to 25 °C (68 to 77 °F)
Manufacturer: Mallinckrodt
NDC number: 0406-9915-01

17. 20 tablets; XX is Roman numeral for 20

18. 3 capsules/day $\times$ 10 days = 30 capsules

19. 48 tablets. Determine number of tablets needed for each part of the prescription: 4 tablets/dose $\times$ 2 doses/day $\times$ 2 days = 16 tablets; 3 tablets/dose $\times$ 2 doses/day $\times$ 2 days = 12 tablets; 4 tablets/dose $\times$ 1 dose/day $\times$ 2 days = 8 tablets; 3 tablets/dose $\times$ 1 dose/day $\times$ 2 days = 6 tablets; 2 tablets/dose $\times$ 1 dose/day $\times$ 2 days = 4 tablets; 1 tablet/dose $\times$ 1 dose/day $\times$ 2 days = 2 tablets. Add the subtotals to determine

the total number to dispense: 16 tablets + 12 tablets + 8 tablets + 6 tablets + 4 tablets + 2 tablets = 48 tablets.

20. 1 oz/day $\times$ 7 days/week = 7 oz for a one week supply

21. 150 capsules; #CL = Roman numeral C (100) plus Roman numeral L (50)

22. 28 capsules/2 daily = 14 days

23. 90 tablets/1 daily = 90 days

24. 120 capsules/4 daily = 30 days; (every 6 hours assumes 4 daily)

25. 120 doses/2 daily = 60 days

3.2 Problem Set

1. bid = twice a day

2. DAW = dispense as written

3. IM = intramuscular

4. IV = intravenous

5. mL = milliliter

6. NKA = no known allergy

7. npo = nothing by mouth

8. q3 h = every 3 hours

9. qid = four times a day

10. tid = three times a day

11. A route of administration is the way the drug is to be given to the patient.

12. Oral, injection, rectal, topical. Additional answers may vary.

13. IM intramuscular; IV intravenous; po by mouth. Additional answers may vary.

14. bid = twice a day; qid = four times a day; q2 h = every 2 hours, etc. Additional answers may vary.

15. IM (intramuscular) administration means medication is injected into a muscle; IV (intravenous) administration means it is injected into a vein.

16. Take two capsules by mouth four times a day as needed for itching.

17. Apply one patch every night at bedtime and remove every morning.

18. Apply one half inch of ointment every six hours.

19. Take two tablets by mouth three times a day before meals.

20. Take one half tablet by mouth twice a day.

21. Instill two drops into the right eye every four hours.

22. Take one tablet by mouth each week, 30 minutes before breakfast with water

23. 6 weeks $\times$ 7 days = 42 days; 42 days $\times$ 1 capsule daily = 42 capsules should be dispensed.

24. 1 capsule $\times$ 3 daily $\times$ 10 days = 30 capsules; 10 remain; 1 daily $\times$ 10 capsules = 10 additional days. 10 days + 10 days = 20 days total.

25. 3 tablets daily/63 tablets = 21 days

Finding Solutions

1. Checksum calculation: 4 + 2 + 9 = 15; 4 + 3 + 2 = 9; 2 $\times$ 9 = 18; 15 + 18 = 33. The last digit is 3, but the DEA number has a 1 in the last place. The DEA number provided is not valid.

2. Take three tablets four times daily or as needed.

3. Norco is the brand name, and hydrocodone APAP is the generic name. Prescribers typically do not write both brand names and generic names on a prescription.

4. Take one tablet by mouth every day in the morning for edema.

5. Take one tablet by mouth twice a day for stomach.

6. Take one tablet by mouth four times a day for five days for shingles.

7. Take one tablet by mouth three times a day for angina.

8. Take one tablet by mouth at bedtime for sleep.

9. Students should have selected the oral syringe. The 1 tsp oral syringe should be filled to the ½ tsp graduation mark.

10. Students should have selected the medicine cup. The 2 tbsp medicine cup should be filled to the 2 tsp graduation mark.

11. Yes.

12. 1 PO QAM

13. 30 days.

14. 90

15. 74.5 kg

16. Take 2 tablets by mouth immediately for 1 dose.

17. You would include "before meals" in the translation.

Chapter 4

4.1 Problem Set

1. mcg

2. mg

3. L

4. g

5. kg

6. m

7. cm

8. mL

9. cc

10. dL

11. 0.6 g

12. 50 kg

13. 0.4 mg

14. 0.04 L

15. 4.2 g

16. 0.005 g

17. 0.06 g

18. 2.6 L

19. 0.03 L

20. 0.02 mL

21. 13,333 doses
Work: 5 kg = 5,000 g = 5,000,000 mg
5,000,000 mg available/375 mg = 13,333.33 doses, rounded to 13,333 doses

22. a. 2 tablets/dose $\times$ 2 doses/day = 4 tablets; 4 tablets + 1 tablet/dose = 5 tablets/day
5 tablets/day $\times$ 30 days = 150 tablets

   b. 150 tablets $\times$ 500 mg/tablet = 75,000 mg/month

23. 0.9 g/3 doses = 0.3 g

24. a. 1.2 g/4 doses = 0.3 g
   b. Convert to milligrams, 0.3 g $\times$ 1,000 mg/ 1 g = 300 mg
   Only the 300 mg tablets can be used.

25. a. x g/100 mL = 1 g/1,000 mL, x g = 0.1 g or 0.1%

   b. August 31, 2017

4.2 Problem Set

1. x mg/1,964 mcg = 1 mg/1,000 mcg; x mg = 1.964 mg

2. x g/418 mg = 1 g/1,000 mg; x g = 0.418 g

3. x mcg/651 mg = 1,000 mcg/1 mg; x mcg = 651,000 mcg

4. x mcg/0.84 mg = 1,000 mcg/1 mg; x mcg = 840 mcg

5. x mcg/0.012 g = 1,000,000 mcg/1 g; x mcg = 12,000 mcg

6. x g/9,213,406 mcg = 1 g/1,000,000 mcg; x g = 9.213406 g

7. x g/284 mg = 1 g/1,000 mg; x g = 0.284 g

8. x mg/9,382.5 mcg = 1 mg/1,000 mcg;
x mg = 9.3825 mg

9. x g/12,321 mcg = 1 g/1,000,000 mcg;
x g = 0.012321 g

10. x kg/184 g = 1 kg/1,000 g;
x kg = 0.184 kg

11. 52 mL × 1 L/1,000 mL = 0.052 L

12. 2.06 g × 1,000 mg/1 g = 2,060 mg

13. 16 mg × 1,000 mcg/1 mg = 16,000 mcg

14. 256 mg × 1 g/1,000 mg = 0.256 g

15. 2,703,000 mcg × 1 g/1,000,000 mcg =
2.703 g

16. 6.9 L × 1,000 mL/1 L = 6,900 mL

17. 62.5 mg × 1 g/1,000 mg = 0.0625 g

18. 15 kg × 1,000 g/1 kg = 15,000 g

19. 2,785,000 mcg × 1 g/1,000,000 mcg =
2.785 g

20. 8.234 mg × 1,000 mcg/1 mg = 8,234 mcg

21. 2 kg × 1,000,000 mg/1 kg = 2,000,000 mg;
or x mg/2 kg = 1,000,000 mg/1 kg,
x mg = 2,000,000 mg

22. 21 L × 1,000 mL/1 L = 21,000 mL; or
x mL/21 L = 1,000 mL/1 L, x mL =
21,000 mL

23. 576 mL × 1 L/1,000 mL = 0.576 L;
or x L/576 mL = 1 L/1,000 mL,
x L = 0.576 L

24. 823 kg × 1,000,000 mg/1 kg =
823,000,000 mg; or x mg/823 kg = 1,000,000
mg/1 kg, x mg = 823,000,000 mg

25. 27 mcg × 1 mg/1,000 mcg = 0.027 mg;
or x mg/27 mcg = 1 mg/1,000 mcg,
x mg = 0.027 mg

26. 5,000 mcg × 1 mg/1,000 mcg = 5 mg;
or x mg/5,000 mcg = 1 mg/1,000 mcg,
x mg = 5 mg

27. 20 mcg × 1 mg/1,000 mcg = 0.02 mg;
or x mg/20 mcg = 1 mg/1,000 mcg,
x mg = 0.02 mg

28. 4.624 mg × 1,000 mcg/1 mg = 4,624 mcg;
or x mcg/4.624 mg = 1,000 mcg/1 mg,
x mcg = 4,624 mcg

29. 3.19 g × 1,000 mg/1 g = 3,190 mg;
or x mg/3.19 g = 1,000 mg/1 g,
x mg = 3,190 mg

30. 8,736 mcg × 1 mg/1,000 mcg = 8.736 mg;
or x mg/8,736 mcg = 1 mg/1,000 mcg,
x mg = 8.736 mg

31. 830 mL × 1 L/1,000 mL = 0.83 L; or
x L/830 mL = 1 L/1,000 mL, x L = 0.83 L

32. 0.94 L × 1,000 mL/1 L = 940 mL;
or x mL/0.94 L = 1,000 mL/1 L, x mL =
940 mL

33. 1.84 g × 1,000 mg/1 g = 1,840 mg; or
x mg/1.84 g = 1,000 mg/1 g, x mg =
1,840 mg

34. 560 mg × 1 g/1,000 mg = 0.56 g; or
x g/560 mg = 1 g/1,000 mg, x g = 0.56 g

35. 1,200 mcg × 1 mg/1,000 mcg = 1.2 mg;
or x mg/1,200 mcg = 1 mg/1,000 mcg,
x mg = 1.2 mg

36. 125 mcg × 1 mg/1,000 mcg = 0.125 mg; or
x mg/125 mcg = 1 mg/1,000 mcg,
x mg = 0.125 mg

37. 0.275 mg × 1,000 mcg/1 mg = 275 mcg; or
x mcg/0.275 mg = 1,000 mcg/1 mg,
x mcg = 275 mcg

38. 480 mL × 1 L/1,000 mL = 0.48 L;
or x L/480 mL = 1 L/1,000 mL, x L =
0.48 L

39. 239 mg × 1 g/1,000 mg = 0.239 g
or x g/239 mg = 1 g/1,000 mg, x g = 0.239 g

40. 1,500 mg × 1 g/1,000 mg = 1.5 g;
or x g/1,500 mg = 1 g/1,000 mg, x g = 1.5 g

41. a. 2 tsp/dose × 5 mL/tsp × 2 doses/day =
20 mL/day

b. 20 mL/day × 7 days/course of treatment
= 140 mL/course of treatment

c. 20 mL/day × 125 mg/5 mL × 1 g/
1,000 mg = 0.5 g

d. Since each bottle contains 100 mL,
two bottles will be needed (200 mL − 140
mL = 60 mL to be discarded).

42. (1) Convert 1.5 g to milligrams: x mg/1.5 g = 1,000 mg/1 g, x mg = 1,500 mg.
    (2) Determine number of capsules: 1,500 mg × 1 capsule/250 mg = 6 capsules

43. a. Convert the prescribed dose to grams, 1,000 mg = 1 g. Since one vial contains 10 g, there are ten 1 g doses in one vial.

    b. x days/10 doses × 1 day/2 doses, x days = 5 days

4.3 Problem Set

1. x tablets/30 mg = 1 tablet/7.5 mg, x tablets = 4 tablets

2. x mL/20 mg = 2 mL/25 mg, x mL = 1.6 mL

3. x mL/125 mg = 5 mL/100 mg, x mL = 6.25 mL, rounded to 6.3 mL

4. x mL/4 mg = 1 mL/5 mg, x mL = 0.8 mL

5. x capsules/1,750 mg = 1 capsule/250 mg, x capsule = 7 capsules

6. x mL/40 mg = 5mL/100 mg; x mL = 2mL

7. x mL/400 mg = 5 mL/200 mg, x mL = 10 mL

8. a. x mL/1,000 mg = 5 mL/250 mg, x mL = 20 mL

   b. x mL/75 mg = 1 mL/15 mg, x mL = 5 mL

   c. x tablets/500 mg = 1 tablet/1,000 mg, x tablets = 0.5 tablet; 0.5 tablet/dose × 4 doses/day = 2 tablets/day

9. Convert 10 mg to 10,000 mcg; x mL/10,000 mcg = 1 mL/40 mcg, x mL = 250 mL

10. x mg/2 mL = 20 mg/2 mL; x mg = 20 mg

11. Convert 400 mcg to 0.4 mg; x mL/1 mg = 1 mL/0.4 mg, x mL = 2.5 mL

12. x mcg/1.2 mL = 400 mcg/1 mL, x mcg = 480 mcg

13. Convert 80 mg to 80,000 mcg; x mcg/0.63 mL = 80,000 mcg/15 mL, x mcg = 3,360 mcg

14. 1.05 kg = 1,050 g = 1,050,000 mg; x capsules/1,050,000 mg = 1 capsule/35 mg, x capsules = 30,000 capsules

15. x doses/880 mg = 2 doses/80 mg, x dose = 22 doses

16. Convert 1,600 mg to 1,600,000 mcg; x mcg/4 mL = 1,600,000 mcg/560 mL, x mcg = 11,428.571 mcg, rounded to 11,428.6 mcg

17. Convert 10 mg to 10,000 mcg; x mL/10,000 mcg = 1 mL/40 mcg, x mL = 250 mL

18. x mL/2,000 units = 1 mL/1,000 units; x mL = 2 mL

19. x mL/900 mg = 1 mL/150 mg; x mL = 6 mL

20. x mg/4 mL = 150 mg/1 mL; x mg = 600 mg

21. x mg/12.5 mL = 50 mg/5 mL, x mg = 125 mg

22. x mL/100 mg = 5 mL/50 mg, x mL = 10 mL

23. x mg/0.5 mL = 10 mg/mL; x = 5 mg

24. 0.8 mL × 10 mg/1 mL; x = 8 mg

25. x mL/150 mg = 5 mL/100 mg; x mL = 7.5 mL

26. 0.5 g = 500 mg; x mL/500 mg = 5 mL/100 mg; x mL = 25 mL

27. x mL/50 mg = 1 mL/5 mg; x = 10 mL

28. x mg/0.8 mL = 5 mg/1 mL, x = 4 mg

29. x mL/100 mg = 5 mL/125 mg, x mL = 4 mL

30. x mg/7.5 mL = 125 mg/5 mL, x mg = 187.5 mg; rounded to 188 mg

31. x mL/20 mg = 5 mL/12.5 mg, x mL = 8 mL

32. x mL/50 mg = 5 mL/12.5 mg, x mL = 20 mL

33. a. Since 150 mg × 1 capsule/25 mg = 6 capsules, 150 mg × 1 capsule/50 mg = 3 capsules, and 150 mg × 1 capsule/75 mg = 2 capsules, the 75 mg/capsule product will result in the fewest capsules taken per day, 2 capsules.

    b. 2 capsules/day × 7 days/week = 14 capsules/week

34. a. 500 mg/dose × 4 doses/day = 2,000 mg/day; 2,000 mg × 5 mL/250 mg = 40 mL

    b. 50 mg × 1 tablet/25 mg = 2 tablets

    c. 480 mg × 5 mL/125 mg = 19.2 mL

    d. 200 mg/dose × 3 doses/day = 600 mg/day; 600 mg × 5 mL/100 mg = 30 mL

4.4 Problem Set

To view the completed Nomogram for Estimating Body Surface Area of Children for questions 1–4, see Figure 4.2.

1. Mosteller: 0.42 m²; nomogram 0.405 m², rounded to 0.41 m²

2. Mosteller: 0.59 m²; nomogram: 0.565 m², rounded to 0.57 m²

3. Mosteller: 0.89 m²; nomogram: 0.89 m²

4. Mosteller: 0.74 m²; nomogram: 0.71 m²

To view the completed Nomogram for Estimating Body Surface Area of Adults for questions 5–10, see Figure 4.3.

5. Mosteller: 1.29 m²; nomogram: 1.275 m², rounded to 1.28 m²

6. Mosteller: 1.82 m²; nomogram: 1.75 m²

7. Mosteller: 1.73 m²; nomogram: 1.72 m²

8. Mosteller: 1.95 m²; nomogram: 1.96 m²

9. Mosteller: 1.53 m²; nomogram: 1.49 m²

10. Mosteller: 2.11 m²; nomogram: 2.15 m²

11. 56 kg × 0.5 mg/kg = 28 mg

12. 87 kg × 125 mg/kg = 10,875 mg per day; for each dose, 10,875 mg/6 doses = 1,812.5 mg

13. 1.4 kg × 4 mL/kg = 5.6 mL

14. a. 80 kg × 0.625 mg/kg = 50 mg

    b. 50 mg/3 doses = 16.6666 mg/dose, rounded to 16.67 mg/dose

15. 6 kg × 5 mg/kg/day = 30 mg/day; 30 mg/2 doses = 15 mg/dose

16. 68.64 kg × 125 mg/kg/day = 8,580 mg/day

17. 10 kg × 10 mg/kg/day = 100 mg/day; 1 day = 24 hr; 100 mg/day = 100 mg/24 hr; 100 mg/2 = 50 mg; 24 hr/2 = 12 hr; 50 mg/12 hr

18. 1.1 m² × 25 mg/m² = 27.5 mg; 27.5 mg/2 doses = 13.75 mg/dose

19. 0.67 m² × 0.75 mg/m² = 0.5025 mg, rounded to 0.50 mg

20. 0.85 m² × 100 mg/m² = 85 mg

21. 0.71 m² × 250 mg/m² = 177.5 mg

22. 0.83 m² × 3.3 mg/m² = 2.739 mg, rounded to 2.7 mg

23. 0.7 m² × 2 mg/m² = 1.4 mg. The physician has ordered a dose higher than the recommended dose. To view the completed Nomogram for Estimating Body Surface Area of Children, turn to page 285.

24. 0.48 m² × 3.3 mg/m² = 1.584 mg, rounded to 1.6 mg. The physician has ordered a dose higher than the recommended dose. To view the completed Nomogram for Estimating Body Surface Area of Children, turn to page 286.

25. 0.47 m² × 250 mg/m² = 117.5 mg. The physician has ordered a dose higher than the recommended dose. To view the completed Nomogram for Estimating Body Surface Area of Children, turn to page 287.

26. 40.9 kg × 50 mg/kg/day = 2,045 mg/day is the recommended dose; order is 300 mg × 3 doses/day = 900 mg/day, which is under the recommended dose per day.

27. a. 36.4 kg × 50 mg/kg = 1,820 mg

 b. 36.4 kg × 100 mg/kg = 3,640 mg

 c. 250 mg × 3 doses/day = 750 mg/day, which is under the minimum recommended dose

 d. 250 mg/dose × 50 mL/500 mg = 25 mL/dose

28. a. 5.45 kg × 20 mg/kg = 109 mg

 b. 5.45 kg × 40 mg/kg = 218 mg

 c. 125 mg × 3 doses/day = 375 mg, which is higher than the maximum recommended dose

 d. 125 mg/dose × 5 mL/125 mg = 5 mL/dose

29. a. 11.8 kg × 0.5 mg/kg = 5.9 mg

 b. 11.8 kg × 1 mg/kg = 11.8 mg

 c. 10 mL × 12 mg/5 mL = 24 mg

 d. No, it is not a safe dose. It is higher than 11.8 mg, the maximum recommended dose.

30. a. 9.32 kg × 5 mg/kg = 46.6 mg; 24 hr/day × 1 dose/8 hr = 3 doses/day; 46.6 mg × 3 doses/day = 139.8 mg/day

 b. 9.32 kg × 10 mg/kg = 93.2 mg; 24 hr/day × 1 dose/6 hr = 4 doses/day; 93.2 mg × 4 doses/day = 372.8 mg/day

 c. 125 mg/dose × 3 doses/day = 375 mg/day, which is higher than the maximum recommended dose

 d. 125 mg × 5 mL/100 mg = 6.25 mL

31. a. 50 kg × 25 mg/kg = 1,250 mg

 b. 50 kg × 50 mg/kg = 2,500 mg

 c. 500 mg × 2 doses/day = 1,000 mg/day, which is under the minimum recommended dose

 d. 500 mg × 5 mL/250 mg = 10 mL

32. a. 28.6 kg × 10 mg/kg = 286 mg

 b. 28.6 kg × 15 mg/kg = 429 mg

 c. It is within the recommended range.

 d. 325 mg × 5 mL/160 mg = 10.156 mL, rounded to 10.2 mL

33. a. [8 years/(8 years + 12 years)] × 600 mg = 240 mg

 b. 68 lb/150 lb × 600 mg = 271.99 mg, rounded down to 271 mg.

Finding Solutions

1. 15 kg × 0.5 mg/kg = 7.5 mg

2. 15 kg × 3 mg/kg = 45 mg

3. 15 mg × 2 doses = 30 mg; dose is in the appropriate range

4. x mL/15 mg = 1 mL/5 mg; x mL = 3 mL

5. 21.8 kg × 10 mg/kg = 218 mg

6. 21.8 kg × 15 mg/kg = 327 mg

7. Prescribed dose of 325 mg is in the appropriate range.

8. x mL/325 mg = 5 mL/160 mg; x mL = 10.2 mL

9. $^{12}/_{24}$ × 600 mg = 300 mg per dose

10. $^{80}/_{150}$ × 600 = 320 mg per dose

11. $^{9}/_{21}$ × 100 = 42.9 or 43 mg per dose

12. $^{62}/_{150}$ × 100 = 41.3 or 41 mg per dose

13. 96 mg × m²/60 mg = 1.6 m2

14. 96 mg × mL/2 mg = 48 mL, select the 100-mL container.

15. 196 lb × kg/2.2 lb × 15 mcg/kg = 1336.4 mcg

16. 1336.4 mcg × mL/400 mcg = 3.3 mL

Chapter 5

5.1 Problem Set

1. 8 cups × 1 pt/2 cups = 4 pt

2. 3 pt × 2 cups/1 pt = 6 cups; 6 cups × 8 fl oz/1 cup = 48 fl oz

3. 1 pt × 2 cups/1 pt = 2 cups; 2 cups × 8 fl oz/1 cup = 16 fl oz; 16 fl oz × 2 tbsp/1 fl oz = 32 tbsp

4. 3 qt × 2 pt/1 qt = 6 pt; 6 pt × 2 cups/
   1 pt = 12 cups; 12 cups × 8 fl oz/1 cup =
   96 fl oz

5. 28 tsp × 1 tbsp/3 tsp = 9.333 tbsp, rounded
   to 9.33 tbsp; 9.33 tbsp × 1 fl oz/
   2 tbsp = 4.665 fl oz, rounded to 4.67 fl oz or
   4 $\frac{2}{3}$ fl oz

6. 1 pt × 1 qt/2 pt = 0.5 qt or $\frac{1}{2}$ qt

7. 6 cups × 8 fl oz/1 cup = 48 fl oz;
   48 fl oz × 2 tbsp/1 fl oz = 96 tbsp;
   96 tbsp × 3 tsp/1 tbsp = 288 tsp

8. 80 mL = 5.3 tbsp; 5$\frac{1}{3}$ tbsp

9. 6 fl oz = 180 mL

10. 90 mL = 3 fl oz

11. 800 mL = 1.67 pt (rounded to 1.7)
    or 1$\frac{2}{3}$ pt

12. 53 mL = 10.6 tsp, about 10$\frac{2}{3}$ tsp

13. 35 mL = 7 tsp

14. 10 L = 10,000 mL; 10,000 mL × 1 gal/
    3840 mL = 2.604 gal, rounded to 2.6 gal

15. 4 tbsp = 60 mL

16. 15 mL × 1 tsp/5 mL = 3 tsp

17. 720 mL × 1 pt/480 mL = 1.5 pt, or 1$\frac{1}{2}$ pt

18. 30 tsp × 5 mL/1 tsp = 150 mL

19. 120 mL × 1 fl oz/30 mL = 4 fl oz

20. $\frac{1}{2}$ gal = 0.5 gal × 3840 mL/
    1 gal = 1920 mL

21. 2 L = 2000 mL; 2000 mL × 1 pt/480 mL =
    4.166 pt, rounded to 4.2 pt

22. 3 tbsp × 15 mL/1 tbsp = 45 mL

23. 1 fl oz × 30 mL/1 fl oz = 30 mL

24. 2 fl oz × 30 mL/1 fl oz = 60 mL

25. 3 fl oz × 30 mL/1 fl oz = 90 mL

26. 4 fl oz × 30 mL/1 fl oz = 120 mL

27. 5 fl oz × 30 mL/1 fl oz = 150 mL

28. 6 fl oz × 30 mL/1 fl oz = 180 mL

29. 7 fl oz × 30 mL/1 fl oz = 210 mL

30. 8 fl oz × 30 mL/1 fl oz = 240 mL

31. 12 fl oz × 30 mL/1 fl oz = 360 mL

32. 16 fl oz × 30 mL/1 fl oz = 480 mL

33. 2 oz × 30 g/1 oz = 60 g

34. 1.5 oz × 30 g/1 oz = 45 g

35. 8 oz × 30 g/1 oz = 240 g

36. 906 g × 1 lb/454 g = 1.995 lb, rounded
    to 2 lb

37. 30 g × 1 lb/454 g = 0.0660 lb, rounded
    to 0.07 lb, about $\frac{1}{16}$ lb

38. 0.8 oz × 30 g/1 oz = 24 g

39. 3.5 lb × 1 kg/2.2 lb = 1.59 kg, rounded to
    1.6 kg

40. 14 lb × 1 kg/2.2 lb = 6.364 kg, rounded to
    6.4 kg

41. 42 lb × 1 kg/2.2 lb = 19.09 kg, rounded to
    19.1 kg

42. 97 lb × 1 kg/2.2 lb = 44.09 kg, rounded to
    44.1 kg

43. 112 lb × 1 kg/2.2 lb = 50.909 kg, rounded
    to 50.9 kg

44. 165 lb × 1 kg/2.2 lb = 75 kg

45. 178 lb × 1 kg/2.2 lb = 80.909 kg, rounded
    to 80.9 kg

46. 247 lb × 1 kg/2.2 lb = 112.27 kg, rounded
    to 112.3 kg

47. 2 pt = 960 mL and 6 fl oz = 180 mL,
    so total milliliters = 960 mL + 180 mL =
    1140 mL; 1140 mL × 1 dose/5 mL = 228
    doses

48. 3 cups = 24 fl oz; 24 fl oz = 720 mL;
    720 mL × 1 dose/10 mL = 72 doses

49. 12 bottles × 16 fl oz = 192 fl oz; 192 fl oz
    = 5760 mL; 5760 mL × 1 dose/15 mL =
    384 doses

50. 5 fl oz = 150 mL; 150 mL × 1 dose/5 mL =
    30 doses

51. 1 pt = 480 mL; 480 mL × 1 dose/15 mL =
    32 doses

52. 1.5 fl oz = 45 mL; 45 mL × 3 times/day =
    135 mL/day

53. 8 fl oz = 240 mL; 240 mL × 1 dose/
    7.5 mL = 32 doses

54. $\frac{1}{2}$ tsp $\times$ 5 mL/1 tsp $\times$ 10 mg/1 mL = 25 mg

55. 4 fl oz $\times$ 30 mL/1 fl oz = 120 mL; 120 mL $\times$ 10 mg/1 mL = 1200 mg; 1200 mg $\times$ 1 day/20 mg = 60 days

56. 2.5 mL $\times$ 1 tsp/5 mL = 0.5 tsp

57. 320 mL $\times$ 1 day/3 tsp $\times$ 1 tsp/5 mL = 21.3 days or 21 full days

58. Conversions: 180 lb $\times$ 1 kg/2.2 lb = 81.8181 kg, rounded to 81.8 kg; 2 tsp $\times$ 5 mL/1 tsp = 10 mL
81.8 kg $\times$ 10 mL/68 kg = 12.029411 mL, rounded to 12 mL
300 mL $\times$ 1 dose/12 mL = 25 doses

59. Conversions: 52 lb $\times$ 1 kg/2.2 lb = 23.636 kg, rounded to 23.6 kg; 1 tsp $\times$ 5 mL/ 1 tsp = 30

5 mL; 4 fl oz $\times$ 30 mL/1 fl oz = 120 mL
23.6 kg $\times$ 5 mL/20 kg = 5.9 mL
120 mL $\times$ 1 dose/5.9 mL = 20.3389 doses, or 20 full doses

60. Conversions: 172 lb $\times$ 1 kg/2.2 lb = 78.181 kg, rounded to 78.2 kg; 2 tbsp $\times$ 15 mL/1 tbsp = 30 mL; 12 fl oz $\times$ 30 mL/1 fl oz = 360 mL
78.2 kg $\times$ 30 mL/50 kg = 46.92 mL, rounded to 46.9 mL
360 mL $\times$ 1 dose/46.9 mL = 7.6759 doses, or 7 full doses

5.2 Problem Set

1. 243 mg

2. 324 mg

3. 405 mg

4. 648 mg

5. 6 lb/(2.2 kg/lb) = 2.727; 2.727 $\times$ 10 = 27.27 mcg; 2.727 $\times$ 15 = 40.905 mcg; rounded dosage: 27.3 mcg to 40.9 mcg

6. 12 oz/x lb = 16 oz/1 lb; x = 0.75; 7 lb 12 oz = 7.75 lb; 7.75 lb/(2.2 kg/lb) = 3.523; 3.523 $\times$ 10 = 35.23; 3.523 $\times$ 15 = 52.845; rounded dosage: 35.2 mcg to 52.9 mcg

7. 23 lb/(2.2 kg/lb) = 10.454; 10.454 $\times$ 6 = 62.724; 10.454 $\times$ 8 = 83.632; rounded dosage: 62.7 mcg to 83.6 mcg

8. 18 lb/(2.2 kg/lb) = 10.454; 8.182 $\times$ 5 = 40.91; 8.182 $\times$ 6 = 49.092; rounded dosage: 40.9 mcg to 49.1 mcg

9. 5 mL $\times$ 80 mg/15 mL = 26.67 mg

10. 60 mg $\times$ 5 mL/120 mg = 2.5 mL or $\frac{1}{2}$ tsp

11. 240 mL $\times$ 24 mg/5 mL = 1152 mg or 1.152 g

12. 120 mL $\times$ 65 mg/15 mL = 520 mg

13. 10 mL $\times$ 2500 mg/60 mL = 417 mg (rounded from 416.67 mg)

14. 15 mL $\times$ 260 mg/600 mL = 6.5 mg

15. 600 mL $\times$ 25 mg/5 mL = 3000 mg = 3 g

16. 30 mg/5 mL = x mg/15 mL
15 $\times$ 30 = 450
450/5 = 90
90 mg

17. 480 mL $\times$ 40 mg/1 mL = 19,200 mg or 19.2 g

18. a. 150 mL $\times$ 1 dose/3.75 mL = 40 doses; 40 doses $\times$ 1 day/3 doses = 13.3 days

    b. 3.75 mL/dose $\times$ 3 doses/day = 11.25 mL/ day $\times$ 10 days = 112.5 mL; 150 mL $-$ 112.5 mL = 37.5 mL

19. a. 1 tsp = 5 mL; 10 mL/day $\times$ 14 days = 140 mL; 150 mL bottle selected

    b. 150 mL $-$ 140 mL = 10 mL

20. 1 tbsp = 15 mL and 12 fl oz/bottle = 360 mL/bottle; 15 mL/dose $\times$ 3 doses/day = 45 mL/day; 360 mL/bottle $\times$ 1 day/45 mL = 8 days/bottle

21. 2 tsp = 10 mL and 1 tbsp = 15 mL, so 25 mL/1 2-day total; 300 mL $\times$ 1 2-day unit/25 mL = 12 2-day units, or 24 days

22. 600 mL $\times$ 25 mg/15 mL = 1000 mg or 1 g

23. 12 fl oz/bottle = 360 mL/bottle and 1 fl oz $\times$ 4 doses/day = 30 mL $\times$ 4 doses/ day = 120 mL/day; 120 mL/day $\times$ 14 days/ treatment = 1680 mL/treatment; 1680 mL/ treatment $\times$ 1 bottle/360 mL = 4.666 bottles, or a total of 5 bottles to be purchased

24. (4 tablets × 2/day) + (3 tablets × 2/day) + (1 tablet × 1/day) = 15 tablets

25. 24 hr/day × 1 dose/3 hr = 8 doses/day; 8 doses/day × 10 days = 80 doses; 80 doses × (1 mL/dose × 2 cheeks) = 160 mL

26. a. 12 fl oz/bottle = 360 mL/bottle, 1 tsp/dose = 5 mL/dose; 360 mL/bottle × 25 mg/5 mL = 1800 mg/bottle

    b. 9 g = 9000 mg; 9000 mg/therapy × 1 bottle/1800 mg = 5 bottles; 5 bottles − 1 initial bottle = 4 refills

27. 2 tsp/dose = 10 mL/dose; 3 doses/day × 10 mL/dose = 30 mL/day; 30 mL/ day × 15 days/treatment = 450 mL/ treatment; 450 mL/treatment × 1 fl oz/30 mL = 15 fl oz/treatment

28. 2 tbsp/dose = 30 mL/dose; 3 doses/day × 30 mL/dose = 90 mL/day; 20 days/treatment × 90 mL/day = 1800 mL/treatment

29. 1 tsp = 5 mL
    Child 1: 5 mL/dose × 3 doses/day = 15 mL/day; 15 mL/day × 4 days = 60 mL
    Child 2: 10 mL/dose × 3 doses/day = 30 mL/day; 30 mL/day × 4 days = 120 mL
    60 mL + 120 mL = 180 mL
    Since 1 bottle = 4 fl oz, 4 fl oz/bottle × 30 mL/1 fl oz = 120 mL/bottle
    The mother will need 2 bottles, or 240 mL.

30. Child 1: 5 mL × 25 mg/5 mL; x mg = 25 mg
    Child 2: 10 mL × 25 mg/5 mL; x mg = 50 mg

31. ³⁄₄ tsp = 0.75 tsp; 0.75 tsp × 5 mL/tsp = 3.75 mL; 3.75 mL × 187 mg/5 mL = 140.25 mg

32. 1¹⁄₂ tsp = 1.5 tsp; 1.5 tsp × 5 mL/tsp = 7.5 mL; 7.5 mL × 187 mg/5 mL = 280.5 mg

33. 125 mg × 5 mL/187 mg = 3.3422 mL, rounded to 3.34 mL

34. 500 mg × 5 mL/187 mg = 13.3689 mL, rounded to 13.37 mL

35. a. 180 g/3 equal parts = 60 g of each

    b. 180 g × 1 oz/30 g = 6 oz; use a 6 oz jar

    c. 1/3/2018 + 6 months = 7/3/2018

36. 12 fl oz bottle × 30 mL/1 fl oz = 360 mL; 360 mL × 1 syringe/60 mL = 6 syringes

5.3 Problem Set

1. (0° − 32°) ÷ 1.8 = -17.777 °C, rounded to -17.8 °C

2. (23° − 32°) ÷ 1.8 = -5 °C

3. (36° − 32°) ÷ 1.8 = 2.222 °C, rounded to 2.2 °C

4. (40° − 32°) ÷ 1.8 = 4.444 °C, rounded to 4.4 °C

5. (64° − 32°) ÷ 1.8 = 17.777 °C, rounded to 17.8 °C

6. (72° − 32°) ÷ 1.8 = 22.222 °C, rounded to 22.2 °C

7. (98.6° − 32°) ÷ 1.8 = 37 °C

8. (100.5° − 32°) ÷ 1.8 = 38.055 °C, rounded to 38.1 °C

9. (102.8° − 32°) ÷ 1.8 = 39.333 °C, rounded to 39.3 °C

10. (105° − 32°) ÷ ÷ 1.8 = 40.555 °C, rounded to 40.6 °C

11. (1.8 × -15°) + 32 = 5 °F

12. (1.8 × 18°) + 32 = 64.4 °F

13. (1.8 × 27°) + 32 = 80.6 °F

14. (1.8 × 31°) + 32 = 87.8 °F

15. (1.8 × 38°) + 32 = 100.4 °F

16. (1.8 × 40°) + 32 = 104 °F

17. (1.8 × 49°) + 32 = 120.2 °F

18. (1.8 × 63°) + 32 = 145.4 °F

19. (1.8 × 99.8°) + 32 = 211.64 °F, rounded to 211.6 °F

20. (1.8 × 101.4°) + 32 = 214.52 °F, rounded to 214.5 °F

21. (1.8 × 130°) + 32 = 266 °F

22. a. (1.8 × -20°) + 32 = -4 °F

    b. 2/1/15 + 6 months = August 1, 2018

23. (300° − 32°) ÷ 1.8 = 148.888 °C, rounded to 148.9 °C

24. a. 2.3 °C
    b. 3.2 °C
    c. 3.9 °C
    d. 2.1 °C
    e. 2.7 °C
    f. 1.6 °C; too cold
    g. 2.4 °C
    h. 2.7 °C
    i. 1.9 °C; too cold
    j. 3.8 °C

5.3 Problem Set, chart for question 24

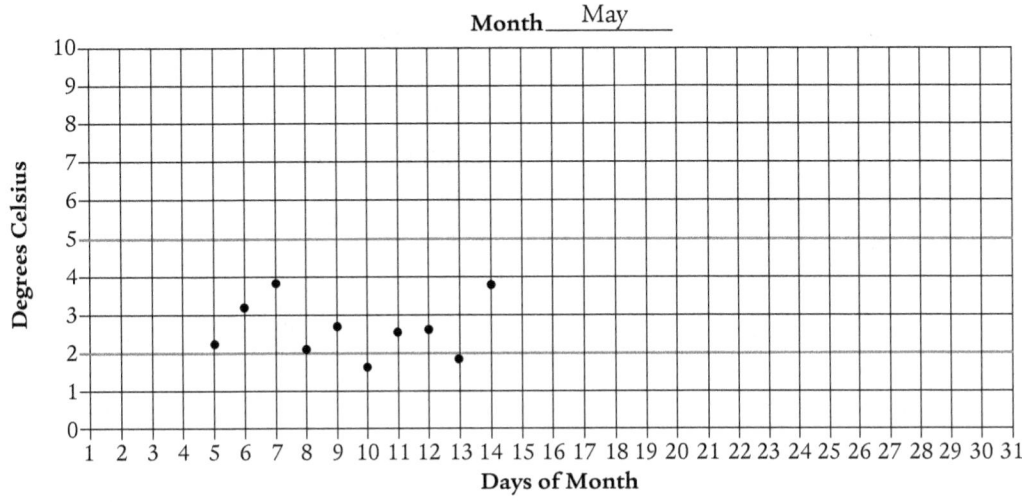

Month ____May____

Degrees Celsius

Days of Month

25. a. 35.2 °F; too cold
    b. 37.6 °F
    c. 37 °F
    d. 37.4 °F
    e. 40.1 °F
    f. 37.8 °F
    g. 39 °F
    h. 36.5 °F
    i. 39.4 °F
    j. 40.5 °F

5.3 Problem Set, chart for question 25

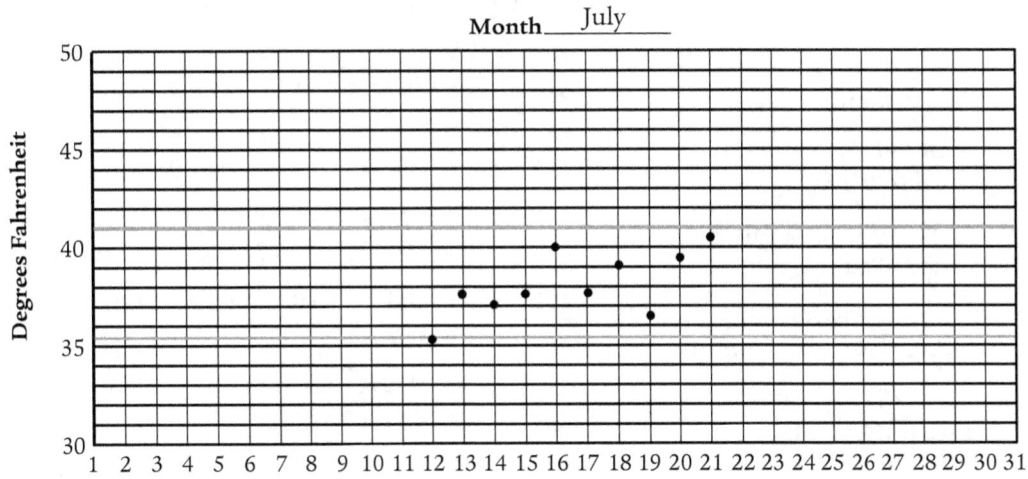

Month ____July____

Degrees Fahrenheit

Finding Solutions

1. 22 lb × 1 kg/2.2 lb = 10 kg

2. 10 kg × 1 mg/kg = 10 mg

3. 10 mg/2 doses = 5 mg

4. x mL/5 mg × 5 mL/40 mg; x = 0.625 mL; the 5 mL oral syringe should be filled to 0.625 mL.

5. less than 1 teaspoon

6. oral syringe

7. 4 g = 4000 mg; 4000 mg divided by 4 doses = 1000 mg/dose

8. x mL/1000 mg = 5 mL/250 mg; x = 20 mL; the medicine cup should be filled to 20 mL (20 cc).

9. x tsp/20 mL = 1 tsp/5 mL; x = 4 tsp

10. 20 mL × 4 doses/day = 80 mL; 80 mL × 10 days = 800 mL

11. 10 mL

12. 60 capsules.

13. 733.3 mg

14. 14.6 mL of the 250 mg/5 mL concentration and 29.3 mL of the 125 mg/5 mL concentration

15. 35.6 degrees to 46.4 degrees Fahrenheit

Chapter 6

6.1 Problem Set

1. x mL/50 mg = 1 mL/10 mg; x mL = 5 mL (5 mL syringe filled to 5 mL)

2. x mL/60 mg = 4 mL/40 mg; x = 6 mL; (10 mL syringe filled to 6 mL)

3. x mL/80 mg = 10 mL/100 mg; x mL = 8 mL; (10 mL syringe filled to 8 mL)

4. x mL/0.75 mg = 1 mL/1 mg; x mL = 0.75 mL (1 mL syringe filled to 0.75 mL)

5. x mL/100 mg = 1 mL/50 mg; x mL = 2 mL; (3 mL syringe filled to 2 mL)

6. x mL/30 mg = 2 mL/20 mg; x mL = 3 mL; (3 mL syringe filled to 3 mL)

7. x mL/40 mg = 2 mL/20 mg; x mL = 4 mL (5 mL syringe filled to 4 mL)

8. Reconstitute to 100 mg/mL; x mL/250 mg = 1 mL/100 mg; x mL = 2.5 mL; (3 mL syringe filled to 2.5 mL)

9. Reconstitute to 100 mg/mL; x mL/400 mg = 1 mL/100 mg; x mL = 4 mL; (5 mL syringe filled to 4 mL)

10. x mL/50 mg = 100 mL/100 mg; x mL = 50 mL (60 mL syringe filled to 50 mL)

11. x mg/0.5 mL = 15 mg/1 mL; x mg = 7.5 mg

12. x mg/1.75 mL = 60 mg/2 mL; x mg = 52.5 mg

13. x mg/3.75 mL = 20 mg/1 mL; x mg = 75 mg

14. x mg/1.3 mL = 2 mg/2 mL; x mg = 1.3 mg

15. x mg/5 mL = 50 mg/10 mL; x mg = 25 mg

16. x mg/5 mL = 25 mg/5 mL; x mg = 25 mg

17. x mg/5 mL = 10 mg/10 mL; x mg = 5 mg

18. x mg/8 mL = 4 mg/1 mL; x mg = 32 mg

19. x mg/1.5 mL = 4 mg/2 mL; x mg = 3 mg

20. x mg/2.5 mL = 50 mg/1 mL; x mg = 125 mg

21. x g/2 mL = 1 g/1,000 mL; x g = 0.002 g = 2 mg

22. x g/1 mL = 1 g/5,000 mL; x g = 0.0002 g = 0.2 mg = 200 mcg

23. x g/1.5 mL = 1 g/10,000 mL; x g = 0.00015 g = 0.15 mg = 150 mcg

24. x g/1.4 mL = 1 g/2,000 mL; x g = 0.0007 g = 0.7 mg = 700 mcg

25. x mg/2.5 mL = 1 g/10,000 mL; x mg = 0.00025 g = 0.25 mg = 250 mcg

26. Convert 500 mg to 0.5 g; x mL/0.5 g = 1,000 mL/1 g; x mL = 500 mL

27. Convert 50 mg to 0.05 g; x mL/0.05 g = 10,000 mL/1 g; x mL = 500 mL

28. Convert 600 mg to 0.6 g; x mL/0.6 g = 300 mL/1 g; x mL = 180 mL

29. Convert 250 mg to 0.25 g; x mL/0.25 g = 500 mL/1 g; x mL = 125 mL

30. x mL/0.01 g = 750 mL/1 g; x mL = 7.5 mL

6.2 Problem Set

1. x mL/30 mEq = 1 mL/4.4 mEq; x mL = 6.81818 mL, rounded to 6.82 mL (10 mL syringe filled to 6.82 mL graduation mark)

2. x mL/45 mEq = 1 mL/4.4 mEq; x mL = 10.22727 mL, rounded to 10.23 mL (10 mL syringe filled to 10 mL graduation mark; 1 mL syringe filled to .23 mL graduation mark)

3. x tablets/32 mEq = 1 tablet/8 mEq; x tablets = 4 tablets

4. x mL/30 mEq = 15 mL/40 mEq; x mL = 11.25 mL; 11.25 mL/ 2 doses = 5.625 mL, rounded to 5.63 mL (10 mL syringe filled to 5.63 mL graduation mark)

5. x mEq/15 mL = 20 mEq/10 mL; x mEq = 30 mEq

6. x mL/30 mEq = 15 mL/20 mEq; x mL = 22.5 mL (20 mL syringe filled to 22.5 mL graduation mark)

7. Select the 20 mEq vial; x mL/14 mEq = 1 mL/2 mEq; x mL = 7 mL (10 mL syringe filled to 7 mL graduation mark)

8. Select the 20 mEq vial; x mL/19 mEq = 1 mL/2 mEq; x mL = 9.5 mL (10 mL syringe filled to 9.5 mL graduation mark)

9. Select the 40 mEq vial; x mL/27 mEq = 1 mL/2 mEq; x mL = 13.5 mL

10. Select the 40 mEq plus the 10 mEq vial; x mL/50 mEq = 1 mL/2 mEq; x mL = 25 mL

11. x mEq/8 mL = 60 mEq/30 mL; x mEq = 16 mEq or x mEq/8 mL = 2 mEq/1 mL; x mEq = 16 mEq

12. x mEq/15 mL = 40 mEq/20 mL; x mEq = 30 mEq or x mEq/15 mL = 2 mEq/1 mL; x mEq = 30 mEq

13. x mL/132 mEq = 1 mL/4 mEq; x mL = 33 mL (60 mL syringe filled to 33 mL graduation mark)

14. x mL/120 mEq = 1 mL/4 mEq; x mL = 30 mL (60 mL syringe filled to 30 mL graduation mark)

15. x mL/4 units = 1 mL/10 units; x mL = 0.4 mL

16.. x units/2.8 mL = 10 units/1 mL; x units = 28 units (30 unit syringe filled to 28 units graduation mark)

17. x mL/3,500 units = 1 mL/1,000 units; x mL = 3.5 mL

18. x units/0.43 mL = 20,000 units/0.8 mL; x units = 10,750 units

19. x mL/7,000 units = 1 mL/10,000 units; x mL = 0.7 mL

20. x mL/24,000 units = 1 mL/10,000 units; x = 2.4 mL

21. x mL/30 mg = 0.8 mL/80 mg; x mL = 0.3 mL

22. x mL/175,000 units = 1 mL/500,000 units; x mL = 0.35 mL

23. x mL/1,200,000 units = 1 mL/600,000 units; x mL = 2 mL

24. x mL/385,000 units = 1 mL/50,000 units; x mL = 7.7 mL

25. x mL/45 units = 1 mL/100 units; x mL = 0.45 mL

26. Calculate morning dose: x mL/18 units = 1 mL/100 units; x mL = 0.18 mL
Calculate evening dose: x mL/10 units = 1 mL/100 units; x mL = 0.1 mL
Add morning and evening doses: 0.18 mL/morning + 0.1 mL/evening = 0.28 mL/day Since the vial shown on the label contains 10 mL, calculate time for 10 mL vial to last: x days/10 mL vial = 1 day/0.28 mL; x days = 35.714 days, rounded to 35 days

27. a. Add morning and evening units: 20 units + 18 units = 38 units/day

b. x mL/38 units = 1 mL/100 units; x mL = 0.38 mL. Calculate the number of days of therapy in a 10 mL vial: 10 mL / 0.38 mL = 26.3 days, rounded down to 26 days for 1 vial. Therefore, 2 vials will be needed for 30 days of therapy.

28. Humulin R: 10 units/dose × 1 dose/day × 30 days = 300 units for month; 300 units × 1mL/100 units = 3mL; 1 vial will be needed Humulin 70/30 Mix: 15 units/dose × 2 doses/day × 30 days = 900 units for month; 900 units × 1mL/100 units = 9mL; 1 vial will be needed

29. x units/0.5 mL = 100 units/1 mL; x units = 50 units

30. 20 units/dose x 2 doses/day = 40 units/day; x mL/40 units = 1 mL/100 units; x mL = 0.4 mL are used daily x days/20 mL = 1 day/0.4 mL; x days = 50 days

6.3 Problem Set

1. Convert 375 mg to 0.375 g. x mL/1.5 g = 1 mL/0.375 g; x mL = 4 mL 4 mL final volume − 3.3 mL diluent volume = 0.7 mL powder volume

2. Convert 250 mg to 0.25 g, and note that 1 tsp = 5 mL. x mL/5 g = 5 mL/0.25 g; x mL = 100 mL final volume 100 mL final volume − 8.6 mL powder volume = 91.4 mL diluent volume

3. Convert 1 g to 1,000 mg. x mL/1,000 mg = 2 mL/125 mg; x mL = 16 mL final volume 16 mL final volume − 14.4 mL diluent = 1.6 mL powder volume

4. Convert 250 mg to 0.25 g. x mL/2 g = 1 mL/0.25 g; x mL = 8 mL final volume 8 mL final volume − 6.8 mL diluent = 1.2 mL powder volume

5. Convert 125 mg to 0.125 g. x mL/2 g = 1 mL/0.125 g; x mL = 16 mL final volume Using the powder volume calculated in #4, 16 mL final volume − 1.2 mL powder volume = 14.8 mL diluent volume

6. Convert 250 mg to 0.25 g. x mL/4 g = 1 mL/0.25 g; x mL = 16 mL final volume 16 mL final volume − 11.7 mL diluent = 4.3 powder volume

7. x mL/6 g = 2.5 mL/1 g; x mL = 15 mL final volume; 15 mL final volume − 12.5 mL diluent volume = 2.5 mL powder volume 2.5 mL powder volume + 2.5 mL diluent volume = 5 mL final volume; 6 g/5mL = 1.2 g/mL = 1200 mg/mL

8. 4 mL final volume − 3.3 mL diluent = 0.7 mL powder volume

9. Using the information from #8, 1 g/4 mL, and converting 1 g to 1,000 mg: x mL/100 mg = 4 mL/1,000 mg; x mL = 0.4 mL

10. x mL/2 g = 1 mL/0.2 g, x mL = 10 mL final volume; 10 mL final volume − 8.8 mL diluent = 1.2 mL powder volume

11. Convert 10 g to 10,000 mg; 45 mL DV + 5 mL PV = 50 mL FV; x mg/1 mL = 10,000 mg/50 mL; x mg = 200 mg, so there will be 200 mg/mL

12. Convert 8 g to 8,000 mg, and remember 1 tsp = 5 mL. x mg/5 mL = 8,000 mg/ 200 mL; x mg = 200 mg, so there are 200 mg/5 mL or 200 mg/tsp

13. x mL/20 g = 6 mL/1 g, x mL = 120 mL FV; 120 mL FV − 106 mL DV = 14 mL PV x mL/20 g = 3 mL/1 g, x mL = 60 mL FV; 60 mL FV − 14 mL PV = 46 mL DV

14. Convert 2 g to 2,000 mg; x mL/2,000 mg = 1 mL/375 mg, x mL = 5.3 mL FV; 5.3 mL FV − 3.5 mL DV = 1.8 mL PV

15. Convert 2.5 g to 2,500 mg; x mL/2,500 mg = 5 mL/300 mg, x mL = 41.7 mL FV; 41.7 mL FV − 9.6 mL PV = 32.1 mL DV

16. Convert 5 g to 5,000 mg; x mL/5,000 mg = 1 mL/250 mg, x mL = 20 mL FV; 20 mL FV − 8.6 mL DV = 11.4 mL PV

17. x mg/10 g = 2.5 mL/1 g, x mL = 25 mL FV; 25 mL FV − 20 mL DV = 5 mL PV; 5 mL PV + 35 mL new DV = 40 mL FV; 10 g/40 mL = 0.25 g/mL or 250 mg/mL

18. 5 mL FV − 4.3 mL DV = 0.7 mL PV

19. 25 mL DV + 5 mL PV = 30 mL FV; convert 5 g to 5,000 mg; x mg/1 mL = 5,000 mg/30 mL; x = 167 mg, so 167 mg/mL

20. 90 mL DV + 10 mL PV = 100 mL FV; convert 20 g to 20,000 mg; x mg/1 mL = 20,000 mg/100 mL; x mg = 200 mg, so 200 mg/mL

21. 20 mL DV + 5 mL PV = 25 mL FV; convert 3 g to 3,000 mg; x mg/1 mL = 3,000 mg/25 mL; x mg = 120 mg, so 120 mg/mL

22. 100 mL FV − 67 mL DV = 33 mL PV

23. Convert 35 g to 35,000 mg; x mg/1 mL = 35,000 mg/100 mL, x mg = 350 mg, so 350 mg/mL

24. (1) 15 mL − 9 mL = 6 mL in bottle; (2) 10 mL + 0.2 mL = 10.2 mL vancomycin; (3) 10.2 mL vancomycin + 6 mL bottle = 16.2 mL FV; x mg/1 mL = 500 mg/16.2 mL; x mg = 30.8641 mg, rounded to 31 mg, so 31 mg/mL

25. a. x mg/1 mL = 1,000 mg/4.4 mL; x mg = 227 mg, so 227 mg/mL; 1 mL + 9 mL = 10 mL, so 227 mg/10 mL, which is simplified to 22.7 mg/mL

    b. x mg /0.1 mL = 22.7 mg/1 mL = 2.27 mg

Finding Solutions

1. x mL/100 mg = 1 mL/50 mg; x = 2 mL

2. The 3 mL syringe should be filled to the 3 mL graduation mark.

3. x mg/50 mL = 50 mg/1 mL; x mg = 2500 mg

4. 2500 mg/100 mg dose = 25 doses

5. x units/30 days = 30 units/1 day; x units = 900 units; x mL/900 units = 1 mL/100 units; x mL = 9 mL; 1 vial will be needed

6. The 30 unit insulin syringe should be selected to deliver 30 units (equivalent to 0.3 mL).

7. 30 units − 6 units = 24 units; the 30 unit syringe should be filled to 24 units (equivalent to 0.24 mL)

8. 40 mEq/x mL = 20 mEq/10 mL; x = 20 mL

9. 4 mEq/x mL = 20 mEq/15 mL; x = 30 mL

10. 15 mL/x mEq = 5 mL/10 mEq; x = 30 mEq

11. 5,000 units/x mL = 10,000 units/mL; x = 0.5 mL

12. 15 mg × 87 kg = 1245 mg, which is typically rounded to 1250 mg in practice

13. Convert 1245 mg to 1.245 g; 1.245 g/x mL = 1 g/20 mL; x = 24.9 mL

Chapter 7

7.1 Problem Set

1. w/v = 10 g/100 mL

2. w/v = 0.45 g/100 mL

3. v/v = 0.25 mL/100 mL

4. v/v = 7 mL/100 mL

5. 10 % = 10 g/100 mL; 10 g /100 mL = x g/500 mL; 10 × 500 = x = 50 g

6. 2% = 2 g/100 mL = x g/1.3 mL; x = 0.026 g = 26 mg

7. 15 g/100 mL = 15%

8. 20 g/500 mL = 4%

9. 0.15 g/1 mL × 100 = 15%

10. 0.03 g/ 1 mL × 100 = 3%

11. 0.005 g/1 mL × 100 = 0.5%

12. $0.002 \text{ g}/1 \text{ mL} \times 100 = 0.2\%$

13. $0.01 \text{ g}/1 \text{ mL} \times 100 = 1\%$

14. $0.02 \text{ g}/1 \text{ mL} \times 100 = 2\%$

15. $3.5\% = 3.5 \text{ g}/100 \text{ mL} = x \text{ g}/2,500 \text{ mL}$;
    $x = 87.5 \text{ g}$

16. $10\% = 10 \text{ g}/100 \text{ mL} = x \text{ g}/1,000 \text{ mL}$;
    $x = 100 \text{ g}$

17. $0.25\% = 0.25 \text{ g}/100 \text{ mL} = x \text{ g}/1,000 \text{ mL}$;
    $x = 2.5 \text{ g}$

18. $0.9\% = 0.9 \text{ g per } 100 \text{ mL}$; 0.9 g

19. $4\% = 4 \text{ g}/100 \text{ mL} = x \text{ g}/500 \text{ mL}$; $x = 20 \text{ g}$

20. $0.45\% = 0.45 \text{ g}/100 \text{ mL} = x \text{ g}/1,000 \text{ mL}$;
    $x = 4.5 \text{ g}$

21. $5\% = 5 \text{ g}/100 \text{ mL} = x \text{ g}/1,000 \text{ mL}$;
    $x = 50 \text{ g}$

22. $0.4\% = 0.4 \text{ g}/100 \text{ mL} = x \text{ g}/500 \text{ mL}$;
    $x = 2 \text{ g}$

23. $4\% = 4 \text{ g}/100 \text{ mL} = x \text{ g}/500 \text{ mL}$; $x = 20 \text{ g}$

24. $2\% = 2 \text{ g}/100 \text{ mL} = x \text{ g}/250 \text{ mL}$; $x = 5 \text{ g}$

25. $7.5\% = 7.5 \text{ g}/100 \text{ mL} = x \text{ g}/5 \text{ mL}$;
    $x = 0.375 \text{ g}$; $0.375 \times 1,000 = 375 \text{ mg}$

26. $0.5\% = 0.5 \text{ g}/100 \text{ mL} = x \text{ g}/50 \text{ mL}$;
    $x = 0.25 \text{ g}$; $0.25 \times 1,000 = 250 \text{ mg}$

27. $1\% = 1 \text{ g}/100 \text{ mL} = x \text{ g}/0.5 \text{ mL}$;
    $x = 0.005 \text{ g}$; $0.005 \times 1,000 = 5 \text{ mg}$

28. $1{:}1,000 = 1,000 \text{ mg}/1,000 \text{ mL} = $
    $x \text{ mg}/1 \text{ mL}$; $x = 1 \text{ mg}$

29. $1{:}5,000 = 1,000 \text{ mg}/5,000 \text{ mL} = $
    $x \text{ mg}/5 \text{ mL}$; $x = 1 \text{ mg}$

30. $100 \text{ g}/1,000 \text{ mL} = x \text{ g}/100 \text{ mL}$; $x = 10 \text{ g}$; 10
    $\text{g}/100 \text{ mL} = 10\%$

31. $100 \text{ g}/1,000 \text{ mL} = x \text{ g}/3000 \text{ mL}$; $x = 300 \text{ g}$

32. NS = 0.9%

33. Rate = 150 mL per hr; $150 \times 24 = $
    3,600 mL in 24 hr period; $0.9\% = $
    $0.9 \text{ g}/100 \text{ mL} = x \text{ g}/3,600 \text{ mL}$; $x = 32.4 \text{ g}$

34. $0.9 \text{ g}/100 \text{ mL} = x \text{ g}/250 \text{ mL}$; $x = 2.25 \text{ g}$

35. $0.9 \text{ g}/100 \text{ mL} = x \text{ g}/500 \text{ mL}$; $x = 4.5 \text{ g}$

36. $0.9 \text{ g}/100 \text{ mL} = x \text{ g}/1,000 \text{ mL}$; $x = 9 \text{ g}$

37. $0.9 \text{ g}/100 \text{ mL} = x \text{ g}/2,225 \text{ mL}$; $x = 20.03 \text{ g}$

38. $0.45 \text{ g}/100 \text{ mL} = x \text{ g}/125 \text{ mL}$; $x = 0.563$,
    rounded to 0.56 g

39. $0.45 \text{ g}/100 \text{ mL} = x \text{ g}/250 \text{ mL}$; $x = 1.125$,
    rounded to 1.13 g

40. $0.45 \text{ g}/100 \text{ mL} = x \text{ g}/750 \text{ mL}$; $x = 3.375$,
    rounded to 3.38 g

41. $0.45 \text{ g}/100 \text{ mL} = x \text{ g}/1,800 \text{ mL}$; $x = 8.1 \text{ g}$

42. $0.45 \text{ g}/100 \text{ mL} = x \text{ g}/2,600 \text{ mL}$; $x = 11.7 \text{ g}$

43. $5 \text{ g}/100 \text{ mL} = x \text{ g}/75 \text{ mL}$; $x = 3.75 \text{ g}$

44. $5 \text{ g}/100 \text{ mL} = x \text{ g}/385 \text{ mL}$; $x = 19.25 \text{ g}$

45. $5 \text{ g}/100 \text{ mL} = x \text{ g}/525 \text{ mL}$; $x = 26.25 \text{ g}$

46. $5 \text{ g}/100 \text{ mL} = x \text{ g}/1,350 \text{ mL}$; $x = 67.5 \text{ g}$

47. $10 \text{ g}/100 \text{ mL} = x \text{ g}/100 \text{ mL}$; $x = 10 \text{ g}$

48. $10 \text{ g}/100 \text{ mL} = x \text{ g}/325 \text{ mL}$; $x = 32.5 \text{ g}$

49. $10 \text{ g}/100 \text{ mL} = x \text{ g}/450 \text{ mL}$; $x = 45 \text{ g}$

50. $10 \text{ g}/100 \text{ mL} = x \text{ g}/875 \text{ mL}$; $x = 87.5 \text{ g}$

7.2 Problem Set

1. $1,000/50 = 20 \text{ hr}$

2. $1,000/100 = 10 \text{ hr}$; 10 hr from 7 PM is
   5 AM

3. $500/30 = 16.666$ rounded to 16.67 hr;
   or approximately 16 hr and 40 min

4. $75 \text{ mL}/45 \text{ min} = x \text{ mL}/60 \text{ min}$;
   $x = 100 \text{ mL/hr}$

5. $100 \text{ mL}/45 \text{ min} = x \text{ mL}/60 \text{ min}$;
   $x = 133 \text{ mL/hr}$

6. $250/5 = 50 \text{ mL/hr}$

7. $1,500/5 = 300 \text{ mg/hr}$

8. Rate is 50 mL over 60 min or 50 mL/hr

9. Rate is 500 mg over 60 min or 500 mg/hr

10. 100 mL/hr

11. $1,000/100 = 10 \text{ hr}$

12. 1 bag = 10 hr; $24/10 = 2.4$; 2.4, rounded up
    to 3 IV bags

13. $20/10 = 2$ mEq/hr

14. $D_5 = 5$ g/100 mL $= x$ g/1,000 mL; $x = 50$; $x = 50$ g

15. NS $= 0.9$ g/100 mL $= x$ g/1,000 mL; $x = 9$ g

16. $1,000/50 = 20$ hr; $24/20 = 1.2$, rounded up to 2 IV bags

17. $1,000/75 = 13.33$ hr; $24/13.33 = 1.8$, rounded up to 2 IV bags

18. $1,000/100 = 10$ hr; $24/10 = 2.4$, rounded up to 3 IV bags

19. $1,000/120 = 8.33$ hr; $24/8.33 = 2.88$, rounded up to 3 IV bags

20. $1,000/125 = 8$ hr; $24/8 = 3$ IV bags

21. $1,000/130 = 7.69$ hr; $24/7.69 = 3.12$, rounded up to 4 IV bags

22. $1,000/150 = 6.66$ hr; $24/6.66 = 3.6$, rounded up to 4 IV bags

23. $1,000/175 = 5.71$ hr; $24/5.71 = 4.2$, rounded up to 5 IV bags

24. $1,000/200 = 5$ hr; $24/5 = 4.8$, rounded up to 5 IV bags

25. $1,000/225 = 4.44$ hr; $24/4.44 = 5.41$, rounded up to 6 IV bags

26. a. $250/4 = 62.5$ mL/hr

    b. $250/4 = 62.5$ mg/hr

27. a. $500/12 = 41.666$, rounded to 41.67 mL/hr

    b. $12,000,000/12 = 1,000,000$ units/hr

28. a. $4\% = 4$ g/100 mL $= x$ g/500 mL; $x = 20$ g; 20 g $= 20,000$ mg; $20,000/500 = 40$; 40 mg/1 mL $= 800$ mg/x mL; $x = 20$ mL/hr

    b. $500/20 = 25$ hr

29. a. 250 mg/500 mL $= 20$ mg/x mL; $x = 40$ mL/hr

    b. 20 mg/1 hr $= 250$ mg/x hr; $x = 12.5$ hr

30. a. $1,600$ mcg/500 mL $= x$ mcg/1 mL; $x = 75$ mL/hr

    b. 4 mcg/1 min $= x$ mcg/60 min; $x = 240$; 240 mcg/hr

31. a. 200 mg/5 mL $= 800$ mg/x mL; $x = 20$ mL

    b. $800/250 = 3.2$ mg/hr; 3.2 mg/1 mL $= 5$ mg/x mL; $x = 1.56$ mL/hr

32. a. 176 lb $= 79.8$ kg; 2 mg $\times 79.8$ kg $= 159.6$ mg; 159.6 mg/x mL $= 40$ mg/mL; $x = 3.99$ mL, rounded to 4 mL

    b. 100 mL/hr

7.3 Problem Set

1. 10 mL/60 min $\times 10 = 1.67$, rounded down to 1 gtt/min

2. 35 mL/60 min $\times 60 = 35$ gtts/min

3. 100 mL/60 min $\times 10 = 16.66$, rounded down to 16 gtts/min

4. 50 mL/30 min $= x$ mL/hr; $x = 100$ mL/hr; $100/60 \times 60 = 100$ gtts/min

5. $500/24 = 20.83$; $20.83/60 \times 15 = 5.21$, rounded down to 5 gtts/min

6. 250 mL/60 min $\times 15 = 62.5$, rounded down to 62 gtts/min

7. 50 mL/60 min $\times 15 = 12.5$, rounded down to 12 gtts/min

8. 95 mL/60 min $\times 20 = 31.67$, rounded down to 31 gtts/min

9. $100 \times 10 = 1,000$ (i.e., 1,000 drops in 100 mL); $40/1,000 = 0.04$ mEq/gtt

10. 25 mL/60 min $\times 15 = 6.25$, rounded down to 6 gtts/min

11. 50 mL/60 min $\times 60 = 50$ gtts/min

12. 10 mL/60 min $\times 20 = 3.33$, rounded to 3 gtts/min

13. mg/gtt $= 450$ mg/250 mL $\times 1$ mL/60 gtts $= 0.03$ mg/gtt

14. mg/gtt $= 8$ mg/250 mL $\times 1$ mL/10 gtts $= 0.0032$ mg/gtt

15. 25 mL/60 min $\times 10$; $25/60 = 0.417 = 4.17$, rounded down to 4 gtts/min

16. mEq/gtt $= 10$ mEq/500 mL $\times 1$ mL/60 gtts $= 0.00033$ mgEq/gtt

Finding Solutions

1. 20 mEq/L × 3 L = 60 mEq

2. 50 g/L × 3 L = 15 g

3. NS = 9,000 mg of sodium/L × 3 L = 27; 27 g in 24 hr

4. 5 g/100 mL = x g/480 mL = 24 g of dextrose

5. 1 g/500 mL = x g/480 mL = 0.96 g = 960 mg of aminophylline

6. 20 mL/1 hr = x mL/24 hr = 480 mL

7. 1,500 mg/x vials = 500 mg/1 vial; x = 3 vials

8. 100 mL/x g = 500 mL/1.5 g; x = 0.3 g; 0.3% w/v

9. Concentration is 1,500 mg/500 mL = 3 mg/mL; this concentration is appropriate since it is less than 5 mg/mL.

10. 1,500 mg/x mins = 500 mg/30 mins; x = 90 mins, or 1.5 hours

11. 0.5 mg/min × 250 mL/450 mg × 60 min/hr = 16.7 mL/hr

12. 16.7 mL/hr × 15 drops/mL × 1 hr/60 mins = 4.18 drops/min, rounded to 4 drops/min

13. Total dose is 0.5 mg/min × 60 min/hr × 18 hr = 540 mg; Each bag contains 450 mg, so 2 bags will be needed.

14. 450 mg/x hr = 30 mg/hr; x = 15, so IV bag will need to be replaced after 15 hours, or at 0900 the next morning.

Chapter 8

8.1 Problem Set

1. 30 g/120 g = 30/120 = ¼ ratio
   Coal tar 4 g = 4/4 = 1 g
   Salicylic acid 1 g = ¼ = 0.25 g
   Triamcinolone 0.1% ung 15 g = 15/4 = 3.75 g
   Aqua-base ointment 100 g = 100/4 = 25 g

You would divide each number by 4 (or multiply by 1/4). Therefore, you will need 1.00 g of coal tar, 0.25 g of salicylic acid, 3.75 g of triamcinolone 0.1% ung, and 25.00 g of aqua-base ointment.

2. 150/30 = 5/1 ratio
   Progesterone 2.4 g × 5 = 12 g
   Polyethylene glycol 3350 30 g ×5 = 150 g
   Polyethylene glycol 1000 90 g × 5 = 450 g

You would multiply each number by 5. Therefore, you will need 12 g of progesterone, 150 g of polyethylene glycol 3350, and 450 g of polyethylene glycol 1000.

3. 120/20 = 6/1 ratio
   Podophyllum resin 25%; 25% = 25 mL/ 100 mL = x mL/20 mL = 5 mL; 5 × 6 = 30 mL
   Benzoin tincture QSAD 120 mL

Therefore, you will need 30 mL of podophyllum resin and QSAD 120 mL of benzoin tincture. *Note:* You could also solve this problem by multiplying 120 × 0.25 = 30 mL; 120-30 = 90 mL.

4. 8 oz = 240 mL
   120/240 = ½ ratio
   Tetracycline 500 mg capsules; 16/2 = 8 capsules Hydrocortisone suspension 15 mL; 15/2 = 7.5 mL
   Lidocaine oral suspension 30 mL; 30/2 = 15 mL
   Mylanta suspension QSAD 240 mL; 240/2 = QSAD 120 mL

Therefore, you will need 8 capsules of tetracycline 500 mg, 7.5 mL of hydrocortisone suspension, 15.0 mL of lidocaine oral suspension, and QSAD 120.0 mL of Mylanta suspension.

5. 4 × 15 = 60 mL
   60/30 = 2/1 ratio
   Antipyrine 1.8 g × 2 = 3.6 g
   Benzocaine 0.5 g × 2 = 1 g
   Glycerin QSAD 30 mL × 2 = QSAD 60 mL

Therefore, you will need 3.6 g of antipyrine, 1.0 g of benzocaine, and QSAD 60 mL of glycerin.

8.2 Problem Set

1.

10		2.5 parts of 10%
	7.5	
5		2.5 parts of 5%

2.5 + 2.5 = 5 parts total

$2.5/5 = x/200 = 100$; $x = 100$ mL of 10% dextrose

$2.5/5 = x/200 = 100$; $x = 100$ mL of 5% dextrose

2.

20		3 parts of 20%
	8	
5		12 parts of 5%

3 + 12 = 15 parts total

$3/15 = x/400 = 80$; $x = 80$ mL of 20%

$12/15 = x/400 = 320$; $x = 320$ mL of 5%

3.

70		7.5 parts of 70%
	12.5	
5		57.5 parts of 5%

7.5 + 57.5 = 65 parts total

$7.5/65 = x/500 = 57.69$; $x = 57.69$, rounded to 58 mL of 70%

$57.5/65 = x/500 = 442.31$; $x = 442.31$, rounded to 442 mL of 5%

4.

10		1 part of 10%
	6	
5		4 parts of 5%

4 + 1 = 5 parts total

$4/5 = x/250 = 200$; $x = 200$ mL of 5%

$1/5 = x/250 = 50$; $x = 50$ mL of 10%

5.

50		2.5 parts of 50%
	7.5	
5		42.5 parts of 5%

2.5 + 42.5 = 45 parts total

$2.5/45 = x/500 = 27.78$; $x = 27.78$, rounded to 28 mL of 50%

$42.5/45 = x/500 = 472.22$; $x = 472.22$, rounded to 472 mL of 5%

6.

20		3 parts of 20%
	8	
5		12 parts of 5%

3 + 12 = 15 parts total

$3/15 = x/250 = 50$; $x = 50$ mL of 20%

$12/15 = x/250 = 200$; $x = 200$ mL of 5%

7.

20		2.5 parts of 20%
	7.5	
5		12.5 parts of 5%

2.5 + 12.5 = 15 parts total

$2.5/15 = x/300 = 50$; $x = 50$ mL of 20%

$12.5/15 = x/300 = 250$; $x = 250$ mL of 5%

8.

20		2.5 parts of 20%
	12.5	
10		7.5 parts of 10%

2.5 + 7.5 = 10 parts total

$2.5/10 = x/500 = 125$; $x = 125$ mL of 20%

$7.5/10 = x/500 = 375$; $x = 375$ mL of 10%

9.

10		2.5 parts of 10%
	7.5	
5		2.5 parts of 5%

2.5 + 2.5 = 5 parts total

$2.5/5 = x/150 = 75$; $x = 75$ mL of 10%

$2.5/5 = x/150 = 75$; $x = 75$ mL of 5%

10.

20		2.5 parts of 20%
	12.5	
10		7.5 parts of 10%

2.5 + 7.5 = 10 parts total

$2.5/10 = x/250 = 62.5$; $x = 62.5$, rounded to 63 mL of 20%

$7.5/10 = x/250 = 187.5$; $x = 187.5$, rounded to 188 mL of 10%

11.

10		2 parts of 10%
	3	
1		7 parts of 1%

2 + 7 = 9 parts total

$2/9 = x/60 = 13.33$; $x = 13.33$, rounded to 13 g of 10%

$7/9 = x/60 = 46.66$; $x = 46.66$, rounded to 47 g of 1%

12.

15		2.5 parts of 15%
	7.5	
5		7.5 parts of 5%

7.5 + 2.5 = 10 parts total

$2.5/10 = x/30 = 7.5$; $x = 7.5$, rounded to 8 g of 15%

$7.5/10 = x/30 = 22.5$; $x = 22.5$, rounded to 23 g of 5%

13. $4 \times 30 = 120$ g

5		2 parts of 5%
	3	
1		2 parts of 1%

$2 + 2 = 4$ parts total

$2/4 = x/120 = 60; x = 60$ g of 5%

$2/4 = x/120 = 60; x = 60$ g of 1%

14.

20		5 parts of 20%
	10	
5		10 parts of 5%

$10 + 5 = 15$ parts total

$5/15 = x/45 = 15; x = 15$ g of 20%

$10/15 = x/45 = 30; x = 30$ g of 5%

15.

10		3 parts of 10%
	8	
5		2 parts of 5%

$3 + 2 = 5$ parts total

$3/5 = x/100 = 60; x = 60$ g of 10%

$2/5 = x/100 = 40; x = 40$ g of 5%

8.3 Problem Set

1. $2.0\% = 2.0$ g/100 g; 2.0 g/100 g $= x$ g/75 g; $2.0 \times 75 = 150$; $150/100 = 1.5$; $x = 1.5$ g

   Therefore, there are 1.5 g of hydrocortisone in 75 g of the cream.

2. 8 g/ 454 g $= x$ g/100 g; $8 \times 100 = 800$; $800/454 = 1.76$; $x = 1.8$ g

   Therefore, the percentage strength of the compound is 1.8%.

3. $2.5\% = 2.5$ g/100 g

   Therefore, 2.5 g of acyclovir will be needed for this preparation.

4. 10 g $+ 50$ g $= 60$ g; 10 g/60 g $= x$ g/100 g; $10 \times 100 = 1{,}000$; $1{,}000/60 = 16.66$ g; $x = 16.7$ g

   Therefore, the percentage strength of the compound is 16.7%.

5. $2\% = 2$ g/100 g; 2 g/100 g $= x$ g/30 g; $2 \times 30 = 60$; $60/100 = 0.6$; $x = 0.6$ g

   Therefore, 0.6 g of triamcinolone will be needed for this prescription.

6. $0.05\% = 0.05$ g/100 g; 0.05 g/100 g $= x$ g/15 g; $0.05 \times 15 = 0.75$; $0.75/100 = 0.0075$ g

   Therefore, 0.0075 g of mometasone fumarate will be needed to prepare the prescription.

7. a. $100 \times 200 = 20{,}000$ mg which is 20 grams, are needed for batch

   b. $20{,}000$ mg $= 0.2$ g; 0.2 g/1 g $= x$ g/100 g; $x = 20$ g; 20%

8. $0.75\% = 0.75$ g/100 g; 0.75 g/100 g $= x$ g/30 g; $0.75 \times 30 = 22.5$; $22.5/100 = 0.225$ g (rounded to 0.23 g) of metronidazole needed for this prescription

9. $0.5\% = 0.5$ g/100 g
   0.5 g/100g $= x$ g/30 g
   $0.5 \times 30 = 15$; $15/100 = 0.15$ g

   0.15 g of clindamycin is needed to prepare this prescription.

10. a. $10\% = 10 \text{ g}/100 \text{ g}$
    $10 \text{ g}/100 \text{ g} = x \text{ g}/50 \text{ g}$
    $10 \times 50 = 500; 500/100 = 5 \text{ g}$

    5 g of acyclovir are needed to prepare this prescription.

    b. 1 dose = 1 g
    $1 \text{ g}/1 \text{ dose} = 50\text{g}/x \text{ doses}$
    $50 \times 1 = 50; 50/1 = 50 \text{ doses}$

    There are 50 doses.

8.4 Problem Set

1. a. $10 \text{ mg}/1 \text{ mL} = x \text{ mg}/10 \text{ mL}; 10 \times 10 = 100; 100/1 = 100; x = 100 \text{ mg}$

   b. $100 \text{ mg/mL} = 1 \text{ mL}$

   c. $10 - 1 = 9 \text{ mL}$

2. a. $10 \text{ mg}/1 \text{ mL} = x \text{ mg}/5 \text{ mL}; 10 \times 5 = 50; 50/1 = 50; x = 50 \text{ mg}$

   b. $40 \text{ mg}/1 \text{ mL} = 50 \text{ mg}/x \text{ mL}; 1 \times 50 = 50; 50/40 = 1.25; x = 1.25 \text{ mL}$

   c. $5 - 1.25 = 3.75 \text{ mL}$

3. a. $10 \text{ mg}/1 \text{ mL} = x \text{ mg}/10 \text{ mL}; 10 \times 10 = 100; 100/1 = 100; x = 100 \text{ mg}$

   b. $500 \text{ mg}/5 \text{ mL} = 100 \text{ mg}/x \text{ mL}; 5 \times 100 = 500; 500/500 = 1; x = 1 \text{ mL}$

   c. $10 - 1 = 9 \text{ mL}$

4. a. $1 \text{ mg}/1 \text{ mL} = x \text{ mg}/5 \text{ mL}; 1 \times 5 = 5; 5/1 = 5; x = 5 \text{ mg}$

   b. $4 \text{ mg}/1 \text{ mL} = 5 \text{ mg}/x \text{ mL}; 1 \times 5 = 5; 5/4 = 1.25; x = 1.25 \text{ mL}$

   c. $5 - 1.25 = 3.75 \text{ mL}$

5. a. $1 \text{ mg}/1 \text{ mL} = x \text{ mg}/10 \text{ mL}; 1 \times 10 = 10; 10/1 = 10; x = 10 \text{ mg}$

   b. $20 \text{ mg}/2 \text{ mL} = 10 \text{ mg}/x \text{ mL}; 2 \times 10 = 20; 20/20 = 1; x = 1 \text{ mL}$

   c. $10 - 1 = 9 \text{ mL}$

6. a. $500 \times 15 = 7,500; 7,500/70 = 107.14 \text{ mL}$ of 70% dextrose

   b. $500 - 107.14 = 392.86$, rounded to 393 mL of sterile water

7. a. $2,000 \times 10 = 20,000; 20,000/50 = 400 \text{ mL}$ of 50% dextrose

   b. $2,000 - 400 = 1,600 \text{ mL}$ of sterile water

8. a. $1,000 \times 10 = 10,000; 10,000/50 = 200 \text{ mL}$ of 50% dextrose

   b. $1,000 - 200 = 800 \text{ mL}$ of sterile water

9. a. $750 \times 8 = 6,000; 6,000/50 = 120 \text{ mL}$ of 50% dextrose

   b. $750 - 120 = 630 \text{ mL}$ of sterile water

10. a. $250 \times 7.5 = 1,875; 1,875/70 = 26.79 \text{ mL}$ of 70% dextrose

    b. $250 - 26.79 = 223.21$, rounded to 223 mL of sterile water

11. a. $1,500/70 \times 17; 1,500/70 = 21.43; 21.43 \times 17 = 364.29 \text{ mL}$ of $D_{70}W$

    b. $1,500/10 \times 3; 1,500/10 = 150; 150 \times 3 = 450.00 \text{ mL}$ of Aminosyn 10%

    c. $1,500/20 \times 2.5; 1,500/20 = 75; 75 \times 2.5 = 187.50 \text{ mL}$ of Liposyn 20%

    d. $20 \times 1.5 = 30; 30/4 = 7.50 \text{ mL}$ of sodium chloride

    e. $15 \times 1.5 = 22.5; 22.5/2 = 11.25 \text{ mL}$ of potassium chloride

    f. $10 \times 1.5 = 15; 15/3 = 5.00 \text{ mL}$ of potassium phosphate

    g. $3 \times 1.5 = 4.5; 4.5/3 = 1.50 \text{ mL}$ of sodium phosphate

    h. $10 \times 1.5 = 15; 15/4.06 = 3.6946$ rounded to 3.69 mL of magnesium sulfate

    i. 10.00 mL of MVI

    j. $364.29 + 450 + 187.5 + 7.5 + 11.25 + 5 + 1.5 + 3.7 + 10 = 1040.74$

    $1,500 - 1040.74 = 459.26 \text{ mL}$ of sterile water

    k. 1,500.00 mL

12. a. $15 \text{ g}/100 \text{ mL} \times 1,500 \text{ mL} \times 100 \text{ mL}/70 \text{ g} = 321.43 \text{ mL}$ of D70W

    b. $4 \text{ g}/100 \text{ mL} \times 1,500 \text{ mL} \times 100 \text{ mL}/10 \text{ g} = 600.00 \text{ mL}$ of Aminosyn 10%

    c. $3 \text{ g}/100 \text{ mL} \times 1,500 \text{ mL} \times 100 \text{ mL}/20 \text{ g} =$

225.00 mL of Liposyn 20%

d. 25 mEq/L $\times$ 1 L/1,000 mL $\times$ 1,500 mL $\times$ 1 mL/4 mEq = 9.38 mL of sodium chloride

e. 12.5 mEq/L $\times$ 1 L/1,000 mL $\times$ 1,500 mL $\times$ 1 mL/2 mEq = 9.38 mL of potassium chloride

f. 10 mM/L $\times$ 1 L/1,000 mL $\times$ 1,500 mL $\times$ 1 mL/3 mM = 5.00 mL of potassium phosphate

g. 2 mM/L $\times$ 1 L/1,000 mL $\times$ 1,500 mL $\times$ 1 mL/3 mM = 1.00 mL of sodium phosphate

h. 10 mEq/L $\times$ 1 L/1,000 mL $\times$ 1,500 mL $\times$ 1 mL/4.06 mEq = 3.69 mL magnesium sulfate

i. 10.00 mL of MVI

j. Sterile water QSAD to 1,500 mL; 1,500 mL − (321.43 mL + 600.00 mL + 225.00 mL + 9.38 mL + 9.38 mL + 5.00 mL + 1.00 mL + 3.69 mL + 10.00 mL) = 315.12 mL sterile water

k. 1500.00 mL

Finding Solutions

1. 20 mEq/L = 20 mEq for one bag

2. 1,000/125 = 8; 24/8 = 3; 3 bags are needed for 24 hours

3. 1,000 $\times$ 12 = 12,000; 12,000/50 = 240 mL of 50% dextrose

4. 1,000 − 240 = 760 mL of sterile water

5. 125 mL/1 hr = x mL/24 hr; 125 $\times$ 24 = 3,000 mL; the patient will receive 3,000 mL of IV fluid in 24 hours

6. 150 mL/1 hr = x mL/24 hr; 150 $\times$ 24 = 3,600 mL; 3,600/1 = 3,600; 3,600.0 mL will be needed for 24 hours

7. 3,600 $\times$ 15 = 54,000; 54,000/70 = 771.43, rounded to 771.4 mL of D70%

8. 3,600 $\times$ 5 = 18,000; 18,000/10 = 1,800.0 mL of AA 10%

9. 3,600 $\times$ 2.5 = 9,000; 9,000/10 = 900.0 mL of Liposyn 10%

10. 10 mEq/1,000 mL = x mEq/3,600 mL; 36,000/1,000 = 36 mEq/bag 4 mEq/1 mL = 36 mEq/x mL; 1 $\times$ 36 = 36; 36/4 = 9.0 mL of NaCl

11. 10 mEq/1,000 mL = x mEq/3,600 mL; 10 $\times$ 3,600 = 36,000/1,000 = 36 mEq/bag

    2 mEq/1 mL = 36 mEq/x mL; 1 $\times$ 36 = 36; 36/2 = 18.0 mL of KCl

12. 2.5 mEq/1,000 mL = x mEq/3,600 mL; 2.5 $\times$ 3,600 = 9,000; 9,000/1,000 = 9 mEq/bag 4.06 mEq/1 mL = 9 mEq/x mL; 1 $\times$ 90 = 9; 9/4.06 = 2.2 mL of MgSO4

13. 20 units/1,000 mL = x units/3,600 mL; 20 $\times$ 3,600 = 72,000; 72,000/1,000 mL = 72 units/ bag 100 units/1 mL = 72 units/x mL; 1 $\times$ 72 = 72; 72/100 = 0.72, rounded to 0.7 mL of insulin 14. 10.0 mL of MVI

15. 771.43 + 1,800.00 + 900.00 + 9.00 + 18.00 + 2.22 + 0.72 + 10.00 = 3,511.37

    3,600 − 3,511.37 = 88.6 mL of sterile water

16. 16 ounces

17. 1.3 ounces

18. 100 mg

19. 120 mg

20. Swish, gargle, and spit 5 mL to 10 mL every six hours as needed for irritation.

Chapter 9

9.1 Problem Set

1. $135,000.00 + $52,000.00 + $23,000.00 + $6,000.00 + $4,000.00 + $2,000.00 + $4,000.00 + $4,000.00 + $750,000.00 = $980,000.00; $980,000.00 $\times$ 0.18 = $176,400.00; $980,000.00 + $176,400.00 = $1,156,400.00; desired income goal for 18% profit is $1,156,400.00

2. $1,401,489.00 − $980,000.00 = $421,489.00; $421,480.00/$1,401,490.00 = 0.30; 0.3 × 100 = 30%; percentage profit is 30%

3. $1,191,692.00 − $980,000.00 = $211,692.00; $211,692.00/$1,191,692.00 = 0.178; 0.178 × 100 = 17.8%; percentage profit is 17.8%

4. $72,000.00 + $52,000.00 + $13,000.00 + $5,500.00 + $2,000.00 + $1,500.00 + $4,000.00 + $3,500.00 + $50,000.00 = $203,500.00; $203,500.00 × 0.2 = $40,700.00; $203,500.00 + $40,700.00 = $244,200.00; Desired income goal for 20% profit is $244,200.00

5. $991,982.00 − $203,500.00 = $788,482.00; $788,482.00/$991,982.00 = 0.79; 0.79 × 100 = 79%; Percentage profit is 79%

6. $1,248,301.00 − $203,500.00 = $1,044,801.00; $1,044,801.00/$1,248,301.00 = 0.837; 0.837 × 100 = 83.7%; percentage profit is 83.7%

7. $54,617.53 − $3700.83 = $50,916.70; the overhead for the week was $50,916.70

8. $13,033.06 × 0.22 = $2867.27; $2867.27 + $13,033.06 = $15,900.33; weekly sales of $15,900.33 are required for a 22% profit

9. $3.96/100 tablets = $0.0396 per tablet, rounded to $0.04 per tablet; $0.04 × 50 tablets = $2; $8.59 − $2 − $4.25 = $2.34 net profit

   $8.59 − $4.25 = $4.34; $4.34 − $2 = $2.34; $2.34/$2 = 1.17 or 117% markup rate

10. $8.50/500 capsules = $0.017 per capsule, rounded to $0.02; $0.02 × 30 capsules = $0.60; $14.80 − $0.60 − $4.25 = $9.95 net profit

    $14.80 − $4.25 = $10.55; $10.55 − $0.60 = $9.95; $9.95/$0.60 = 16.58 or 1658% markup rate

11. $118.50/100 tablets = $1.185 per tablet, rounded to $1.19; $1.19 × 30 tablets = $35.70; $45.50 − $35.70 − $4.25 = $5.55 net profit

    $45.50 − $4.25 = $41.25; $41.25 − $35.70 = $5.55; $5.55/$35.70 = 0.1554 or 15.5% markup rate

12. $83.50/500 tablets = $0.167 per tablet, rounded to $0.17; $0.17 × 100 tablets = $17.00; $23.16 − $17.00 − $4.25 = $1.91 net profit

    $23.16 − $4.25 = $18.91; $18.91 − $17.00 = $1.91; $1.91/$17.00 = 0.1123 or 11.2% markup rate

13. $41.20/100 tablets = $0.412 per tablet, rounded to $0.41; $0.41 × 90 tablets = $36.90; $41.70 − $36.90 − $4.25 = $0.55 net profit

    $41.70 − $4.25 = $37.45; $37.45 − $36.90 = $0.55; $0.55/$36.90 = 0.015, or 1.5% markup rate

14. $37.50/480 mL = $0.078 rounded to 0.08 per mL; $0.08 × 240 mL = $19.20; $25.34-$19.20 = $6.14 (net profit).

    $25.34-$4.25 = $21.09; $21.09-19.20 = $1.89; $1.89/$19.20 = 0.098, 9.8% markup rate.

15. $62.30/6 packs = $10.38 per pack; $10.38 × 1 pack = $10.38; $17.90 − $10.38 − $4.25 = $3.27 net profit

    $17.90 − $4.25 = $13.65; $13.65 − $10.38 = $3.27; $3.27/$10.38 = 0.315, or 31.5% markup rate

16. $5.89 × 0.2 = $1.18; $5.89 − $1.18 = $4.71; discounted selling price is $4.71

17. $1.19 × 0.15 = $0.18; $1.19 − $0.18 = $1.01; discounted selling price is $1.01

18. $7.29 × 0.30 = $2.19; $7.29 − $2.19 = $5.10; discounted selling price is $5.10

19. $5.69 × 0.15 = $0.85; $5.69 − $0.85 = $4.84; discounted selling price is $4.84

20. $3.89 × 0.25 = $0.9725, rounded to 0.97; $3.89 − $0.97 = $2.92; discounted selling price is $2.92

21. $4.26 × 0.30 = $1.28; $4.26 − $1.28 = $2.98; discounted selling price is $2.98

22. $8.70 × 0.5 = $4.35; $8.70 − $4.35 = $4.35; discounted selling price is $4.35

23. $2.99 × 0.40 = $1.20; $2.99 − $1.20 = $1.79; discounted selling price is $1.79

24. $12.50 × 0.3 = $3.75; $12.50 + $3.50 = $16.00; $16.00 × 12 tubes = $195.00; the total selling price is $195.00

25. $111.60/36 = $3.10 (purchase price per bottle); $3.10 + $1.75 = $4.85; selling price is $4.85 per bottle

26. $15.60 × 0.25 = $3.9; the markup amount is $3.90; $15.60 + $3.90 = $19.50; the selling price is $19.50

27. $30.75 − $24.80 = $5.95; $5.95/$24.80 × 100; $5.95/$24.80 = 0.2399; 0.2399 × 100 = 23.99, rounded to 24%; markup rate is 24%

28. $650.00 − $520.00 = $130.00; gross profit is $130.00

29. $2.05/100 = 0.0205; 0.0205 × 100 = 2.05; $650.00-$520.00 = $130.00; $130.00-$2.05 = $127.95; $127.95/1000=$0.127 (rounded to $0.13); net profit is $0.13 per tablet.

30. $120.50 × 0.25 = $30.13; markup amount is $30.13; $120.50 + $30.13 = $150.63; selling price is $150.63

31. $24.00 × 0.15 = $3.60; markup amount is $3.60; $24.00 + $3.60 = $27.60; selling price is $27.60

32. $200.00 × 0.27 = $54.00; markup amount is $54.00; $200.00 + $54.00 = $254.00; selling price is $254.00

33. $27.50 × 0.21 = $5.78; markup amount is $5.78; $27.50 + $5.78 = $33.28; selling price is $33.28

34. $67.50 × 0.18 = $12.15; markup amount is $12.15; $67.50 + $12.15 = $79.65; selling price is $79.65

35. $840.00 × 0.32 = $268.80; markup amount is $268.80; $840.00 + $268.80 = $1108.80; selling price is $1108.80

36. $550.00 × 0.30 = $165.00; markup amount is $165.00; $550.00 + $165.00 = $715.00; selling price is $715.00

37. $120.50 + $24.00 + $200.00 + $27.50 + $67.50 + $840.00 + $550.00 = $1829.50; the total amount that the pharmacy spent

on the shipment was $1829.50; $150.63 + $27.60 + $254.00 + $33.28 + $79.65 + 1108.80 + $715.00 = $2368.96; $2368.96 − $1829.50 = $539.46; the total amount made by the pharmacy was $539.46; $549.46/$1829.50 × 100; $549.46/$1829.50 = 0.3003; 0.3003 × 100 = 30.03 rounded to 30; the total markup rate was 30%

9.2 Problem Set

1. $48.90 × 0.13 = $6.36; $48.90 − $6.36 = $42.54; $42.54/60 tablets × 20 tablets; $42.54/60 tablets = $0.71 per tablet; $0.71 × 20 tablets = $14.20 for the prescription; the pharmacy will submit for $14.20 reimbursement

2. $84.07 × 0.13 = $10.93; $84.07 − $10.93 = $73.14; $73.14/100 tablets × 30 tablets; $73.14/100 tablets = $0.73 per tablet; 0.73 × 30 tablets = $21.90 for the prescription; the pharmacy will submit for $21.90 reimbursement

3. $30.25 × 0.13 = $3.93; $30.25 − $3.93 = $26.32; $26.32/1000 tablets × 100 tablets; $26.32/1000 tablets = $0.02632 per tablet, rounded to 0.03; 0.03 × 100 tablets = $3.00 for the prescription; the pharmacy will submit for $3.00 reimbursement

4. $120.68 × 0.04 = $4.83; $120.68 + $4.83 = $125.51; $125.51/500 tablets × 30 tablets; $125.51/500 = $0.25 × 30 = $7.50; $7.50 + $6.25 = $13.75; the pharmacy will submit for $13.75 reimbursement

5. $39.78 × 0.04 = $1.59; $39.78 + $1.59 = $41.37; $41.37/100 tablets × 60 tablets; $41.37/100 = $0.41 × 60 = $24.60; $24.60 + $6.25 = $30.85; the pharmacy will submit for $30.85 reimbursement

6. $317.50 × 0.04 = $12.70; $317.50 + $12.70 = $330.20; $330.20/30 tablets × 20 tablets; $330.20/30 = $11.01; $11.01 × 20 = $220.20; $220.20 + $6.25 = $226.45; the pharmacy will submit for $226.45 reimbursement

7. a. $71.35/100 × 50; $71.35/100 = $0.7135 rounded to $0.71; $0.71 × 50 = $35.5; the pharmacy cost is $35.50

7. b. $71.35 × 0.035 = $2.50; $71.35 + $2.50 = $73.85; $73.85/100 tablets × 50 tablets; $73.85/100 = $0.7385 rounded to $0.74 × 50 = $37.00; $37.00 + $4.50 = $41.50; the pharmacy will submit for $41.50 reimbursement

7. c. $41.50 − $35.50 = $6.00; the pharmacy will make a profit of $6.00 on this prescription

8. a. $36.35 × 0.03 = $1.09; $36.35 − $1.09 = $35.26; $35.26 × 2 = $70.52; the pharmacy cost is $70.52

b. $36.35 × 0.05 = $1.82; $36.35 + $1.82 = $38.17 per inhaler × 2 = $76.34; the pharmacy will submit this for $76.34 reimbursement

c. $76.34 − $70.52 = $5.82; the pharmacy will make $5.82 on this prescription

9. a. $302.35/30 × 10; $302.35/30 = $10.08; $10.08 × 10 = $100.80; the pharmacy cost is $100.80

b. $100.80 × 0.03 = $3.02; $100.80 − $3.02 = $97.78; $97.78 + $7.00 = $104.78; the pharmacy will submit this for $104.78 reimbursement

c. $104.78 − $100.80 = $3.98; the pharmacy will make $3.98 on this prescription

10. a. $117.35/50 × 30; $117.35/50 = $2.35; $2.35 × 30 = $70.5; the pharmacy cost is $70.50

b. $70.50 × 0.03 = $2.12 (rounded to hundredths); $70.50 + $2.12 = $72.62; $72.62 + $4.00 = $76.62; the pharmacy will submit this for $76.62 reimbursement

c. $76.62 − $70.50 = $6.12; the pharmacy will make $6.12 on this prescription

11. a. $85.35/80 × 15; $85.35/80 = $1.07; $1.07 × 15 = $16.05; the pharmacy cost is $16.05

b. $16.05 × 0.045 = $0.72; $16.05 + $0.72 = $16.77; the pharmacy will submit this for $16.77 reimbursement

c. $16.77 − $16.05 = $0.72; the pharmacy will make $0.72 on this prescription

12. a. $310.00 × 6 = $1860.00; the pharmacy will be reimbursed $1860.00 for the capitation fee

b. $15.75 + $106.50 + $27.80 + $210.00 + $47.50 + $105.25 + $160.00 + $52.00 + $150.00 + $210.00 + $76.00 + $10.50 + $28.00 + $62.50 + $210.00 + $210.00 + $17.00 = $1698.80; the pharmacy cost is $1698.80

c. The pharmacy made a profit

d. $1860.00 − $1698.80 = $161.20

13. a. $15.75 + $106.50 + $27.80 + 210.00 + 47.50 + 105.25 + 160.00 + $52.00 + $150.00 + $210.00 + $76.00 + $10.50 + $28.00 + $62.50 + $210.00 + $210.00 + $17.00 = $1698.80; the pharmacy cost is $1698.80

b. $1698.80 × 0.03 = $50.96; $1698.80 + $50.96 = $1749.76; $2.00 per prescription × 17 = $34.00; $1749.76 + $34.00 = $1783.76; the pharmacy will submit this for $1783.76 reimbursement

c. The pharmacy made a profit

d. $1783.76 − $1698.80 = $84.96; the pharmacy made a profit of $84.96

e. The pharmacy made more money under Mountain HMO's capitation plan

f. $161.20 − $84.96 = $76.24; the pharmacy made $76.24 more under the capitation plan

14. a. $275.00 × 10 = $2750.00; the total amount that the HMO reimbursed for capitation fees is $2750.00

b. $89.63 + $126.54 + $420.45 + $117.50 + $46.75 = $729.87; the total pharmacy cost is $800.87

c. The pharmacy made a profit

d. $2750.00 − $800.87 = $1949.13; the pharmacy made a profit of $1949.13

15. a. $275.00 × 12 = $3300.00; the total amount that the HMO reimbursed for capitation fees is $3300.00

b. $78.26 + $75.23 + $25.48 + $128.46 + $21.86 + $61.89 + $41.20 + $16.59 + $5.80 + $3.87 + $21.67 + $58.24 = $538.55; the total pharmacy cost is $538.55

c. the pharmacy made a profit

d. $3300.00 − $538.55 = $2761.45; the pharmacy made a profit of $2761.45

16. a. $225.00 × 40 = $9000.00; $9000.00 + $60.00 = $9060.00; the total amount the HMO will reimburse the pharmacy is $9060.00

b. the pharmacy made a profit

c. $9060.00 − $1867.50 = $7192.50; the pharmacy made a profit of $7192.50

17. a. $210.00 × 42 = $8820.00; $4.25 × 54 = $229.50; $8820.00 + $229.50 = $9049.50; the total amount that the insurance company reimbursed is $9049.50

b. The pharmacy lost money

c. $9049.50 − $9634.73 = −585.23; the pharmacy lost $585.23

9.3 Problem Set

1. 1 bottle of 500

2. 2 bottles of 100

3. 1 bottle of 500

4. 1 bottle of 60

5. 1 bottle of 100

6. no purchase necessary

7. 1 bottle of 50

8. no purchase necessary

9. no purchase necessary

10. 3 of the 15 g; 4 of the 80 g

11. 1 of the 15 g; 1 of the 60 g; 2 of the 80 g

12. 1 of the 60 mL

13. 1 of the 15 g; 1 of the 60 g

14. 3 of the 60 g;

15. 1 of the 15 g; 1 of the 60 g; 0 of the 4 oz

16. 2 of the 15 g; 1 of the 60 g

17. 0 of the 15 g; 0 of the 45 g

18. 0 of the 15 g; 1 of the 30 g; 0 of the 60 g; 1 of the 120 g

19. 0 of the 15 g; 0 of the 30 g; 1 of the 60 g

20. 01 of the 15 g; 0 of the 30 g; 1 of the 60 g; 0 of the 120 g

21. 1 of the 20 mL; 1 of the 60 mL

22. 1 bottle of 100

23. 1 bottle of 100

24. 1 bottle of 100

25. 2 bottle of 60

26. 1 bottle of 100

27. 1 bottle of 1000

28. 0 (or 1) bottles of 100

29. 1 bottle of 1000

30. 1 bottle of 100

31. 1 bottle of 300

32. 1 bottle of 100

33. 0 (or 1) bottles of 100

34. 1 bottle of 1000

35. 1 bottle of 100

36. 0 bottles of 100

37. a. 7 jars

b. 3 bottles of 1000

c. 20 bottles

d. 3 bottles

e. 11 bottles

38. a. $38,207.00/7 = $5458.14, rounded to $5458.00; $183,445.00/$5458.00 = 33.61, rounded to 34; they have approximately a 34 day supply

b. 34 − 28 = 6; they are 6 days over their goal; $5458.00 × 6 = $32,748.00; they are $32,748.00 over their goal

39. a. $26,504.00/7 = $3786.29, rounded to $3786.00; $123,490.00/$3786.00 = 32.62, rounded to 33; they have approximately a 33 day supply

   b. 33 – 26 = 7; they are 7 days over their goal; $3786.00 × 7 = $26,502.00; they are $26,502.00 over their goal

40. $147,210.00/24 = $6133.75; the approximate cost of goods sold in one day was $6133.75; $6133.75 × 7 days = $42936.25; the cost of products sold last week is $42936.25

41. $51,280.00 + $5000.00 = $56,280.00; $56,280.00/7 = they must average $8,040.00 per day

42. $1,612,00.00/$132,936.00 = 12.123, rounded to 12.13; their turnover rate was 12.13

43. $1,768,000.00/$156,200.00 = 11.318, rounded to 11.32; their turnover rate was 11.32

44. $20,800.00/$520.00 = 40; turnover rate is 40

45. $5760.00/$178.00 = 32.36; turnover rate is 32.36

46. $7213.00/$360.00 = 20.04; turnover rate is 20.04

47. $5060.00/$320.00 = 15.81; turnover rate is 15.81

48. $6000.00/$385.00 = 14.58; turnover rate is 15.58

49. $52,500.00/$5,000.00 = 10.5; turnover rate is 10.5

50. $8294.00 − $2138.00 = $6156.00; $6156.00/6 = $1026.00; the annual depreciation is $1026.00

51. $18,350.00 × 2 = $36,700.00; $1567.00 × 2 = $3134.00; $36,700.00 – $3134.00 = $33,566.00; $33,566.00/12 = $2797.17; the annual depreciation is $2797.17

Finding Solutions

1. 1000-count bottle at $10.00 per bottle = $0.01 per capsule

2. one bottle

3. $10.00

4. $149.00 × 127 = $18,923.00; $3.50 × 52 = $182.00; $18,923.00 + $182.00 = $19,105.00. The amount the HMO reimbursed the pharmacy was $19,105.00

5. $6,283.24

6. The pharmacy made a profit

7. $19,105.00 – $6,283.24 = $12,821.76; the pharmacy made a profit of $12,821.76

Common Pharmacy Abbreviations and Acronyms

The abbreviations with red lines through them are ones that are still in use but are discouraged by Institute for Safe Medication Practices (ISMP). The ISMP recommends the use of the correct words instead. Many of these discouraged abbreviations are also on The Joint Commission's Official "Do Not Use" List of Abbreviations.

Abbreviation	Meaning
A-B-C	
aaa	apply to affected area
ACA	Affordable Care Act (Patient Protection and Affordable Care Act)
~~ac; a.c.; AC~~	before meals
ACE	angiotensin-converting enzyme inhibitors
~~ad; a.d.; AD~~	right ear
ADD	attention-deficit disorder
ADH	antidiuretic hormone
ADHD	attention-deficit hyperactivity disorder
ADME	absorption, distribution, metabolism, and elimination
ADR	adverse drug reaction
AIDS	acquired immune deficiency syndrome
AM; a.m.	morning
ANDA	Abbreviated New Drug Application
APAP	acetaminophen; Tylenol
AphA	American Pharmacy Association
ARBs	angiotensin receptor blockers
~~as; a.s.; AS~~	left ear
ASA	aspirin
~~au; a.u.; AU~~	both ears; each ear
b.i.d.; BID	twice daily
BMI	Body Mass Index
BP	blood pressure
BUD	beyond-use date
°C	degrees centigrade; temperature in degrees centigrade
Ca^{++}	calcium

Abbreviation	Meaning
Cap, cap	capsule
CDC	Centers for Disease Control and Prevention
CF	cystic fibrosis
CHF	congestive heart failure
CNS	Central Nervous System
COPD	chronic obstructive pulmonary disease
CPR	cardio pulminary resuscitation
CSP	compounded sterile preparation
CV	cardiovascular
D-E-F	
D_5; D_5W; D5W	dextrose 5% in water
D_5 ¼; D5 1/4	dextrose 5% in ¼ normal saline; dextrose 5% in 0.225% sodium chloride
D_5 ⅓; D5 1/3	dextrose 5% in ⅓ normal saline; dextrose 5% in 0.33% sodium chloride
D_5 ½; D5 1/2	dextrose 5% in ½ normal saline; dextrose 5% in 0.45% sodium chloride
D_5LR; D5LR	dextrose 5% in lactated Ringer's solution
D_5NS; D5NS	dextrose 5% in normal saline; dextrose 5% in 0.9% sodium chloride
DAW	dispense as written
D̶C̶; d̶/̶c̶	discontinue
D/C	discharge
DCA	direct compounding area
Dig	digoxin
disp	dispense
EC	enteric-coated
Elix	elixir
eMAR	electronic medication administration record
EPO	epoetin alfa; erythropoietin
ER; XR; XL	extended-release
°F	degrees Fahrenheit; temperature in degrees Fahrenheit
$FeSO_4$	ferrous sulfate; iron
G-H-I	
g, G	gram
gr	grain
GI	gastrointestinal
GMP	good manufacturing practice
gtt; gtts	drop; drops
h; hr	hour
HC	hydrocortisone
HCTZ	hydrochlorothiazide
HIPAA	Health Insurance Portability and Accountability Act
HIV	human immunodeficiency virus
HMO	Health Maintenance Organization
HRT	hormone replacement therapy

Abbreviation	Meaning
h.s.; HS	bedtime (comes from Latin *hora somni* meaning "hour of sleep"); hs should also not be used
IBU	ibuprofen; Motrin
ICU	intensive care unit
IM	intramuscular
IND	Investigational New Drug Application
Inj, IJ	injection
IPA	isopropyl alcohol
ISDN	isosorbide dinitrate
ISMO	isosorbide mononitrate
ISMP	Institute for Safe Medication Practices
IV	intravenous
IVF	intravenous fluid
IVP	intravenous push
IVPB	intravenous piggyback
J-K-L	
K; K+	potassium
KCl	potassium chloride
kg	kilogram
L	liter
LAFW	laminar airflow workbench; hood
lb	pound
LD	loading dose
LVP	large-volume parenteral
JCAHO	Joint Commission on the Accreditation of Healthcare Organizations
M-N-O	
Mag; Mg; MAG	magnesium
MAR	medication administration record
mcg	microgram
MDI	metered-dose inhaler
MDV	multiple-dose vial
mEq	milliequivalent
mg	milligram
MgSO$_4$	magnesium sulfate; magnesium
mL	milliliter
mL/hr	milliliters per hour
mL/min	milliliters per minute

Abbreviation	Meaning
MMR	measles, mumps, and rubella vaccine
MRSA	methiciliin-resistant S. aureaus
MOM; M.O.M.	milk of magnesia
M.S.	morphine sulfate (save MS for multiple sclerosis)
MU†; mu	million units
MVI; MVI-12	multiple vitamin injection; multivitamins for parenteral administration
Na⁺	sodium
NABP	National Association of Boards of Pharmacy
NaCl	sodium chloride; salt
NDA	New Drug App
NDC	National Drug Code
NF; non-form	nonformulary
NKA	no known allergies
NKDA	no known drug allergies
NPO, npo	nothing by mouth
NR; d.n.r.	no refills; do not repeat
NS	normal saline; 0.9% sodium chloride
½ NS	one-half normal saline; 0.45% sodium chloride
¼ NS	one-quarter normal saline; 0.225% sodium chloride
NSAID	nonsteroidal anti-inflammatory drug
NTG	nitroglycerin
OC	oral contraceptive
od; o.d.; OD	right eye
ODT	orally disintegrating tablet
OPTH; OPHTH; Opth	ophthalmic
os; o.s.; OS	left eye
OTC	over the counter; no prescription required
ou; o.u.; OU	both eyes; each eye
oz	ounce
P-Q-R	
p.c.; PC	after meals
PCA	patient-controlled anesthesia
PCN	penicillin
pH	acid-base balance
PHI	protected health information
PM; p.m.	afternoon; evening
PN	paternal nutrition

Abbreviation	Meaning
PNS	peripheral nervous system
PO; po	orally; by mouth
PPE	personal protective equipment
PPI	proton pump inhibitor
PR	per rectum; rectally
PRN; p.r.n.	as needed; as occasion requires
PTSD	Post Traumatic Stress Disorder
PV	per vagina; vaginally
PVC	polyvinyl chloride
q	every
q.h.; qhour	every hour
q2h	every 2 hours
q4h	every 4 hours
q6h	every 6 hours
q8h	every 8 hours
q12h	every 12 hours
q24h	every 24 hours
q48h	every 48 hours
QA	quality assurance
QAM; qam	every morning
qDay; QD, Qrd	every day
q.i.d.; QID	four times daily
QOD; Q other day; Q.O. Day	every other day
QPM; qpm	every evening
qs; qsad	quantity sufficient; a sufficient quantity to make
QTY; qty	quantity
qwk; qweek	every week
RA	rheumatoid arthritis
RDA	recommended daily allowance
Rx	prescription; pharmacy; medication; drug; recipe; take
S-T	
sig	write on label; signa; directions
SL; sub-L	sublingual
SMZ-TMP	sulfamethoxazole and trimethoprim; Bactrim
SNRI	serotonin nonrepinephrine reuptake inhibitor
SPF	sunburn protection factor

Abbreviation	Meaning
SR	sustained-release
SS; ss	one-half
SSRI	selective serotonin reuptake inhibitor (don't use for sliding scale insulins)
STAT, Stat	immediately; now
STD	sexually transmitted disease
Sub-Q; SC; SQ; sq, subcut, SUBCUT	subcutaneous
SUPP; Supp	suppository
susp	suspension
SVP	small-volume parenteral
SW	sterile water
SWFI	sterile water for injection
Tab; tab	tablet
TB	tuberculosis
TBSP; tbsp	tablespoon; tablespoonful; 15 mL
TDS	transdermal delivery system
t.i.d.; TID	three times daily
t.i.w.; TIW	three times a week
TKO; TKVO; KO; KVO	to keep open; to keep vein open; keep open; keep vein open (a slow IV flow rate)
TNA	Total Nutrition Admixture
TPN	total parenteral nutrition
TSP; tsp	teaspoon; teaspoonful; 5 mL
U-V-W	
U or u	unit
u.d., UD, ut dictum	as directed
ung	ointment
USP	U.S. Pharmacopoeial Convention
USP-NF	*U.S. Pharmacopoeia-National Formulary*
UTI	urinary tract infection
UV	ultraviolet light
VAG; vag	vagina; vaginally
Vanco	vancomycin
VO; V.O.; V/O	verbal order
w/o	without
X-Y-Z	
Zn	zinc, but *ZnSO₄*—should not be used for zinc sulfate
Z-Pak	azithromycin; Zithromax

Measures and Conversions

Metric	*Volume* 1 L = 1000 mL 1 mL = 1 cc		
	Weight 1 g = 1000 mg 1 mg = 1000 mcg		

Household	*Volume* 1 gal = 4 qt 1 qt = 2 pt 1 pt = 2 cups = 16 fl oz 1 fl oz = 2 tbsp = 6 tsp	*Weight* 1 lb = 16 oz *Length* 1 yd = 3 ft 1 ft = 12 in

CONVERSIONS

	Household	Apothecary	Metric
Volume	1 qt = 32 fl oz		0.96 L
	1 pint = 16 fl oz		480 mL *
	1 cup = 8 fl oz		240 mL
	2 tbsp = 1 fl oz	6 fʒ = 1 fℨ	30 mL *
	1 tbsp	3 fʒ	15 mL
	1 tsp	1 fʒ	5 mL †
		1 ♏	0.0625 mL
Weight	2.2 lb		1 kg
	1 lb		454 g
	1 oz	8 ʒ	30 g
Length	1 in		2.5 cm

* There are actually 29.57 mL in 1 fl oz, but 30 mL is usually used. When packaging a pint, companies will typically include 473 mL, rather than the full 480 mL, thus saving money over time.

† There are actually 3.75 mL in an apothecary fʒ. However, convention dictates that 1 fʒ = 5 mL = 1 tsp.

INDEX

Locators for figures are indicated by *f,* tables by *t,* and photos by *p* following the page number.

IMAGE CREDITS

Chapter 1   1© Paradigm Publishing, 2© Paradigm Publishing, 9 Reprinted with permission of Mylan Pharmaceuticals Inc. All rights reserved, 10 Reprinted with permission of Mylan Pharmaceuticals Inc, 18 © Paradigm Publishing, 19© Paradigm Publishing, 20© Paradigm Publishing, 22© Paradigm Publishing, 23© Paradigm Publishing, 17© Paradigm Publishing, 16© Paradigm Publishing, 17© Paradigm Publishing, 17© Paradigm Publishing, 39© Paradigm Publishing

Chapter 2   42© Paradigm Publishing, 42© Paradigm Publishing, 43© Paradigm Publishing, 45© Copyright Eli Lilly and Company. All Rights Reserved. Used with Permission, 45 Copyright Pfizer Inc. Used with permission, 45© Paradigm Publishing, 48© Paradigm Publishing, 48 Images used with permission from Fresenius Kabi USA, LLC, 50© Paradigm Publishing, 52© Paradigm Publishing, 54 Images used with permission from Fresenius Kabi USA, LLC, 55© Paradigm Publishing, 60 Images used with permission from Fresenius Kabi USA, LLC, 61 Images used with permission from Fresenius Kabi USA, LLC, 54 Images used with permission from Fresenius Kabi USA, LLC, 61 Images used with permission from Fresenius Kabi USA, LLC, 61© Paradigm Publishing, 62 Images used with permission from Fresenius Kabi USA, LLC, 62 Courtesy of Apothecary Products, Inc., 63 Courtesy of Apothecary Products, Inc.

Chapter 3   72© Paradigm Publishing, 73© Paradigm Publishing, 76 Copyright Pfizer Inc. Used with permission, 76 Reprinted with permission of Mylan Pharmaceuticals Inc. All rights reserved, 76 Images used with permission from Fresenius Kabi USA, LLC, 77 Image courtesy of American Regent, Inc., 78 Courtesy of Apothecary Products, Inc., 78 Copyright Nipon Laicharoenchokchai/Shutterstock, 86 Courtesy of Tova Wiegand-Green, 86 Copyright Paul Orr/Shutterstock, 86 Copyright: PANYA KUANUN/Shutterstock, 79 Image courtesy of Optimer, 80 © Paradigm Publishing, 81 Macrobid container label used with permission. Macrobid is a registered trademark of Almatica Pharma, Inc., 81 © Copyright Eli Lilly and Company. All Rights Reserved. Used with Permission. Prozac is a trademark of Eli Lilly and Company, 82 © Copyright Eli Lilly and Company. All Rights Reserved. Used with Permission. 82 Reprinted with permission of Mylan Pharmaceuticals Inc. All rights reserved, 82 Copyright Pfizer Inc. Used with permission., 82 Mallinckrodt LLC, 83 © Paradigm Publishing, 83© Paradigm Publishing, 83© Paradigm Publishing, 83© Paradigm Publishing, 83©, Paradigm Publishing, 83© Paradigm Publishing, 83© Paradigm Publishing, 83© Paradigm Publishing, 83©, Paradigm Publishing, 87© Paradigm Publishing, 87© Paradigm Publishing, 87© Paradigm Publishing, 87© Paradigm Publishing,

87© Paradigm Publishing, 87© Paradigm Publishing, 87© Paradigm Publishing, 87© Paradigm Publishing, 87© Paradigm Publishing, 87© Paradigm Publishing, 91© Paradigm Publishing, 80© Paradigm Publishing

Chapter 4   94© Paradigm Publishing, 94© Paradigm Publishing, 94© Paradigm Publishing, 95© Paradigm Publishing, 97© Paradigm Publishing, 97© Paradigm Publishing, 97© Paradigm Publishing, 103© Paradigm Publishing, 103© Paradigm Publishing, 103© Paradigm Publishing, 103 Images used with permission from Fresenius Kabi USA, LLC, 105© Paradigm Publishing, 105© Paradigm Publishing, 106© Paradigm Publishing, 107© Paradigm Publishing, 108© Paradigm Publishing, 109© Paradigm Publishing, 109 Mallinckrodt LLC , 109© Paradigm Publishing, 110© Paradigm Publishing, 110 Images used with permission from Fresenius Kabi USA, LLC, 110© Paradigm Publishing, 110 Images used with permission from Fresenius Kabi USA, LLC, 111 Copyright Pfizer Inc. Used with permission., 111© Paradigm Publishing, 111© Paradigm Publishing, 111© Paradigm Publishing, 111 Images used with permission from Fresenius Kabi USA, LLC, 112© Paradigm Publishing, 112© Paradigm Publishing, 112© Paradigm Publishing, 116 Copyright © Novartis Pharmaceuticals Corp. Used with permission., 117 Copyright © Novartis Pharmaceuticals Corp. Used with permission., 128© Paradigm Publishing

Chapter 5   130 © Paradigm Publishing, 131© Paradigm Publishing, 135© Paradigm Publishing, 135 ©burwellphotography/istockphoto 136© Paradigm Publishing, 136 Mallinckrodt LLC, 141 © Paradigm Publishing, 141© Paradigm Publishing, 144 Mallinckrodt LLC, 144©, Paradigm Publishing, 147© Paradigm Publishing, 147© Paradigm Publishing, 149© Paradigm Publishing, 149©, Paradigm Publishing, 150© Paradigm Publishing, 150© Paradigm Publishing, 150© Paradigm Publishing, 153© Paradigm Publishing, 154© Paradigm Publishing, 155© Paradigm Publishing, 156© Paradigm Publishing, 157©, Paradigm Publishing, 158© Paradigm Publishing, 158© Paradigm Publishing, 158© Paradigm Publishing, 158© Paradigm Publishing, 158© Paradigm Publishing, 159© Paradigm Publishing, 159© iStockphoto/malerapaso, 162© Paradigm Publishing, 162© Paradigm Publishing, 163© Paradigm Publishing, 146© Paradigm Publishing, 147©, Paradigm Publishing, 139© Paradigm Publishing, 144© Paradigm Publishing, 150© Paradigm Publishing, 154© Paradigm Publishing

Chapter 6   170 Images used with permission from Fresenius Kabi USA, LLC, 171© Paradigm Publishing, 171 Images used with permission from Fresenius Kabi USA, LLC, 172 (top and bottom) © Paradigm Publishing, 172 (center) Images used with permission from Fresenius Kabi USA, LLC, 172© Paradigm Publishing, 173 Images used with permission from Fresenius Kabi USA, LLC, 173 Images used with permission from Fresenius Kabi USA, LLC, 174 Images used with permission from Fresenius Kabi USA, LLC, 178 Images used with permission from Fresenius Kabi USA, LLC, 178 Images used with permission from Fresenius Kabi USA, LLC, 178 Images used with permission from Fresenius Kabi USA, LLC, 178 Images used with permission from Fresenius Kabi USA, LLC, 178 Images used with permission from Fresenius Kabi USA, LLC, 178 Images used with permission from Fresenius Kabi USA, LLC, 179 Images used with permission from Fresenius Kabi USA, LLC, 179 Images used with permission from Fresenius Kabi USA, LLC, 179 Images used with permission from Fresenius Kabi USA, LLC. 179 Images used with permission from Fresenius Kabi USA, LLC, 179 Images used with permission from Fresenius Kabi USA, LLC, 179 Images used with permission from Fresenius Kabi USA, LLC, 180 Images used with permission from Fresenius Kabi USA, LLC, 180 Images used with permission from Fresenius Kabi USA, LLC, 180 Images used with permission from Fresenius Kabi USA, LLC, 180 Images used with permission from Fresenius Kabi USA, LLC, 180 Images used with permission from Fresenius Kabi USA, LLC, 180 Images used with permission from Fresenius Kabi USA, LLC, 180 Images used with permission from Fresenius Kabi USA, LLC, 183© Paradigm Publishing, 183 Images used with permission from Fresenius Kabi USA, LLC, 184 Images used with permission from Fresenius Kabi USA, LLC, 184 Images used with permission from Fresenius Kabi USA, LLC, 184 Images used with permission from Fresenius Kabi USA, LLC, 186© Paradigm Publishing, 187 Images used with permission from Fresenius Kabi USA, LLC, 188© Paradigm Publishing, 192© Copyright Eli Lilly and Company. All Rights Reserved. Used with Permission, 191© Copyright Eli Lilly and Company. All Rights Reserved. Used with Permission, 193© Copyright Eli Lilly and Company. All Rights Reserved. Used with Permission, 194 Illustrations (c) Paradigm Publishing, 197© Copyright Eli Lilly and Company. All Rights Reserved. Used with Permission, 197© Copyright Eli Lilly and Company. All Rights Reserved. Used with Permission, 197© Copyright Eli Lilly and Company. All Rights Reserved. Used with Permission, 194© Copyright Eli Lilly and Company. All Rights Reserved. Used with Permission., 195 Images used with permission from Fresenius Kabi USA, LLC, 195 Images used with permission from Fresenius Kabi USA, LLC, 195 Images used with permission from Fresenius Kabi USA, LLC, 195 Images used with permission from Fresenius Kabi USA, LLC, 195 Images used with permission from Fresenius Kabi USA, LLC, 195© Paradigm Publishing, 196 Images used with permission from Fresenius Kabi USA, LLC, 196 Images used with permission from Fresenius Kabi USA, LLC, 196 Images used with permission from Fresenius Kabi USA, LLC, 196 Image courtesy of Sanofi-Aventis, 196© Copyright Eli Lilly and Company. All Rights Reserved. Used with Permission, 197© Copyright Eli Lilly and Company. All Rights Reserved. Used with Permission, 197© Copyright Eli Lilly and Company. All Rights Reserved. Used with Permission, 197© Copyright Eli Lilly and Company. All Rights Reserved. Used with Permission, 197© Copyright Eli Lilly and Company. All Rights Reserved. Used with Permission., 197 Image courtesy of Sanofi-Aventis, 197 Image courtesy of Sanofi-Aventis, 203©

Paradigm Publishing, 203© Paradigm Publishing, 206 Images used with permission from Fresenius Kabi USA, LLC, 178 Images used with permission from Fresenius Kabi USA, LLC, 178 Images used with permission from Fresenius Kabi USA, LLC, 179 Images used with permission from Fresenius Kabi USA, LLC, 179 Images used with permission from Fresenius Kabi USA, LLC, 180 Images used with permission from Fresenius Kabi USA, LLC, 180 Images used with permission from Fresenius Kabi USA, LLC, 180 Images used with permission from Fresenius Kabi USA, LLC, 180 Images used with permission from Fresenius Kabi USA, LLC, 178 Images used with permission from Fresenius Kabi USA, LLC, 183 Images used with permission from Fresenius Kabi USA, LLC, 196 Images used with permission from Fresenius Kabi USA, LLC, 196 Image courtesy of Sanofi-Aventis , 197 Image courtesy of Sanofi-Aventis, 197 Image courtesy of Sanofi-Aventis, 184 Images used with permission from Fresenius Kabi USA, LLC, 183 Images used with permission from Fresenius Kabi USA, LLC, 184 Images used with permission from Fresenius Kabi USA, LLC, 186 © Paradigm Publishing, 189 © Copyright Eli Lilly and Company. All Rights Reserved. Used with Permission. , 189 © Copyright Eli Lilly and Company. All Rights Reserved. Used with Permission, 189© Copyright Eli Lilly, 189© Copyright Eli Lilly, 190© Copyright Eli Lilly and Company. All Rights Reserved. Used with Permission. , 191© Copyright Eli Lilly and Company. All Rights Reserved. Used with Permission, 194© Paradigm Publishing, 1940© Paradigm Publishing

Chapter 7 215 Images used with permission from Fresenius Kabi USA, LLC, 216 Images used with permission from Fresenius Kabi USA, LLC, 216© Pfizer Inc., 216 Images used with permission from Fresenius Kabi USA, LLC, 217 Images used with permission from Fresenius Kabi USA, LLC, 216 Images used with permission from Fresenius Kabi USA, LLC, 217 Images used with permission from Fresenius Kabi USA, LLC, 216 Image courtesy of American Regent, Inc., 217 Image courtesy of American Regent, Inc., 218 Image courtesy of Baxter Healthcare Corporation. All rights reserved, 218 Image courtesy of Baxter Healthcare Corporation. All rights reserved., 223© Paradigm Publishing, 224© Paradigm Publishing, 224© Paradigm Publishing, 224© Paradigm Publishing, 227© Paradigm Publishing, 231© Paradigm Publishing, 231© Paradigm Publishing, 231© Paradigm Publishing, 232© Paradigm Publishing, 235© Paradigm Publishing, 235© Paradigm Publishing, 217 Images used with permission from Fresenius Kabi USA, LLC, 217 Images used with permission from Fresenius Kabi USA,, 216 Images used with permission from Fresenius Kabi USA, LLC, 213 Image courtesy of Baxter Healthcare Corporation. All rights reserved, 217 Images used with permission from Fresenius Kabi USA, LLC, 231© Paradigm Publishing, 236 Images used with permission from Fresenius Kabi USA, LLC, 236© Paradigm Publishing

Chapter 8 241© Paradigm Publishing, 241© Paradigm Publishing, 242© Paradigm Publishing, 252© Paradigm Publishing, 252© Paradigm Publishing, 253© Paradigm Publishing, 253© Paradigm Publishing, 260 Images used with permission from Fresenius Kabi USA, LLC, 266© Paradigm Publishing, 266© Paradigm Publishing, 266© Paradigm Publishing, 261© Paradigm Publishing, 261© Paradigm Publishing, 267© Paradigm Publishing

CPSIA information can be obtained
at www.ICGtesting.com
Printed in the USA
LVHW060152190621
690594LV00004B/4